W9-BSI-501

EATING ON THE WILD SIDE

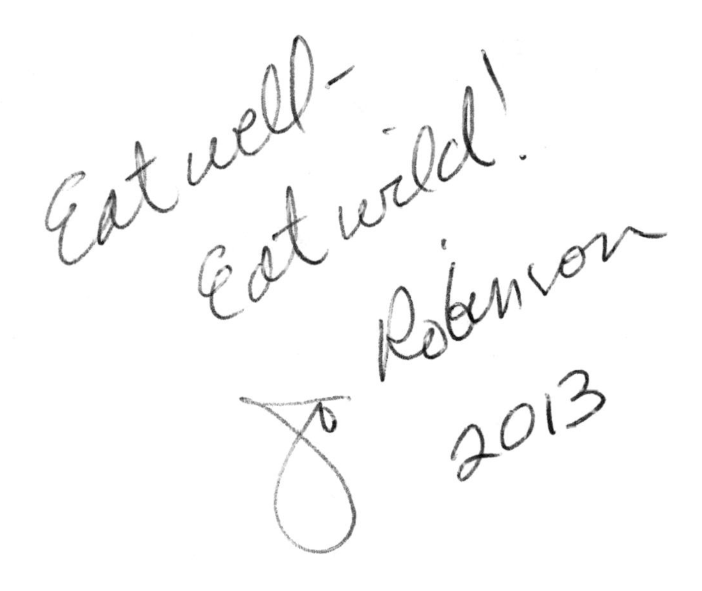

EATING
ON THE
WILD SIDE

THE MISSING LINK TO OPTIMUM HEALTH

JO ROBINSON

Illustrations by Andie Styner

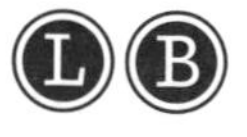

LITTLE, BROWN AND COMPANY
New York Boston London

Little, Brown and Company
Hachette Book Group
237 Park Avenue, New York, NY 10017
littlebrown.com

First Edition: June 2013

Little, Brown and Company is a division of Hachette Book Group, Inc. The Little, Brown name and logo are trademarks of Hachette Book Group, Inc.

Illustrations by Andie Styner of Roobiblue Studios

ISBN 978-0-316-22794-0
LCCN 2013934815

10 9 8 7 6 5 4 3 2 1

RRD-C

Printed in the United States of America

I dedicate this book to all the researchers, food activists, and plant breeders who are working to preserve the genetic diversity of our fruits and vegetables and to enhance their nutritional content. Through their efforts, we can begin to reclaim a wealth of nutrients that we, unwittingly, removed from our diet over a period of ten thousand years.

CONTENTS

Wild Nutrients: Lost and Found 3

PART ONE: VEGETABLES

1 | From Wild Greens to Iceberg Lettuce: Breeding Out the Medicine 21

2 | Alliums: All Things to All People 47

3 | Corn on the Cob: How Supersweet It Is! 74

4 | Potatoes: From Wild to Fries 96

5 | The Other Root Crops: Carrots, Beets, and Sweet Potatoes 111

6 | Tomatoes: Bringing Back Their Flavor and Nutrients 137

7 | The Incredible Crucifers: Tame Their Bitterness and Reap the Rewards 158

8 | Legumes: Beans, Peas, and Lentils 177

9 | Artichokes, Asparagus, and Avocados: Indulge! 195

CONTENTS

PART TWO: FRUITS

10 | Apples: From Potent Medicine to Mild-Mannered Clones 215

11 | Blueberries and Blackberries: Extraordinarily Nutritious 239

12 | Strawberries, Cranberries, and Raspberries: Three of Our Most Nutritious Fruits 260

13 | Stone Fruits: Time for a Flavor Revival 276

14 | Grapes and Raisins: From Muscadines to Thompson Seedless 303

15 | Citrus Fruits: Beyond Vitamin C 318

16 | Tropical Fruits: Make the Most of Eating Globally 345

17 | Melons: Light in Flavor and Nutrition 359

Acknowledgments 373

Scientific References 375

Index 401

EATING ON THE WILD SIDE

INTRODUCTION

WILD NUTRIENTS

LOST AND FOUND

Where do our fruits and vegetables come from? Not from the supermarket, of course. That's just where they are sold. Nor do they come from large commercial farms, local farms, or even our backyard gardens. That's where they are planted, tended, and harvested. The fruits and vegetables themselves came from wild plants that grow in widely scattered areas around the globe. Most of our blueberries are descended from wild "swamp blueberries" that are native to the Pine Barrens of New Jersey. The wild ancestor of our beefsteak tomato is a berry-size fruit that grows on the flanks of the Andes Mountains. Our hefty orange carrots are related to scrawny purple roots that grow in Afghanistan. When our distant ancestors invented farming ten thousand or so years ago, they began altering these and other wild plants to make them more productive, easier to grow and harvest, and more enjoyable to eat. To date, four hundred generations of farmers and tens of thousands of plant breeders have played a role in redesigning native plants. The combined changes are so monumental that our present-day fruits and vegetables seem like modern creations.

Consider the banana, our most popular fruit. The wild ancestor of the banana grows in Malaysia and parts of Southeast Asia. The bananas come in a multitude of shapes, colors, and sizes. Most of them are chock-full of large, hard seeds. Their skins are so firmly attached that you have to cut them off with a knife. Take a bite of the dry, astringent flesh and you'd wonder why you went to the trouble. Over several thousand years, we clever humans have transformed this barely edible fruit into the Cavendish banana, the yellow, long-fingered banana that is sold in all our supermarkets. We love the Cavendish for its zip-off peels, sweet and creamy flesh, and the fact that its seeds have been downsized to mere dots. The seeds are not viable, of course, but seeds are not needed when plants are grown from cuttings, which is how all our bananas are propagated. Generation after generation, we have reshaped native plants and made them our own.

THE LOSS OF VITAMINS, MINERALS, PROTEIN, FIBER, AND HEALTHFUL FATS

Unwittingly, as we went about breeding more palatable fruits and vegetables, we were stripping away some of the very nutrients we now know to be essential for optimum health. Compared with wild fruits and vegetables, most of our man-made varieties are markedly lower in vitamins, minerals, and essential fatty acids. A wild plant called purslane has six times more vitamin E than spinach and fourteen times more omega-3 fatty acids. It has seven times more betacarotene than carrots.

Most native plants are also higher in protein and fiber and much lower in sugar than the ones we've devised. The ancestor of our modern corn is a grass plant called teosinte that is native to central Mexico. Its kernels are about 30 percent protein and 2 percent sugar. Old-fashioned sweet corn is 4 percent protein and 10 percent sugar. Some of the newest varieties of supersweet corn are as high as 40 percent sugar. Eating corn this sweet can have the same impact on your blood sugar as eating a Snickers candy bar or a cake doughnut.

Today, most health experts agree that the most healthful diet is one that is high in fiber and low in sugar and rapidly digested carbohydrates. This regimen is referred to as a low-glycemic diet because it helps keep our blood glucose at optimum levels. A low-glycemic diet has been linked to a reduced risk of cancer, cardiovascular disease, chronic inflammation, obesity, and diabetes—our five modern scourges. Wild fruits and vegetables are the original low-glycemic foods.

A DRAMATIC LOSS OF PHYTONUTRIENTS

Within the past two decades, plant scientists around the world have discovered another major difference between wild plants and our modern varieties: the plants that nature made are much higher in polyphenols, or phytonutrients. (In this book, I will use the terms *phytonutrients* and *bionutrients* interchangeably. *Phyton* is the Greek word for "plant.") Plants can't fight their enemies or hide from them, so they protect themselves by producing an arsenal of chemical compounds that protect them from insects, disease, damaging ultraviolet light, inclement weather, and browsing animals.

More than eight thousand different phytonutrients have been identified to date, and each plant produces several hundred of them. Many of the compounds function as potent antioxidants. When we consume plants that contain high amounts of bioavailable antioxidants, we get added protection against noxious particles called free radicals that can inflame our artery linings, turn normal cells cancerous, damage our eyesight, increase our risk of becoming obese and diabetic, and intensify the visible signs of aging. Other phytonutrients are involved in the communication between our cells, and yet others alter our genes. A number of small-scale studies have shown that select bionutrients in plants can also enhance athletic performance, reduce the risk of infection, fight the flu, lower blood pressure, lower LDL cholesterol, speed up weight loss, protect the aging brain, improve mood, and boost immunity.

Because of these many potential health benefits, phytonutrients have become one of the hottest new areas of research. More than thirty thousand scientific papers have been published on the topic since the year 2000. Some of the research has been appearing in the popular press. Many health-conscious consumers can now talk knowledgeably about the resveratrol in red wine, the lycopene in tomatoes, and the anthocyanins in blueberries. The nutraceutical industry has been quick to capitalize on the research. Browse the Internet and you will find thousands of high-priced pills, energy bars, juice drinks, and powders that contain phytonutrient extracts. Have you had your lycopene capsule today?

If we were still eating wild plants, there would be no need for these supplements. One species of wild tomato, for example, has *fifteen times* more lycopene than the typical supermarket tomato. Some of the native potatoes that grow in the foothills of the Andes have twenty-eight times more phytonutrients than our russet potatoes. One species of wild apple that grows in Nepal has an amazing one hundred times more bionutrients than our most popular apples; just a few ounces of the fruit provide the same amount of phytonutrients as six large Fujis or Galas.

AN APPLE A DAY DID *NOT* KEEP THE DOCTOR AWAY

Remarkably, some varieties of produce in our supermarkets are so relatively low in phytonutrients and high in sugar that they can *aggravate* our health problems, not alleviate them. In an eye-opening study that took place in 2009, forty-six overweight men with high cholesterol and triglycerides agreed to participate in an eating experiment. Twenty-three of the men stayed on their regular diets and served as a control group; the other twenty-three men added one Golden Delicious apple to their daily fare. The goal of the project was to see if eating more fruit would reduce the men's high risk of cardiovascular disease. At the end of the two-month study, the researchers measured the blood fats of both groups of men and compared the results with tests that had been taken when the study began. To the researchers' surprise, the men who had eaten an apple a day had higher levels of triglycerides and LDL cholesterol than they had at the beginning of the study, giving them an *increased* risk of heart attack and stroke.

As the investigators puzzled over this finding, they concluded that the results had to do with the variety of apple they had chosen for the study. The Golden Delicious, they discovered, was too low in phytonutrients to lower the men's cholesterol and so high in sugar that it raised their triglycerides. The results of this study have a direct bearing on the health of Americans, because the sweet and juicy Golden Delicious is one of our most popular apples. The universal health advice to "eat more fruits and vegetables" is woefully out of date. We need good advice on *which* fruits and vegetables to eat.

There is another notion that needs to be revised. Many people in this country believe that the varieties of fruits and vegetables that were raised by our grandparents and great-grandparents are better for our health than the ones we grow today. According to this view, we should consume more heirloom fruits and vegetables. But the latest research shows that many modern varieties are more nutritious than our coveted heirlooms. The Golden Delicious apple, for example, is a one-hundred-year heirloom. The Liberty apple, which was released seventy-five years later, has twice the antioxidant value. It is now clear that the date that a variety is created is not a good predictor of how it will influence our health.

No domesticated apple, however, whether modern or heirloom, has as many phytonutrients as wild apples. As you will see in the pages to come, we will not experience optimum health until we recover a wealth of nutrients that we have squandered over ten thousand years of agriculture, not just the last one hundred or two hundred years.

FROM HUNTER-GATHERERS TO FARMERS

Until the invention of farming, all the people on the planet lived on wild plants and animals. Anthropologists tell us that these long-ago ancestors lived in small clans of twenty to forty people and moved from camp to camp throughout the year in search of food. They timed their journeys to coincide with the annual migration of game and the ripening of wild nuts, seeds, fruits, and vegetables. By necessity, all their food was local, organic, and seasonal. Because they hunted or foraged all their food, they are referred to as hunter-gatherers.

Our distant relatives continued to dine at nature's café until roughly five thousand to twelve thousand years ago. Then, for reasons not fully understood, groups of people in a handful of areas around the world broke ties with the past and began to raise their own food. In addition to hunting for wild game, they began to tame wild goats, pigs, and sheep so they could have a ready supply of meat. They milked the goats and sheep and turned their milk into cheese and fermented drinks.

They also began to create the very first gardens. In the beginning, gardening was a simple affair. The first farmers gathered seeds and cuttings from wild plants and grew them in one location to make them easier to tend and harvest. For many generations, the farmers raised too little food to meet all their needs, so they continued to gather wild plants. As the centuries passed, however, our ancestors became such skilled farmers that they were able to stop wandering in search of food and settle down in the first permanent settlements. Our species had made the epic transition from being hunters and gatherers to being herders and gardeners. The Agricultural Revolution—the great-grandmother of all food revolutions—had begun.

WE ARE THE FOOD MAKERS

As we humans set off on our excellent adventure in agriculture, all the other creatures on the planet remained true to their original diets—and do so to this day. Zebras, lemurs, elephants, eagles, rodents, weasels, bats, wombats, and the great apes eat the same food today as they did eons ago, provided we've left them enough habitat. Although animal handlers report that captive chimpanzees prefer M&M's to bananas, the chimps have yet to make any candy. Out of an estimated seven million species of animals, we alone had the intelligence, dexterity, and ability to plan for the future that allowed us to walk away from our native diet and create a brand-new menu that was more to our liking.

Therein lies the problem. Starting with the very first gardens, our farming ancestors chose to cultivate the wild plants that were the most pleasurable to eat. As a rule, the chosen plants were tender, low in bitterness and astringency, and high in sugar, starch, or oil. Plants that were bitter, tough, thick-skinned, dry, devoid of sugar, or too seedy were left behind in the wilderness. Why go to the trouble of cultivating plants that are unpleasant to eat?

Archaeologists have gathered detailed evidence about those earliest food choices. Wild figs and dates were two of the first plants to be cultivated, and they are among the sweetest of all native fruits. Although hunter-gatherers had consumed only small amounts of grain, the first farmers made starchy cereal grains a central part of their diet. Farmers in the Middle East grew wheat, barley, and millet. African farmers raised pearl millet and sorghum. Corn was king throughout the Americas, and rice became the staple crop of Asia. The era of carbs had begun.

Oil-rich plants were also highly favored. Archaeologists have unearthed the charred remains of an olive orchard in Palestine that was in production seven thousand years ago. Sesame seeds were domesticated for their oil about five thousand years ago. Oil-rich avocados were one of three staple crops in some parts of Mexico three thousand years ago.

Then as now, people knew what they wanted to eat—sweet, starchy, and fatty food. Because of our ancestors' extraordinary efforts, they were able to produce an abundant supply of these "must-have" plants within a short walking distance of their dwellings. For the first time in our long history on the planet, we humans no longer had to eat bitter or fibrous food or spend hours every day processing our food to make it fit to eat. We were creating the food supply of our dreams.

We now know that one of the consequences of cultivating the sweetest and mildest-tasting wild plants was a dramatic loss in phytonutrients. Many of the most beneficial bionutrients have a sour, astringent, or bitter taste. Unwittingly, when our ancestors rejected strong-tasting fruits and vegetables, they were lowering their protection against a long list of diseases and troubling conditions. Throughout our history of agriculture, our ability to transform our diet has far exceeded our understanding of the way those changes impact our health and well-being.

By the time of the Roman Empire, 250 generations of farmers had already played a role in reshaping the human diet. The differences between wild plants and our man-made varieties had, even then, become marked. The roots of domesticated beets, carrots, and parsnips were twice as large as the roots of their wild ancestors, and they contained less protein, more sugar, and more starch. Most domesticated fruits were several times larger than wild fruits, and they had thinner skins, more sugar, less fiber, more pulp, and fewer antioxidants. Cultivated greens were less bitter and, as a direct consequence, had fewer health-enhancing phytonutrients.

By the end of the nineteenth century, people around the world had created hundreds of thousands of new varieties designed to satisfy their needs and wishes. In the twentieth century, science-based breeding techniques speeded up the process. A plant breeder could start out with an idea for a new variety of plum or corn and make it a reality in just ten years, not several generations. Now, plant geneticists can insert foreign genes into corn or beets or potatoes and create a new variety in a matter of hours.

To this day, the nutritional content of our man-made varieties has been an afterthought. A plant researcher for the United States

Department of Agriculture (USDA) can spend years perfecting a new variety of blackberry or apple without ever measuring its phytonutrient content or its effect on blood sugar. If the variety is attractive, pleasing to eat, productive, and disease resistant, it is considered a triumph. Meanwhile, our bodies hunger for the nutrients that we have left by the wayside.

THE LOSS OF FLAVOR—A MODERN CALAMITY

We have been breeding the medicine out of our food for thousands of years, but the loss of flavor has been a relatively new exploit. It came about because of another agricultural revolution—the industrialization of our food supply. In the late nineteenth and early twentieth centuries, the introduction of mechanized plowing, planting, and harvesting equipment made it possible for farmers to manage much larger tracts of land. These large farms produced more food than was needed by the people in the surrounding community, so the fruits and vegetables began to be shipped to distant locations on the new railways and highways, bringing an abrupt end to ten thousand years of local production.

Growing food on megafarms greatly increased productivity, but it caused a marked loss of flavor. Fruits and vegetables now spent days or weeks in transport and storage, which used up their phytonutrients and natural sugars and made them more acidic and bitter. Ironically, after having spent ten thousand years making fruits and vegetables ever more palatable, we had reversed course and begun making them less enjoyable to eat.

By the mid-twentieth century, every aspect of farming had become mechanized. One of the unforeseen consequences was that our fresh produce was being subjected to much rougher handling than ever before. For millennia, farmers had harvested their produce by hand. Now, enormous machines lumbered over five-hundred-acre farms, tossing the fruits and vegetables into waiting trucks. The trucks dumped their cargo onto conveyor belts to be washed, sorted, and packed. The boxes of produce were jostled onto more trucks and then spent days in transit to warehouses, where they were stored anywhere from a few days to six months. The USDA and state agricultural schools began to throw their efforts into breeding industrial-strength varieties that were able to survive the ordeal. Our fruits and vegetables now had to be extra durable, as uniform as widgets, and be able to retain the illusion of freshness after spending weeks or even months in a warehouse.

Apples, potatoes, and a number of other fruits and vegetables store relatively well and were well adapted to these changing conditions. Soft fruits, however, could not be made durable enough for industrial agriculture, so the fruit industry had to find a workaround. The twentieth-century solution was to harvest the fruit while it was still green and firm enough to be handled without bruising or splitting. If the immature produce did not ripen during transport, it could be force-ripened in climate-controlled warehouses once it reached its destination.

By now it has become abundantly clear that fruit picked while still green and then artificially ripened is not as flavorful or juicy as fruit that ripens under the sun. Large supermarkets stage elaborate displays of fruits and vegetables, but the produce no longer tastes as good as it looks. The strawberries are twice as large as old-fashioned varieties, but they have half the flavor. All too often, the peaches, plums, and nectarines turn out to be mealy and bland. In some instances, our so-called "fresh" fruits and vegetables are not just less appealing to eat—they are downright distasteful. In 2008, a panel of professional food tasters sampled carrots that had been stored in a warehouse for several weeks, which is a typical amount of time. The panelists reported that the vegetables had "a strong, burning, turpentine-like flavor most clearly perceived at the back of the throat during and after chewing."

No wonder the USDA and private health agencies have spent hundreds of millions of dollars encouraging Americans to eat more fruits and vegetables and gotten such dismal results. Government statistics show that only 25 to 30 percent of US adults consume the recommended amount of fruits and vegetables. When people are disappointed time and again by the flavor of the produce available in the supermarkets, they stop buying it. It takes more than a media campaign to change their ways.

What can we do to restore the long-lost nutrients and flavor of our fruits and vegetables? Clearly, we can't go back to foraging for wild plants — there are too many of us and not enough wilderness. Imagine, for a moment, the 1.6 million inhabitants of Manhattan trekking up to the Adirondacks to gather wild roots and berries; it's not going to happen. Just as important, few of us would choose to eat wild plants, even if they were growing in our own backyards. Some varieties of sour crabapples have five times the cancer-fighting capacity of a Honeycrisp, but most of us would choose the sweeter, juicier fruit all the same. We are no longer accustomed to eating our bitter medicine.

EATING ON THE WILD SIDE

This book presents a new and radical solution to the dramatic loss of nutrients and flavor in our modern fruits and vegetables. Although living on wild plants is no longer feasible, we can "eat on the wild side." To do this, we can choose those select varieties of fruits and vegetables that have retained much of the nutritional content of their wild ancestors. One of the most important discoveries of twenty-first-century food science is that there are vast nutritional differences among the many varieties of a given fruit or vegetable. For example, some of the varieties of tomatoes sold in a typical supermarket have ten times more phytonutrients than other varieties that are displayed on the same table. The old idea that a tomato is a tomato is a tomato no longer holds. You'd have to eat ten of the least nutritious variety to get the same amount of lycopene as you would from one tomato of the most nutritious variety. Surprisingly, some supermarket tomatoes come close to the nutritional payload of their wild Peruvian ancestors. These jewels of nutrition have been hiding in plain sight. Now, for the first time, food chemists are providing the information we need to know which ones they are.

A similar range in phytonutrient content has been found among all the fruits and vegetables we eat, including corn, asparagus, onions, lettuce, beans, blueberries, grapes, plums, oranges, peaches, kale, broccoli, watermelons, and apples. Pungent-tasting onions have eight times more phytonutrients than sweet ones. A Granny Smith apple gives you three times move bionutrients than a Golden Delicious and thirteen times more than a Ginger Gold. Some of the uncommon varieties of apples sold in farmers markets and "U-pick" orchards are two to three times higher in antioxidants than the Granny Smith.

In addition to phytonutrients, our modern produce has a wide range of other nutrients, including fiber, protein, vitamins, minerals, essential fatty acids, and sugar. Eating a baked russet potato can boost your blood sugar as much as eating two slices of white bread. By contrast, some heirloom and hybrid varieties of potato can help *stabilize* your blood sugar. Some will even lower the blood pressure of people with hypertension. When you choose these stellar varieties, you will increase your protection against a host of diseases and debilitating conditions without spending any more time or money. You will also come closer to enjoying optimum health.

You may be surprised by some of the varieties that have proven to be nutritionally superior to others. One of the new food rules states that we should shop by color, selecting varieties that are red, orange, purple, dark green, and yellow. Although richly colored fruits and vegetables are among the most nutritious, there are dozens of exceptions to the rule. White-fleshed peaches and nectarines, for example, have twice as many bionutrients as yellow-fleshed varieties. Two different varieties of apples can have equally bright red skin, but one will give you three times more antioxidant protection than the other. The globe artichoke, despite its drab color, is one of the most nutritious vegetables in the grocery store. Its ghostly pale heart—even when canned—is almost as good for you as the leaves themselves. These choices are not intuitive. In order to reclaim the most lost nutrients, you need to shop with a list.

TWENTY-FIRST-CENTURY KITCHEN NUTRITION

Once you've brought your fruits and vegetables home from the store or harvested them from your garden, their nutritional fate is in your hands. Depending on how you store, prepare, and cook them, you can either destroy their beneficial bionutrients or retain or even enhance them. This, too, is a relatively new discovery. Until this century, little was known about the health benefits of phytonutrients or how to preserve them during storage and cooking. In the past two decades, food researchers have discovered hundreds of new ways to retain the bionutrients in our fresh produce and make them more bioavailable. It doesn't matter how many nutrients are in a fruit or vegetable if we can't absorb them.

Some of the findings to come out of the high-tech food labs are so different from conventional wisdom that you might feel as though you were tumbling down a rabbit hole. Most berries, for example, increase their antioxidant activity when you cook them. Believe it or not, canned blueberries have more phytonutrients than fresh ones—provided you consume the canning liquid. Simmering a tomato sauce for hours—the traditional Italian method—does more than blend its flavors; it can triple its lycopene content. Cooking carrots whole and then slicing or dicing them *after* they've been cooked makes them taste sweeter and increases their ability to fight cancer.

Our understanding of how to store fruits and vegetables is undergoing a sea change as well. Watermelons become more nutritious if you leave them out on the counter for several days before you eat them. Potatoes can be stored for weeks or even months without losing any of their nutritional value, but broccoli begins to lose its cancer-fighting compounds within twenty-four hours of harvest. In order to get all the vegetable's much-touted benefits, you have to grow it yourself or purchase it directly from a farmer and then eat it as soon as possible. Many foods do not lend themselves to centralized production and long-distance shipping, and broccoli is one of them. When we stopped eating locally grown produce and abandoned our home gardens, we lost at least half the protective properties of our fruits and vegetables as well as much of their flavor.

A ROAD MAP TO THIS BOOK

This book is divided into two sections. Part I is devoted to vegetables, and part II focuses on fruits. Each chapter features a different fruit or vegetable or an entire family of fruits or vegetables. At the beginning of each chapter, you will read about the wild ancestors of those particular foods and the role they played in the lives of hunter-gatherers. (Whipped fermented fish oil on stewed crabapples, anyone?) Then you will discover why, when, and how four hundred generations of farmers and modern plant breeders have whittled away at the nutritional content of their food—a whodunit with no clear villains.

The second half of each chapter focuses on solutions. You will learn the names of some of the most nutritious varieties of fruits and vegetables available today. I have gleaned this information from more than one thousand research journals published in the United States and abroad. These discoveries are so new and come from such a multitude of scientific disciplines that few of the varietal names have become public knowledge until now.

You will learn that it is possible to find many highly nutritious varieties of fruits and vegetables in a conventional supermarket. Still more are available in farmers markets, farm stands, natural-food stores, and ethnic markets. When you buy these select varieties directly from a farmer, you get to enjoy fresh-picked flavor as well as added health benefits. The most uncommon varieties of produce must be grown from seed. This is no hardship if you live in one of the nation's thirty-five million households that has a home garden. Growing the most delectable and nutritious fruits and vegetables in your own backyard or nearby community garden is the wave of the future.

You will also learn new ways to store, prepare, and cook fruits and vegetables to enhance their flavor and retain or increase their health benefits. Most of the techniques are simple and easy to remember. Each chapter concludes with a summary to help you recall key points.

The information in this book is useful to anyone who eats fruits and vegetables. Whether you are an omnivore, vegetarian, or vegan, you will discover new ways to make your diet more flavorful and nutritious. If you're on a specific regimen to lose weight, control allergies, or curb inflammation, choosing the varieties recommended in this book will further your goals. If you cook for young children, picky eaters, an older person with a flagging appetite, or people who swear by fast food or meat and potatoes, you will learn how to make "stealth" substitutions that will improve your loved ones' chances of enjoying robust good health.

Finally, if you or someone you know is struggling with a serious medical condition or illness, eating on the wild side will swell your kitchen medicine chest with a host of healing compounds that have been bred out of our food during our ten-thousand-year history of agriculture. Hippocrates's famous saying "Let food be thy medicine and medicine be thy food" will be more than inspirational words; it will become your daily reality.

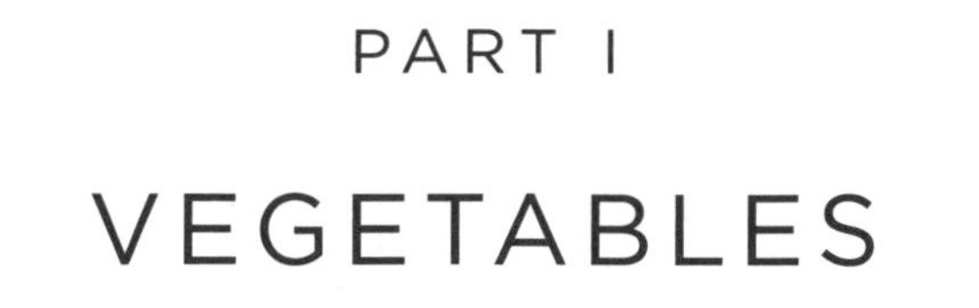

PART I

VEGETABLES

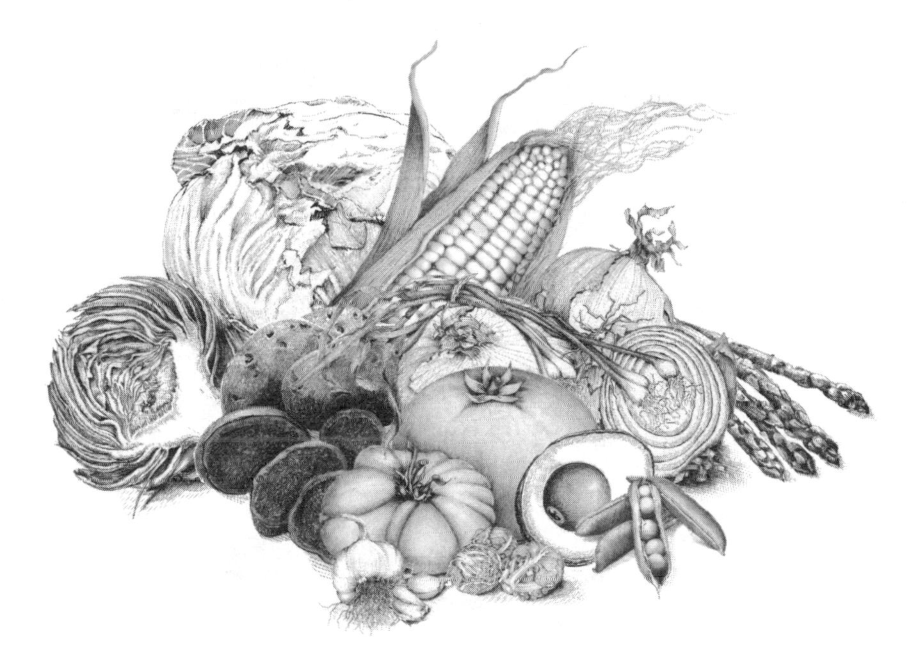

CHAPTER 1

FROM WILD GREENS TO ICEBERG LETTUCE

BREEDING OUT THE MEDICINE

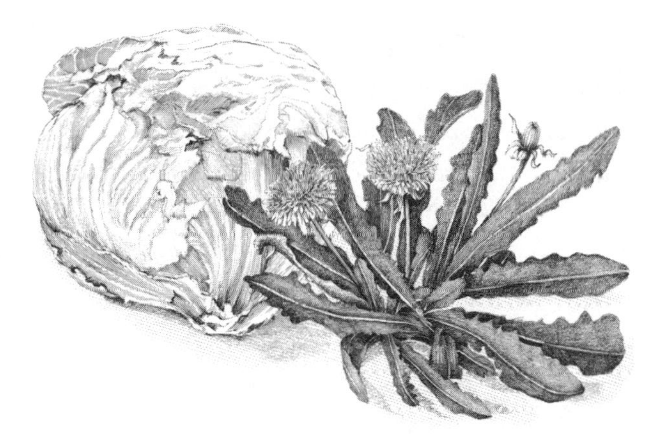

Iceberg lettuce and wild dandelion

Today, we can purchase fresh fruits and vegetables twelve months of the year. When they are out of season in one region of the country, they are shipped in from another or imported from as far away as Chile or China. This seamless supply allows us to forget the seasonal cycle of plants and their brief harvest seasons. We can buy fresh greens in December, apples in April, and grapes all year round.

The people who first inhabited this land did not have that luxury. During the winter months, hunter-gatherers had to make do with their caches of dried meat, fish, roots, fruit, and herbs. When spring finally arrived, they were hungry for fresh food. Even then, however, their choices were limited. The wild berry bushes and fruit trees had yet to blossom. Root plants—such as camas (a type of lily), wild carrots, onions, and groundnuts—were too small to be harvested. The wild grasses and legumes had yet to form seeds. To satisfy their craving for something live and growing, they consumed large quantities of spring greens and shoots, the only fresh food on their strictly local and seasonal menu.

WILD GREENS—BOTH FOOD AND MEDICINE

The wild greens that hunter-gatherers consumed were so rich in phytonutrients that they used them as medicine as well as food. The leaves of wild lamb's-quarters (*Chenopodium album*), also known as goosefoot and fat hen, were consumed by hunter-gatherers from North America to Africa. The greens were eaten raw, fried in fat, dried, added to soups, or mixed with meat. The Pomo people, who lived in northern California, steamed the leaves and used them to treat stomachaches. The Potawatomi of the upper Mississippi region used lamb's-quarters to cure a condition that we now know to be scurvy, a nutritional deficiency caused by a lack of vitamin C. The Iroquois made a paste of the fresh greens and applied it to burns to relieve pain and speed healing. Many tribes consumed the seeds of the plant as well as the leaves, even though the seeds were very small and tedious to gather. Americans are now eating the seeds of domesticated varieties of lamb's-quarters, which are unusually high in protein. They go by the name quinoa.

Lamb's-quarters may prove to be a potent healer in twenty-first-century medicine as well. Recent studies show that the greens are rich in phytonutrients, fight viruses and bacteria, and block the growth of human breast cancer cells. More investigations are under way.

Dandelions, the plague of urban lawns, were a springtime treat for the Navajo, Cherokee, Iroquois, and Apache. The leaves were eaten raw, steamed, or boiled, and they were added to soups and stews. Compared to spinach, one of our present-day "superfoods," dandelion leaves have eight times more antioxidants, two times more calcium, three times more vitamin A, and five times more vitamin K and vitamin E. Our modern superfoods would have been substandard fare for hunter-gatherers.

Wild greens may be excellent for our health, but how do they taste? I suggest you find out. You can begin with dandelions. First, locate some dandelion leaves that are pesticide-free and have not been visited by neighborhood pets. Rinse a leaf and take a bite. As you will discover, the leaf is relatively thick and chewy and it is covered with tiny hairs, top and bottom. For a second or two, the leaves will taste rather bland. Then, in a flash, a bloom of bitterness will start at the roof of your mouth and spread down the back of your throat. If you pay close attention, you will note that your tongue and mouth are becoming faintly numb—undeniable proof of the plant's painkilling properties. Nothing in the grocery store has prepared you for this riot of sensations.

Over the course of ten thousand years of agriculture, our farming ancestors managed to remove the bitterness from most of our greens. Unwittingly, though, when they removed the bitterness, they were also stripping away a host of highly beneficial phytonutrients that happen to have a bitter, astringent, or sour taste. Our mild-to-a-fault iceberg lettuce, for example, has one-fortieth as many bionutrients as bitter dandelion greens. Calcium is bitter as well, so the calcium content of our modern greens is also relatively low. This could be one of the reasons that osteoporosis now afflicts so many older Americans. In 2011, forty-four million individuals were diagnosed with low bone density or with osteoporosis, placing them at high risk for fractures. Hunter-gatherers who consumed calcium-rich wild greens had much denser bones than we do today, despite the fact that they consumed no dairy products.

As a group, we Americans are more averse to eating bitter greens than people living in other parts of the world. Iceberg lettuce is our most popular variety of leafy green by far, despite the fact that legions of chefs, health seekers, and foodies have moved on to arugula and mesclun. According to the USDA, Americans consume more servings of iceberg lettuce per week than all other fresh vegetables *combined,* with the exception of white potatoes. Half the population has never purchased any salad greens other than iceberg lettuce. To meet this demand, farms in California and a few other locations produce four million metric tons of the bland lettuce every year.

An excellent way to begin eating on the wild side is to add more nutrient-rich greens to your diet. You will find many highly nutritious varieties at supermarkets, salad bars, and some restaurants. You will find even more healthful greens when you shop in natural-food stores, farmers markets, or buy seeds for your garden. In this chapter, you will learn how to select the most nutritious greens wherever you shop, even when certain recommended varieties are not available. You will also learn new ways to prepare, store, and serve them that will enrich their flavor and health benefits.

LETTUCE

When you shop for fresh fruits and vegetables in a conventional supermarket, you will see that some items have labels showing their varietal name but others do not. When you shop for apples, for example, the name of each variety is usually posted on a sign. You know if you are buying a Gala, Red Delicious, or Honeycrisp. Typically, varietal names are also supplied for pears, cherries, grapes, avocados, oranges, onions, plums, mushrooms, and a number of other fruits and vegetables. This is not always true of lettuce and other greens, however. When you buy salad greens, you may have no way of knowing if that head of green looseleaf lettuce on display is Black-Seeded Simpson, Green Ice, or Salad Bowl. The produce manager is likely to be equally in the dark.

Fortunately, there are other ways to select the most nutritious greens in the store. Let's begin with lettuce. The lettuce varieties that have the most phytonutrients share two easily recognizable traits.

The first is color. As a general rule, the most intensely colored salad greens have the most phytonutrients. There is also a hierarchy to the colors. Ironically, the most nutritious greens in the supermarket are not green at all but red, purple, or reddish brown. These particular hues come from phytonutrients called anthocyanins, which also make blueberries blue and strawberries red. Anthocyanins are powerful antioxidants that show great promise in fighting cancer, lowering blood pressure, slowing age-related memory loss, and even reducing the negative effects of eating high-sugar and high-fat foods.

The next most nutritious greens are dark green in color. Dark green varieties are rich in a phytonutrient called lutein, which is another potent antioxidant and has been shown to protect eye health and calm inflammation. As a general rule, lettuce varieties with light green leaves give you the fewest health benefits.

The second trait to look for is more surprising. The arrangement of the individual leaves on a lettuce plant plays a major role in determining its phytonutrient content. When a lettuce plant has leaves that are tightly wrapped like a cabbage's, the phytonutrient content tends to be very low. This is true of iceberg lettuce and other crisphead varieties. Plants with loose and open leaves, particularly the looseleaf varieties, contain many times more bionutrients. As a rule, plants that have a combination of open and wrapped leaves, such as romaine and Bibb lettuce, have moderate amounts.

Why does the arrangement of the leaves on a plant influence its phytonutrient content? The reason is that all leaves have a love-hate relationship with the sun: they need sunlight to grow and produce carbohydrates, but the sun's UV rays can destroy them. In order to survive, they have to manufacture their own botanical sunscreen—pigmented antioxidants that block the harmful effects of UV light. Looseleaf lettuce is the most vulnerable to UV rays because most of its leaves are exposed to direct sunlight. As a result, the leaves have to produce extra quantities of phytonutrients. When we eat looseleaf lettuce, we absorb those compounds, which then become part of our *own* self-defense system—not only against UV rays but against cancer, chronic inflammation, and cardiovascular disease as well. The plant's protection becomes our protection.

When leaves—such as the ones inside crisphead and romaine lettuce—are sheltered from the sun, they are not exposed to UV rays and can slack off on the production of phytonutrients. Remarkably, the leaves on the inside of iceberg lettuce have *1 percent* of the antioxidant activity of the leaves on the sun-exposed outside of the plant. Location, location, location.

Now you have the information you need to select the most nutritious salad greens in the supermarket. *Choose the most intensely colored lettuces—preferably red or dark green—that also have the loosest arrangement of leaves.* Red looseleaf lettuce is the best choice; lab tests confirm that it is extra-rich in antioxidants and vitamins. Next comes dark green looseleaf lettuce, followed by red or dark green Bibb and romaine lettuces. Iceberg and other head lettuces may be crisp and refreshing, but they have very few phytonutrients to offer. Their light green leaves and high percentage of sheltered leaves are the reason for their low-nutrient status.

As a rule, the most nutritious greens in the grocery store have a more intense flavor than greens that are lower in food value. Some are hot and spicy, some are bitter, and some are sour. If a particular variety of lettuce is a bit intense for your taste, combine it with a milder variety, such as butterhead or romaine. You can also mellow its flavor by adding dried or fresh fruit to the salad. Avocado has a moderating effect as well. (Fat is one of the best antidotes to bitterness.) Adding a small amount of honey to a vinaigrette will also mask strong flavors. (See the recipe for honey mustard vinaigrette on page 39.)

CHOOSING THE FRESHEST LETTUCE

The freshness of lettuce and other salad greens also influences their nutritional benefits. The longer the greens have been in transit or stored in a warehouse or displayed in the store, the lower their antioxidant value and the more bitter they taste. Knowing how to pick the freshest greens in the supermarket is especially important in the winter months, when up to 12 percent of our lettuce is imported from Mexico—adding days to the average transit time.

As a rule, whole heads of lettuce are fresher than packaged greens or lettuce that is sold precut, because it takes time to process the greens. Also, cut leaves spoil more rapidly than whole heads of lettuce. (When the heads are separated into individual leaves, the plant produces chemicals that speed the leaves' decay.) When you examine the lettuce, look for crisp leaves with no sign of yellowing or wilting. The lettuce should also feel heavy for its size, an indication that it has preserved its internal moisture and will be crisp and inviting.

Why Do Some People Like Bitter Foods and Others Reject Them?

All people dislike intensely bitter, acidic, sour, or astringent flavors. It's a part of our basic survival kit. This built-in repulsion protects us from eating poisonous plants, which are characterized by those flavors. We take one bite and spit them out.

Our response to moderately bitter food is more varied. Surveys show that, among the US population, about 25 percent enjoy bitter foods and seek them out. Fifty percent tolerate bitter foods but do not favor them. The remaining 25 percent find most bitter flavors very unpleasant.

The people who are highly sensitive to bitter flavors are most likely to avoid coffee or drink it with cream or sugar. Green tea and soy products are distasteful to them. If they drink wine, they prefer white to red. They find that white grapefruit tastes unpleasantly bitter. Even though they know they "should" eat more kale, spinach, and broccoli, they prefer corn, potatoes, and peas.

This wide range of responses to bitter flavors is influenced by many factors, including culture, childhood diet, and the availability of different types of foods. Children in some cultures enjoy food that would taste very bitter to adults living in other parts of the world. Hunter-gatherers relished food that most of us would find repellent.

As a group, we Americans are more averse to bitter flavors than people from other countries. For example, most Americans prefer sweet apples to tart ones, caffe latte to espresso, and milk chocolate to dark chocolate.

Nothing reveals our national aversion to bitterness, however, as much as our choice of beer. The bitterness of beer is ranked in terms of international bitterness units, or IBUs, a scale that ranges from 1 to 100. The higher the number, the more bitter the brew. The Irish brand Guinness, a relatively bitter-tasting beer, ranges between 45 and 60 IBUs. German pilsners approach 100. Budweiser, a light American lager, is only 8 IBUs. Although hundreds of new US microbreweries are now producing full-flavored beer, our bestselling brand continues to be Bud Light, which is a mere 6.4 IBUs. When it comes to beer, we are the world's wimps.

There is a biological component to the bitter response that can override all other factors. Each of us inherits a unique set of genes that governs our response to flavors. One set of genes, for example, determines the size and number of taste buds on your tongue and the lining of your mouth. People born with genes that code for large numbers of small taste buds are more sensitive to bitter flavors and to all other taste sensations as well. Physiologists call them supertasters.

Many supertasters have grown up being accused of being picky, squeamish, or "fussy eaters." In reality, they are *better* tasters than the rest of the population and need a smaller amount of a given flavor to get the same response. What tastes slightly bitter to other people tastes far more bitter to them.

Being a supertaster can make it more difficult to enjoy nutritious vegetables that have an astringent, sour, or bitter taste. Throughout this book, I describe ways to mask bitter flavors or to prevent them from developing in the first place. I also highlight the foods that have a mild flavor and are also unusually rich in nutrients.

PREPACKAGED GREENS

Since the 1990s, packages of "triple-washed" salad greens have been very popular in US markets. Forty percent of the salad greens now grown in California are cut up and packed into bags. To make a salad from packaged greens, all you have to do is rip open the bag, dump the greens into a bowl, and anoint them with a ready-made salad dressing. People have been eating more salads as a result.

"California salad" is a general term for a mix of different kinds of lettuce and salad vegetables. Typically, it is sold in a plastic bag or lidded container. The mix can contain hot and spicy greens (arugula, radicchio, mustard greens, and Asian greens), mild lettuces (Bibb lettuce, baby spinach, and oak leaf lettuce), or a combination of the two. Some contain as many as fifteen different vegetables, including less familiar greens and herbs such as chervil, mâche (corn salad), beet greens, and cilantro. All bags of mixed greens, no matter their exact composition, have more phytonutrients than salads made from iceberg or romaine lettuce alone. For maximum health benefits, choose the mix with the highest proportion of red, dark green, or purple-tinged leaves.

To pick the freshest bagged greens, examine them carefully. The cut edges of the leaves are the first to discolor. Limp or yellow leaves are another indication of long storage. For added confirmation of freshness, look for the "use-by" date on the packaging. By law, food producers must display the last day that the produce can be expected to maintain a reasonable quality for consumption. (Note that "reasonable" quality is not the same as "excellent" quality.) Packages with the most distant "use-by" dates are the freshest. At any given time, you will be able to find bagged salad vegetables that are a week or two fresher than others.

HOW TO STORE LETTUCE

Most people store their salad greens in the plastic bags they get from the store. Others store them in sealed bags or containers. None of these practices does an adequate job of preserving the phytonutrients, crispness, and flavor of the vegetables. If you spend ten minutes prepping the greens for the fridge and then store them in the right kind of bag, they will stay crisp and retain their fresh flavor and health benefits days longer.

As soon as you bring the greens home, pull off the leaves, rinse them, and soak them for about ten minutes in very cold water. The cold water lowers their temperature, which slows the aging process. It also increases the internal moisture of the greens, which keeps them crisp longer. Next, dry them with a towel or in a salad spinner. Any moisture left on the surface hastens their decay. For optimum storage, you want the moisture *inside* the greens, not on the outside.

Here's a surprise. If you tear up the lettuce before you store it, you can *double* its antioxidant value. The living plant responds to the insult as if it were being gnawed by an insect or eaten by an animal: it produces a burst of phytonutrients to fend off the intruders. Then when you eat the greens, you benefit from the added antioxidant protection. There's one caveat. Eat the greens within a day or two, because the tearing also hastens their decay.

There is a surprisingly simple way to preserve the phytonutrients in lettuce and other greens while they are being stored in your refrigerator. Put the greens in a resealable plastic bag, squeeze out as much air as possible without crushing the leaves, seal the bag, and then use a needle or a pin to prick it with between ten and twenty evenly spaced holes. (Make ten pinpricks in quart-size bags and twenty in larger bags.) Put the bag in the crisper drawer of your refrigator, which is the coolest, most humid location.

Why the holes? The tiny, almost invisible pinpricks provide the ideal level of humidity inside the bag and enable the beneficial exchange of gases. When fruits and vegetables are harvested, they do not die in the customary sense of the word, even though they are detached from the plant. They continue to consume oxygen and produce carbon dioxide; in other words, they "breathe." If you store the greens in a tightly sealed bag without the pinpricks, the carbon dioxide levels rise and the oxygen declines. After a few days, the lettuce leaves will begin to die from lack of oxygen. As a result, their fresh flavor and most of their phytonutrients will disappear.

The opposite problem occurs when you put the greens in an unsealed bag or in the crisper drawer of your refrigerator without any covering. In this case, the lettuce is exposed to so much oxygen that it begins to respire very rapidly. As it does, it uses up its stored sugar and antioxidants, making them unavailable for you. The lettuce will also go limp because the humidity inside the refrigerator is too low to maintain the internal moisture of the leaves.

The solution is to store the lettuce inside a sealed bag pricked with holes. The humidity remains high and the greens get enough oxygen to stay alive, but not so much that they respire too rapidly. To reuse the bags, mark them so you can identify them later. (The holes are invisible.) As you will see in later chapters, this inexpensive, novel storage technique helps preserve the nutrients and fresh flavor of many other fruits and vegetables as well. I will be referring to the pinpricked bags as "microperforated" bags throughout this book.

BEYOND THE SUPERMARKET

When you shop at a farmers market or farm stand, you will see a greater variety of fresh salad vegetables than you do in the supermarket. What's more, you will be able to shop for specific varieties because the names will be displayed along with the greens, or, if they're not, the farmer will be able to give you that information. Look around and you'll find looseleaf varieties that are as dark as red wine, such as the aptly named Merlot. You will see red-colored varieties of romaine, Bibb, and iceberg lettuce that are much higher in antioxidants than the conventional green varieties. Just as important, the vegetables will be impeccably fresh. Most farmers pick their produce within twenty-four hours of bringing it to market. Bring along the list of recommended varieties at the end of this chapter to help guide your choices.

If you are a home gardener, you're in lettuce heaven. Some seed catalogs list fifty or more varieties. Leaf through the pages and you'll find heirloom varieties with evocative names such as Flashy Troutback, Devil's Tongue, and Drunken Woman Frizzy-Headed. You will also be able to find all the varieties listed on pages 42–44.

OTHER SALAD GREENS

Some of the most nutritious greens in the store are not from the lettuce family. Some belong to the cabbage family, some are herbs, and others are close cousins of lettuce. Many of them are slightly bitter or spicy hot, which goes hand in hand with their many health benefits. The more of them you add to your salads, the more wild nutrients you reclaim.

ARUGULA

Wild arugula is a favorite springtime green in Greece, southern Italy, and France, where people head to the woods each April to gather baskets of the greens. The wild varieties are more nutritious and more intensely flavored than the varieties sold in our stores, but even supermarket arugula is rich in phytonutrients. Arugula (*Eruca vesicaria* M.) is a member of the cabbage family, and, like most crucifers, it is rich in a family of phytonutrients called glucosinolates, compounds with strong anticancer properties. The common name for arugula is rocket. Arugula is higher in antioxidants than most green lettuces, including dark green leafy varieties. Only red lettuce tops it. Arugula is also higher in calcium, magnesium, folate, and vitamin E than most salad greens. If you're not acquainted with arugula, search the produce section of the supermarket for a dark green, leafy vegetable with deeply cut leaves that resemble those of a dandelion. Arugula has a shorter shelf life than most greens, so take the time to choose the freshest in the store. Fresh arugula is firm, dark green, and has little odor. Place the greens in a microperforated bag and store in the crisper drawer of your refrigerator.

According to a 2011 Colorado State University survey, adults are evenly divided between arugula likers and arugula haters. Arugula is more peppery than bitter. If you're a supertaster (see page 28) or do not like arugula, look for younger plants with leaves that are no more than five inches long. They are milder than more mature plants. You can tone down the assertiveness of arugula even more by mixing it with milder greens. Eat the greens raw for the most health benefits. You can also sauté them or use them as a substitute for spinach in many of your recipes and still get most of their anticancer properties. If you boil them, however, as much as 60 percent of their glucosinolates will leach into the water.

Many restaurants now serve arugula salads on a regular basis. Typically, young leaves are tossed in a vinaigrette, topped with slices of fruit or vegetables, and then adorned with feta or some other type of cheese. Make your own variations at home. Substitute slices of hard-boiled eggs or artichoke hearts for the cheese and sprinkle the salad with sunflower seeds, walnuts, or toasted pecans. Serve slices of cooked beets on a bed of arugula and top with slivers of raw red onion and crumbled feta or blue cheese.

If you have a garden, access to a community garden, or enough space on your deck or fire-escape landing for a large pot, consider growing arugula. True to its name, arugula "rockets" out of the ground in early spring. You will be feasting on the leaves in just thirty to forty days. Two months after you plant it, however, it can turn hot, spicy, and go to seed, or "bolt." To have a continuous supply of young, mild-tasting arugula, plant seeds every few weeks. Adagio, a new variety, does not flower until long after other varieties have gone to seed, making it a good choice for the home gardener.

RADICCHIO

Radicchio (*Cichorium intybus*) is from the chicory family. Europeans enjoy its frankly bitter flavor more than we do. But the bitterness comes with rewards. Compared to romaine, it has four times more antioxidants. Eating more radicchio is good for your health.

Radicchio comes in red and green varieties, the most familiar being the Italian Rosso di Chioggia. This variety forms a loose head of bright magenta leaves set off with white veins and ribs. You can't miss it. Rosso di Treviso is the same color as Rosso di Chioggia, but does not form a head. It has three times more bionutrients than Rosso di Chioggia and ten times more than green varieties of radicchio.

SPINACH

Spinach (*Spinacia oleracea* L.) is our most popular dark green vegetable and is higher in antioxidants than most lettuce greens. Like other dark green plants, it is rich in lutein, a phytonutrient that helps protect the eyes and reduce inflammation. Lutein may have antiaging properties as well. In a study of older rats, a daily dose of spinach extract improved the rodents' strength, balance, and mental abilities. Closer examination showed that the spinach had made their brain neurons more responsive. Popeye, if you recall, had a quick wit in addition to his bulging biceps.

Spinach has become a popular salad green in recent years and large quantities are being grown for this purpose. Typically, the plants are harvested when they are young and tender and then bagged as loose greens. Many people who find mature spinach too bitter for their tastes love the baby greens. A consumer survey determined that most people like baby spinach as much as lettuce when used in hamburgers, tacos, and sandwiches. This is one of those "stealth" substitutions you can try with teenagers and young children.

For the freshest flavor and most health benefits, however, buy whole spinach in bunches rather than as bagged leaves. The longer the spinach is stored in a bag, the lower its antioxidant properties. Spinach leaves that have been stored for just one week give you half the antioxidant benefits of freshly harvested greens. Spinach plants with midsize leaves have more phytonutrients than baby spinach or plants with larger leaves. When you bring spinach home from the store, soak it in cold water and then spin or pat it dry. Spinach spoils even more rapidly than lettuce greens, so eat it as soon as possible. If you plan to store it for a few days, use a microperforated bag.

When cooking spinach, steam it or cook it in the microwave. Do not boil. After ten minutes of boiling, three-quarters of its phytonutrient content will have leached into the cooking water. The greener the color of the water, the more nutrients you have lost. As you can see by the graph below, you would be better off drinking the water and discarding the greens.

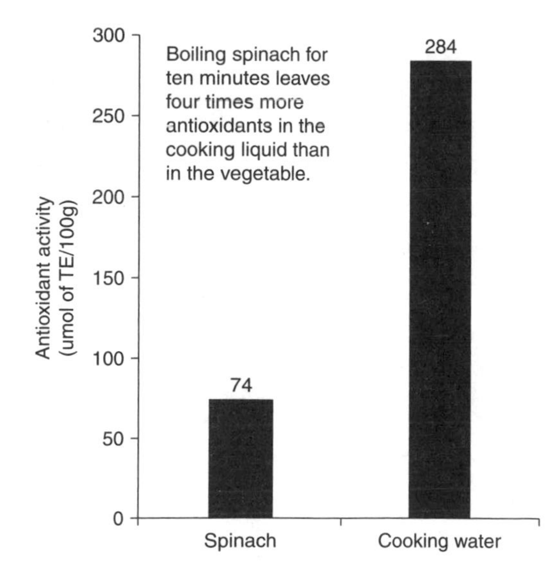

Going Wild at the Salad Bar

Choose from the following ingredients and you will create a wonderfully nutritious salad. Top your salad with a dressing made from extra virgin olive oil and either vinegar or lemon juice.

Artichoke hearts
Arugula
Bell peppers—any color
Cabbage—preferably red
Cherry tomatoes
Looseleaf lettuce—preferably red or dark green
Nuts and seeds—not croutons
Onions—red, yellow, or green
Radicchio—any variety
Spinach
Sprouts

SALAD DRESSINGS

Your salad is not complete until you dress it up. Prepared salad dressings are ultraconvenient to use. Before you buy them, however, read the list of ingredients. Most dressings have a significant amount of salt and either sugar or high-fructose corn syrup. Be wary of the term "natural flavors," too, because it means that the salad dressing can contain up to 20 percent MSG, a chemical flavor enhancer that many people want to avoid. Look for salad dressings that are made from wholesome ingredients with no unwanted additives.

Low-fat and nonfat salad dressings are not as good for your health as once believed. A decade or two ago, the medical profession advised people to cut back on all types of fat, including salad dressings. Diet gurus chimed in with the slogan that "Only fat can make you fat!" Adding a fat-free dressing to a salad made from raw vegetables created a nonfat salad—the holy grail of nutrition. Some purists sprinkled their salads with vinegar or lemon juice and left it at that.

Now it is known that we cannot absorb some of the most important nutrients in salad greens unless the dressing or the meal it's eaten with contains some type of fat. Olive oil, according to a 2012 Purdue University study, does the best job of making those compounds more bioavailable. It takes almost seven times more soybean oil, by contrast, to get the same results. Soybean oil is the most common oil in commercial salad dressings.

I recommend that you make your own salad dressing whenever possible. You can make a fresh, wholesome, and flavorful salad dressing in five minutes. Extra virgin olive oil is the best oil to use. For even more health benefits, look for a newcomer on the supermarket shelves—*unfiltered* extra virgin olive oil. The fact that most of our extra virgin olive oil has been filtered may come as a surprise; one assumes that terms such as "first pressing" and "cold pressed" mean that the oil has not been refined in any way. In reality, most of the extra virgin olive oil sold in this country has been decanted, centrifuged, and filtered before it is bottled. These processing steps turn a murky oil into a clear one, which US consumers have come to expect. Hold up a glass bottle of extra virgin olive oil to the light. If the oil is clear, it's been filtered. Clarifying extra virgin olive oil, it is now known, filters out half its bionutrients. One of those beneficial compounds is squalene, which has been proven to help fight cancer and protect the skin from UV damage.

Another advantage to buying unfiltered olive oil is that it retains its nutritional value and low acidity three months longer than filtered oil. This is because its greater antioxidant content protects the oil from oxidizing and turning rancid. If you can't find unfiltered oil in your area, order it on the Internet. The prices range from affordable to ridiculous. Expect to see more brands of unfiltered extra virgin olive oil in supermarkets in the near future. The word is getting out.

Apple cider vinegar, red wine vinegar, balsamic vinegar (especially naturally aged balsamic vinegar), and fresh lemon juice are also good sources of antioxidants. The flavor of the oil and the vinegar you use has the most influence on the overall flavor of the dressing. Sample different brands and types of olive oil and vinegar to find out which ones you like best.

How you store your olive oil is the key to maintaining its fresh flavor and antioxidant content. The first step is to purchase only the amount you plan to use in one or two months; olive oil may be cheaper by the gallon, but it is likely to be rancid before you use it up. The next step is to store your olive oil in a sealed container in a dark, cool location. This defeats the three main destroyers of antioxidants in your food—oxygen, light, and heat. If you invest in a premium brand of olive oil, treat it as you would an expensive wine. Pour the oil into an empty dark-colored wine bottle and seal it with a vacuum stopper that allows you to pump out some of the oxygen. The stoppers are sold in wine stores, kitchen stores, and on the Internet.

The traditional Greek salad dressing, the simplest of all, is one of the most nutritious. Drizzle your salad with extra virgin olive oil and finish with a few squirts of lemon juice and a dash of salt and pepper. I also recommend the following salad dressing because it does a good job of masking the flavor of bitter greens. Two of its ingredients—honey and mustard—have been proven to tone down assertive flavors. The pungency of the garlic also distracts you from the bitterness of the greens.

HONEY MUSTARD VINAIGRETTE

You can alter this basic recipe by adding any of the following ingredients: ½ teaspoon sweet paprika, 1 teaspoon grated lemon or orange peel, or 1 teaspoon dried herbs, such as tarragon, basil, mint, or oregano. If you prefer fresh herbs, use 1 tablespoon of the finely chopped leaves.

TOTAL TIME: 5–10 MINUTES YIELD: 1½ CUPS

¼ cup vinegar of your choice
1–2 tablespoons freshly squeezed lemon juice, lime juice, or orange juice
1 tablespoon honey
1–2 garlic cloves, finely minced or pushed through a garlic press
1 tablespoon prepared mustard or 1 teaspoon powdered mustard
¾ teaspoon salt, or more or less to taste
Freshly ground black pepper to taste
1 cup extra virgin olive oil, preferably unfiltered

Combine all ingredients except the oil and mix until well blended. You can beat with a spoon or wire whisk or blend for ten seconds in a food processor on medium-high speed. Then add the oil in a thin drizzle, whisking constantly. If you're using a food processor, process on medium speed as you add the oil. Pour enough dressing over the salad to coat the greens, but not so much that it pools in the bottom of the salad bowl. Store in the refrigerator for up to two weeks. Bring to room temperature before using.

ABOUT THE CHARTS OF RECOMMENDED VARIETIES

Each chapter in parts I and II ends with a chart listing some of the most nutritious and delicious varieties of fruits and vegetables available in the United States. Each one of the recommended varieties has been tested for nutritional content, and the results have been published in a peer-reviewed scientific journal. The varieties are in the top 10 percent in terms of their phytonutrient content. Many of them are also relatively high in fiber, vitamins, and minerals and have a low glycemic index.

The varieties are sorted into two categories according to availability. Each chart begins with varieties or types of fruits and vegetables that can be found in most supermarkets. The next section lists varieties that are more likely to be found in local farmers markets, specialty stores, U-pick farms, or seed catalogs. An updated list of recommended varieties is available at my website, http://www.eatwild.com.

If you want to grow some of the least common varieties of fruits and vegetables, you may have difficulty locating the seeds or plants. To find them, search the Internet for their varietal names. Also, The Mother Earth News website has a helpful search engine called the Seed and Plant Finder (http://www.motherearthnews.com/Find-Seeds-Plants.aspx). Enter the variety you are looking for and the program will search for it in a dozen or more seed catalogs, including ones that specialize in rare plants.

I have specified USDA plant hardiness zones for most of the varieties recommended in the book. The zones tell you whether or not a given plant will survive typical winter conditions in your area. The country is divided into zones based on average annual minimum winter temperatures. Zones with lower numbers have lower average minimum temperatures. If you live in zone 5, for example, and a given plant is recommended for zones 6–8, the plant may not survive the coldest nights in your area. If you do not know your zone, you can go to the USDA website (http://www.planthardiness.ars.usda.gov/) and either refer to the map or enter your zip code in the box provided.

As you will see, I have not included detailed nutritional data for each variety. One reason is that I gathered the data from a large number of studies, and each of them used a slightly different set of procedures or units of measurement. Just as you can't compare apples to oranges, you can't compare apples to apples if one study lists their phytonutrient content in terms of "grams of phenolics per 100 grams of dry weight" and the other expresses it as "micromoles per liter of juice." To provide precise numbers would be meaningless and confusing. Also, the phytonutrient content of a plant does not factor in how much you will absorb. If you want more specific details, you will find them in the studies listed in the Scientific References section, pages 375–400.

RECOMMENDED VARIETIES OF SALAD VEGETABLES

IN THE SUPERMARKET

VARIETY OR TYPE	COMMENTS
Arugula	A member of the cabbage family, arugula has a peppery taste and is often added to other greens in a salad. Arugula is high in lutein and overall antioxidant value.
California salad, or mixed greens	"California salad" is another term for mixed lettuce greens. Typically, it comes in a plastic bag or box. Select mixtures that are the freshest and have the greatest quantity of dark green, purple, or red leaves.
Frisée (also called curly endive)	Frisée, also known as curly endive, is a spiky salad vegetable that is mildly bitter. There are fine and coarse leaf types.

VARIETY OR TYPE	COMMENTS
Looseleaf Lettuce	As a general rule, the most nutritious looseleaf lettuces have red leaves, followed by those with dark green leaves and then those with lighter-colored leaves.
Rosso di Chioggia	Rosso di Chioggia, a variety of radicchio with magenta leaves and white ribs, is compact, resembling a head of cabbage in shape. It is very high in antioxidant value.
Rosso di Treviso	Rosso di Treviso, also a radicchio, is the same color as Rosso di Chioggia, but it does not form a head. It has three times more bionutrients than di Chioggia and ten times more than most salad greens. An antioxidant superstar.

FARMERS MARKETS, SPECIALTY STORES, U-PICK FARMS, AND SEED CATALOGS

VARIETY	TYPE	DESCRIPTION	INFORMATION FOR GARDENERS
Blackjack (also called Black Jack)	Looseleaf	Slightly ruffled leaves are dark burgundy at the early, baby-leaf stage. One of the highest in antioxidant value.	Slow to bolt.
Cimarron	Romaine	Mix of green, red, and bronze leaves. More nutritious than green romaine lettuce. Stiff-ribbed, but with a tender heart.	Grows 10–12 inches tall. Does well in hot and cold climates. High-yielding. Slow to bolt.
Cocarde	Oak leaf	Large green leaves edged in red or bronze. Smooth, almost waxy, with a delicate texture. Sweet yet flavorful.	Slow to bolt.
Concept	Batavian	Thick, juicy, medium-green leaves. Flavorful and rarely bitter. (Batavian lettuce has characteristics of romaine and looseleaf.) High in lutein.	Slow to bolt.

VARIETY	TYPE	DESCRIPTION	INFORMATION FOR GARDENERS
Dazzle	Romaine	Miniature romaine with burgundy outer leaves and crunchy, sweet, pale green hearts. One small head makes one salad.	Small size makes it suitable for containers and window boxes.
Eruption	Romaine	Intensely red miniature romaine lettuce. Glossy, savoyed (curled and wrinkled) leaves are crisp and mild. Much more nutritious than green varieties of romaine.	Small size makes it suitable for containers and window boxes. Slow to bolt. Resistant to tip burn.
Fire Mountain	Looseleaf	Large, frilled, deep burgundy leaves.	Slow to turn bitter in hot weather.
Flame	Looseleaf	Mild flavor, with intensely red, shiny leaf tips that add great color to salads.	Slow to bolt.
Galactic (also called Red Galactic)	Looseleaf	Glossy, dark red, lightly frilled, slightly bitter leaves; firm but pliable, which makes them ideal for using as a food wrap. Very high in anthocyanins and antioxidants.	Can be harvested when immature and used as baby greens. Slow to bolt.
Lollo Rosso (also called Lolla Rossa)	Looseleaf	Ruffled, fan-shaped, 5–8-inch leaves are dark magenta with a pale green base. Crisp, semisucculent, with a hardy texture and a mild, slightly bitter, nutty taste. Extra-high in antioxidant activity.	Slow-growing. Does best in warm days and cool nights. Harvesting an entire outer layer of leaves encourages regrowth.
Merlot	Looseleaf	A deep maroon lettuce with crisp leaves. Very high in anthocyanins. A bit tart.	Bolt-resistant.
Merveille des Quatre Saisons (also called Marvel of Four Seasons and Continuity)	Butterhead	This tasty French heirloom is one of the most widely grown lettuces in the world but is less well known in the United States. It has thin, magenta-colored outer leaves and a pale green heart.	Early-maturing.

VARIETY	TYPE	DESCRIPTION	INFORMATION FOR GARDENERS
Outredgeous	Romaine	One of the reddest romaines on the market. Its upright, slightly ruffled, glossy leaves are bright red on top and light green at the base. Much higher in anthocyanins and other phytonutrients than green romaines.	High-yielding lettuce.
Prizehead	Looseleaf	Bronze-tipped outer leaves over frilled, light green inner leaves. Crisp, sweet, and tender. An heirloom rich in antioxidants.	Fast grower. Early harvest.
Red Iceberg	Crisphead	Copper-colored outer leaves surround green-to-white inner head. Medium-size. Mild flavor. Good for salads or sandwiches. More nutritious than traditional iceberg lettuce.	Requires very fertile, loose soil. Pick outside leaves for a continuous harvest.
Red Oak Leaf	Looseleaf	Oak-shaped leaves mature to a deep burgundy color.	Maintains a mild flavor all season long. Resistant to late-season mildew.
Red Sails	Looseleaf	Heavily savoyed red-bronze leaves. Mild flavor. Higher in lutein and beta-carotene than all other lettuces tested in a recent study.	Resists tip burn. All-American selection.
Red Velvet	Looseleaf	Solid, deep red leaves with green-tinted backs. Pleasant, chewy texture.	Plants form loose heads that are slow to bolt. Makes a stunning border planting.
Revolution	Looseleaf	Deep red leaves are thick and frilly and stay crunchy, even after refrigerating.	Plant is 10–12 inches tall. Bolt-resistant.
Rouge d'Hiver	Romaine	Large, smooth, with outer leaves in shades from medium red to bronze.	Tolerates cold but not hot weather.
Ruby Red	Looseleaf	Delicately frilled, with intense red color that does not fade in hot weather. Sweet and succulent. Works well as a garnish and adds color to salads.	Matures early in the season. Heat-tolerant and bolt-resistant.

SALAD GREENS: POINTS TO REMEMBER

1. ***Choose red, red-brown, purple, or dark green looseleaf varieties.***
   The most nutritious lettuce cultivars are deeply colored and have a loose arrangement of greens. Pale-colored varieties that form a tight head are the least nutritious. Whole heads of lettuce are fresher than bagged greens.
2. ***Spend ten minutes preparing your lettuce to preserve its flavor and nutrients.***
   Separate a head of lettuce into its individual leaves or open a bag of loose greens and soak them in very cold water for ten minutes. Dry in a salad spinner or with a towel to remove the surface water. If you tear your lettuce into bite-size pieces, you will increase its antioxidant content. But if you do, be sure to eat it within one or two days. Place the greens in a resealable plastic bag that you have pricked with between ten and twenty tiny holes. Squeeze out the air, seal, and store in the crisper drawer of your refrigerator.
3. ***Enrich your salads with extra-nutritious nonlettuce varieties.***
   Arugula, radicchio, endive, and spinach are higher in phytonutrients than most lettuce varieties and will enrich the nutritional content of your salads.
4. ***Choose bags of mixed greens with the most colorful, freshest leaves.***
   If you buy packaged salad greens, look for mixtures that contain red and dark green varieties. Reject bags of greens that have yellow, brown, or withered leaves. Check the "use-by" date for added confirmation of freshness.

5. ***Extra virgin olive oil is one of the best oils to use in a salad dressing.***
   Fat-free dressings limit your absorption of the fat-soluble vitamins in salad greens. Extra virgin olive oil is an excellent oil to use because it makes the nutrients in the greens more bioavailable. Unfiltered extra virgin olive oil is even better because it has more antioxidants and will stay fresh longer.

6. ***Tame the bold flavors of bitter greens.***
   Many of the most healthful salad vegetables are high in beneficial but bitter-tasting phytonutrients. If you are extra-sensitive to bitterness, mix small amounts of bitter greens with milder lettuce. Add avocados or dried or fresh fruit. A honey mustard salad dressing further masks the bitterness.

CHAPTER 2

ALLIUMS

ALL THINGS TO ALL PEOPLE

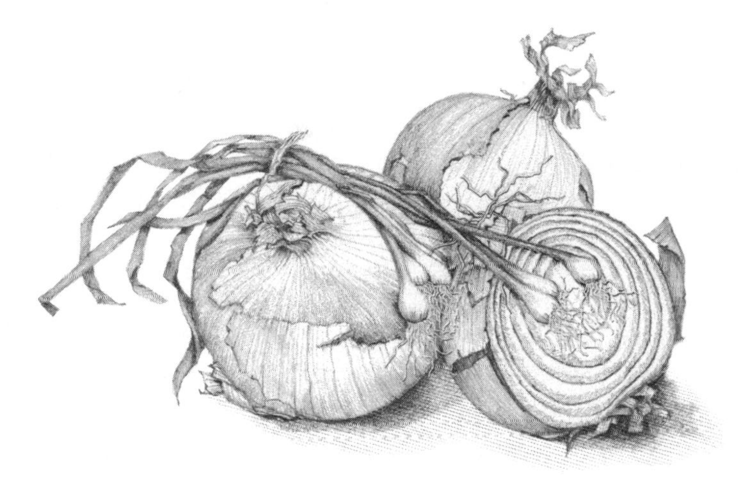

Wild and modern onions

When Hippocrates said, "Let food be thy medicine and medicine be thy food," he was probably giving a toast with a goblet of red wine during a meal that was redolent with onions and garlic. Garlic, onions, shallots, scallions, chives, and leeks—the allium family—have been celebrated throughout history as savory vegetables, essential condiments, and lifesaving medicine.

Hunter-gatherers the world over were keenly aware of these multiple benefits. Native Americans gathered more than one hundred different kinds of wild alliums for food and medicinal purposes, according to Daniel E. Moerman, a recognized expert on the diets of North American hunter-gatherers. The tribes used them to treat infected wounds, restore appetites, boost energy, repel scorpions, soothe bee stings, relieve colic and croup, lower fevers, and as a general tonic for colds, sore throat, and earaches.

Because the bulbs had so many important uses, tribes could be very protective of their allium fields. The Menominee Nation of the Great Lakes region laid claim to an extensive field of wild garlic, or ramps, that was located on the southern tip of Lake Michigan. The area was so rife with ramps that their odor perfumed the air for miles. The Menominee called their prized field Shikako, or "skunk place." The name lives on today in its anglicized form, Chicago.

Wild alliums are more pungent than their domesticated cousins, which we eat today. To tame their bite, hunter-gatherers mixed them with other foods or cooked them in soups and stews, much as we do. They steamed onions by wrapping them in fresh leaves and placing them close to a fire, which made them taste sweet and mild.

Interestingly, some tribes were as worried about "onion breath" as we are today, according to Erna Gunther, a noted twentieth-century anthropologist. Members of the Puget Sound Songish tribe consumed raw onions on long canoe voyages to increase their endurance. But, she added, they did this "only when traveling alone."

It is believed that the first people to domesticate wild alliums lived thousands of years ago in the mountainous regions of Pakistan. The wild onions in that area have tiny bulbs about the size of our modern scallions, and they are blazingly hot. The heat is generated by sulfur-based nutrients called thiosulfinates, which play a number of beneficial roles in our bodies, including fighting cancer and reducing the risk of artery-blocking blood clots. As is true in many other plant families, the more bite, the more benefits.

Over time, alliums became part of the medical arsenal of people around the world. An Egyptian papyrus dating from approximately 1500 BC gave instructions on how to concoct twenty-two different garlic preparations to treat conditions ranging from fatigue to cancer. The Great Pyramid of Cheops at Giza was built by slaves who were fed onions and garlic to increase their stamina.

Alliums were the first "performance-enhancing" substance. Athletes competing in the early Olympic Games around 700 BC relied on them to increase their strength and endurance. Before the competition, they consumed pounds of onions, drank onion juice, and rubbed olive oil and cut onions over their bodies.

During outbreaks of the Black Death in the Middle Ages, French priests added garlic and onions to their meals in the hopes of fending off the horrific disease. Church records show that French priests were more resistant to the plague than English priests, who had turned up their noses at the malodorous "peasant food."

Onions were a fundamental part of the diet of Union troops during the Civil War. They were also used as field dressings. The onions were finely chopped and made into poultices to treat infected wounds and amputated limbs. Onions were so important to the welfare of the soldiers that a shortage was viewed as a military emergency. In May of 1864, General Ulysses S. Grant discovered that his troops had run out of alliums. He sent an urgent telegram to the war department: "I will not move my army without onions!" Three railroad cars full of onions arrived within a few days.

During World War II, before penicillin became widely available, Russian medics applied raw garlic to the infected wounds of their soldiers. The English military began referring to garlic as "Russian penicillin." As recently as 2009, the war department in the Republic of Moldova, a small country in eastern Europe, issued a daily ration of one onion and several cloves of garlic to each member of its army to protect them from the H1N1 flu.

All these uses and more are now being backed by medical science. The term "Russian penicillin" turns out to be surprisingly accurate. One milligram of allicin, the main active ingredient in garlic, is equivalent to 15 international units of penicillin. Each clove has from seven to thirteen milligrams of allicin, so three cloves contain the same antibacterial activity as a standard dose of penicillin. (Eating the garlic, however, does not produce the same results as being injected with penicillin.) In one important respect, garlic has the edge on penicillin. Common bacteria are one thousand times more likely to become resistant to our modern antibiotics than to garlic. The researchers who made this discovery concluded: "It is clear that garlic appears to satisfy all of the criteria for antibacterial agents, and it is also cheap and safe. The historical view that garlic can 'cure all' may not be unjustified."

Alliums may also help fend off the flu. In a 2009 test-tube study, quercetin, the main phytonutrient in onions, killed a type A flu virus better than the prescription drug Tamiflu, which at the time was the state-of-the art remedy.

Garlic has another important health benefit. In medieval times, people wore garlic around their necks to ward off werewolves. Cancer is our modern werewolf—lethal, frightening, and seemingly uncontrollable. Eating more garlic may be one of the best natural remedies against the disease. In a test-tube study measuring the anticancer properties of a number of vegetables, including Brussels sprouts, kale, broccoli, and cabbage, garlic was the most effective. According to the Canadian investigators who conducted the study, "Garlic was by far the strongest inhibitor of tumor cell growth." They reported that it blocked 100 percent of the growth of human cancers of the stomach, pancreas, breast, prostate, lungs, kidneys, and brain.

Because of all its proven and promising "anti" properties (antioxidant, antibacterial, antiviral, anticlotting, and anticancer), garlic has been dubbed the Allicin Wonderland Drug.

GARLIC

In the history of agriculture, no one has mounted a concerted campaign to make garlic bulbs larger, sweeter, or milder tasting. For this reason, they have retained most of their wild nutrients. You can walk into a grocery store and buy the first variety you see and be assured of making a healthful choice.

Whether or not you get all the health benefits of the garlic, however, depends on how you prepare and cook it. In 2001, a group of Israeli food chemists discovered that conventional ways of preparing garlic can destroy most of its health benefits. Raw garlic contains the ingredients needed to make allicin, its most active ingredient, but not the compound itself. Allicin is created when two substances in garlic come into contact with each other. One is a protein fragment called alliin and the other is a heat-sensitive enzyme called alliinase. In an intact clove of garlic, these compounds are isolated in separate compartments. They do not commingle until you slice, press, or chew the garlic and rupture the barriers between them. Then the combustion begins.

The Israelis discovered that heating garlic immediately after crushing it or slicing it destroys the heat-sensitive enzyme that triggers the reaction. As a result, no allicin is created. It takes only two minutes in a frying pan to reduce garlic to little more than a flavoring ingredient. If you microwave freshly chopped garlic for just thirty seconds, 90 percent of its cancer-fighting ability is gone. Nuke it for sixty seconds and none remains. Garlic's proven ability to thin the blood, one of its most important benefits, is also compromised by heat.

You can cook garlic and reap all its benefits if you make a simple change in the way you prepare it. Chop, mince, slice, or mash the garlic and then *keep it away from the heat for ten minutes.* During this time, the maximum amount of allicin is created so the heat-sensitive enzyme is no longer needed. You can sauté, bake, or fry the garlic and still get all its medicine. Garlic has so many healing properties that waiting those critical ten minutes could reduce your risk of a number of worrisome diseases.

To follow this ten-minute rule, you will need to adapt some recipes. For example, the first step in many Asian dishes is to slice a garlic clove and fry it in hot oil. As the toasty flavor develops, the health benefits disappear. To salvage the allicin in the garlic, slice or chop it and let it rest for ten minutes *before* putting it in the frying pan. Give garlic a rest before adding it to hot sauces, soups, and stir-frys as well.

If you eat garlic raw, you don't have to worry about short-circuiting the production of allicin. Slice or mash the garlic and add it to prepared and homemade foods that do not require cooking, such as pesto, hummus, mayonnaise, aioli, garlic bread, bruschetta, salad dressings, dips, salsas, and spreads.

TO PRESS OR NOT TO PRESS

Some well-known chefs disdain the garlic press. "The garlic press will do the job," Julia Child intoned in her 1996 publication, *In Julia's Kitchen with Master Chefs,* "but a garlic press, at least among certain of the food cognoscenti, is absolutely a no-no-non-object used only by non-people and non-cooks." Julia taught "real" cooks how to smash the cloves with the broad blade of a chef's knife and then slice and dice with dazzling precision.

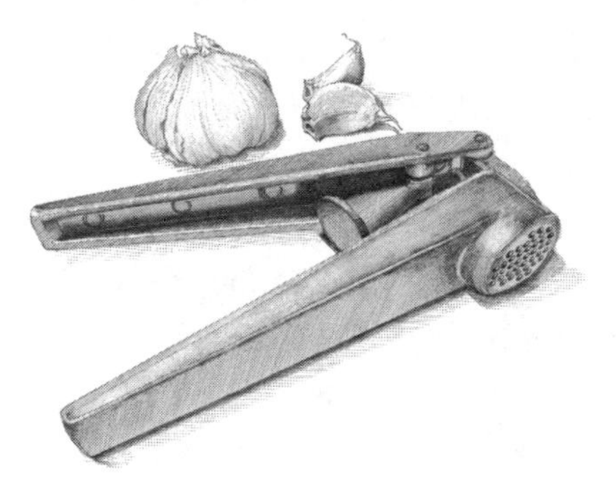

Garlic and garlic press

With all due respect to Julia, I recommend that you use a garlic press most of the time. The press minces the clove so finely that its flavor is suffused throughout the dish; you won't get a nubbin of garlic in one bite and nothing in the next. It is also the quickest and easiest way to prepare garlic. The talented chefs on the PBS television program *America's Test Kitchen* can slice and dice with the best of them, but, most of the time, you will see them reaching for a garlic press.

Finally, a garlic press does the best job of intermarrying the alliin and the alliinase, maximizing the production of allicin. If you want to get all garlic's protective properties, remember this mantra: *Press, then rest.* If you don't have a garlic press, or if you have one that is awkward or difficult to use, treat yourself to a new one. Look for a press that has a large bowl and enough leverage to enable you to crush several cloves at once or crush a large clove without removing the skin. A well-designed press is also a great aid for cooks with weak or arthritic hands. Some of the newer presses have two sides, one for pressing garlic and the other for slicing it.

SHOPPING FOR GARLIC IN THE SUPERMARKET

Most supermarkets carry only one kind of garlic, the California Silverskin. This plump, white-skinned garlic has come to represent "garlic" for most Americans. There are scores of other varieties, but they don't make it into conventional stores. The reason that the silverskin has commandeered the market is that it is the ideal made-for-industry garlic. First, it is highly productive: plant one clove and you get a new head of garlic with sixteen cloves, an impressive sixteen-to-one rate of return. Second, the cloves have tightly wrapped skins, which keep them from drying out and provide an effective barrier against insects, mold, and disease. As a result, they have a long shelf life.

The silverskin does have a few drawbacks, however. The cloves can be very pungent, especially those that are harvested late in the year. Their pungency intensifies the longer they're stored. The California garlic you buy in June may have been stoking its fire in a warehouse for seven months and can be hot enough to sting your tongue.

Another consideration is that the silverskin has a less complex flavor than other varieties. The first time I compared the flavor of a California Silverskin with an heirloom variety called Spanish Roja, I was stunned by the contrast. The Roja had a rich, garlicky flavor and a pleasing amount of heat. I went back for more. The silverskin had only one flavor: hot! One bite was more than enough.

In terms of health benefits, however, the silverskin is on a par with other varieties. It is also widely available and relatively inexpensive. Eating this ubiquitous allium will strengthen your defense against a long list of troubling conditions and diseases. To get the most flavor and medicine from the silverskins, choose the freshest garlic in the store. Look for plump bulbs that are tightly encased in their papery outer wrapping. Bulbs with frayed or loose outer skins are more likely to be dried out or moldy. The bulbs should be firm to the touch, with no brown spots, dampness, softening, or mildew. There should be no sign of sprouting.

BEYOND THE SUPERMARKET

A new and more redolent world opens up for you when you shop for garlic away from the supermarket. Specialty produce stores and farmers markets offer garlic in a wide array of colors, shapes, and sizes. Their pungency ranges from sweetly mild to blistering hot. Up for a challenge? Bite into a raw clove of Purple Cauldron. During peak harvest season, which is from May to September, you will have dozens of cultivars to choose from. Another way to become better acquainted with the many varieties is to attend a garlic festival. Most of them are held in July or August. Search the Internet for the words "garlic festival" (in quotation marks) along with the name of your city, county, or state.

The mother of all garlic festivals takes place in Gilroy, California, the self-proclaimed garlic capital of the world. The Gilroy festival is an extravaganza that features celebrity chefs, crafts, cooking demonstrations, food booths, and frequent sightings of Miss Gilroy Garlic. The festival attracts more than one hundred thousand visitors each year, which translates into large crowds and long lines. The main drawback, however, is that it celebrates only one variety of garlic, the California Silverskin. If you want less festivity and more variety, visit a smaller festival in your area.

TWO KINDS OF GARLIC

You will see two kinds of garlic in farmers markets and seed catalogs: softneck garlic (*Allium sativum* var. *sativum*) and hardneck garlic (*Allium sativum* var. *ophioscorodon*). Both types of garlic are excellent for your health, but, as a general rule, hardneck garlic has a bit of an edge. The hardneck has closer genetic ties with wild garlic and therefore has retained more of its medicinal properties. (The California Silverskin is a softneck variety.)

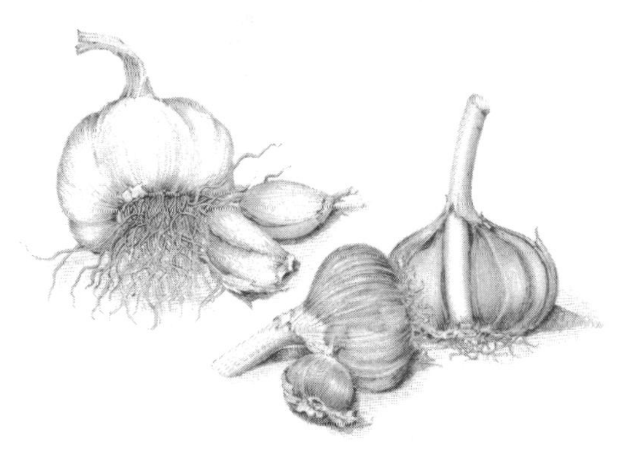

Softneck and hardneck garlic

To distinguish between the two kinds of garlic, examine the tops of the bulbs. Hardneck garlic, shown on the right in the drawing above, has a hollow stub projecting from the top that resembles a twig. True to its name, it has a hard neck. When you open the bulb, you will see a single row of cloves circling the stem, which extends down to the roots.

Softneck garlic, on the left in the drawing, has what appears to be a stem but is actually a twisted, flexible bundle of papery skin. Inside, there are several concentric rows of cloves, with the smaller cloves in the center. Softneck garlic has more individual cloves than hardneck varieties, making it heavier and plumper.

Hardneck varieties cost more than the softneck varieties for a number of good reasons. Growing hardneck varieties requires more hand labor. They also mature more slowly, have a smaller yield per acre, and spoil more rapidly. In short, they are poorly designed for mass production and distribution. For this reason, expect to pay two to ten times more for them. But don't let the price scare you away. Even though the hardneck variety Spanish Roja might cost eight dollars per pound, each head of garlic weighs only two ounces. For your eight dollars, you get eight heads of garlic that will last for weeks. The recommended varieties on pages 69–70 have earned high marks for flavor and nutrition. Look for them in specialty stores, farmers markets, farm stands, and seed catalogs. Garlic ships well, so you can also order it online.

CONVENIENCE PRODUCTS

There are a number of garlic preparations in the grocery store that are designed for your convenience. You can buy prepeeled garlic, powdered garlic, garlic salt, and minced garlic in a jar. All of them cost more than fresh garlic. What's more, they save you very little time. You can squeeze a clove of fresh garlic through a garlic press in the same amount of time it takes to find the bottled garlic in the back of your refrigerator. Compare the taste of fresh garlic with prepared products and you'll have another reason to use whole cloves. Try this taste test. Mix one pat of soft butter with a small amount of freshly squeezed garlic. Then mix another pat of soft butter with a small amount of prepared garlic. Spread on crackers or bread. Let your taste buds be the judge.

There is only one kind of prepared garlic that is worth its salt: freeze-dried garlic. When garlic and other alliums are freeze-dried, they retain most of their beneficial nutrients. Look for these products at select grocery stores or on the Internet. Freeze-dried garlic maintains its potency and flavor as long as you keep it in a sealed container to keep out the moisture. It costs more than fresh garlic, however, so using fresh garlic is still your best choice.

HOW TO STORE GARLIC

You can store garlic for one or two months if you pay attention to details. Begin by selecting fresh garlic bulbs. To store them outside the refrigerator, wrap the heads in netting or an open paper bag to allow good air circulation. Keep them out of the light. Do not store them in areas next to heat-generating appliances. One option is to store garlic in a garlic keeper, which is a pot with side holes for ventilation and a lid to block the light. There are hundreds of different types of garlic keepers available on the Internet.

Garlic stays fresh longer in the refrigerator than at room temperature, provided you don't put it in the crisper drawer, where the high humidity, like spring rain, will induce it to sprout. Instead, place the garlic on one of the shelves. (Until garlic is chopped, it has no odor.) Interestingly, when you store garlic, its pungency and allicin content can increase tenfold. Over time, it may become too hot for your taste. After a few months, even the mildest garlic can turn rogue.

ONIONS

Until about seventy years ago, all the varieties of onions sold in this country were pungent and potent, giving consumers a wide range of phytonutrients and antioxidant protection. Around the middle of the twentieth century, new varieties of onions were introduced that had more sugar and a lot less medicine. The first of the sweet orbs was created by a French soldier named Peter Pieri, who discovered an unusually large, mild, and sweet variety of onions growing on the Mediterranean island of Corsica. In 1900, he gathered their seeds and brought them with him when he settled in the Walla

Walla Valley in Washington State. Pieri began a breeding program to make the Italian imports even milder, sweeter, and larger. Each year he selected the onions that came closest to his vision and saved their seeds for the next planting. With the aid of his sons and other growers, he achieved his goal in the 1940s. Washingtonians loved Pieri's sweet, juicy onions, and the variety was soon outselling more robust onions throughout the state. In the 1960s, a marketer gave them the appealing name Walla Walla Sweets, and the meek onions found a ready market across the country.

In the 1950s and '60s, other varieties of extra-mild, extra-large onions began to appear in the nation's grocery stores, including Vidalia, Texas 101, and Bermuda onions. Americans snapped up these mild-mannered alliums, which motivated growers to create even larger and sweeter varieties. Today we can dine on onions named Jumbo Sweet, Sweetie Sweet, and Candy Cane that have as much as 16 percent sugar, the same percentage found in our sweetest apples. If you go to an onion festival, you can buy a raw sweet onion that has been skewered on a stick and dunked in caramel—a candied allium. One California supermarket chain with 155 stores sells only sweet onions during the summer months. Its customers don't complain. In fact, they are willing to pay 30 percent more per pound to buy them.

Our love of mild, sweet onions may have left us more vulnerable to disease, including cancer. In a 2004 test-tube study, extracts of strongly flavored onions destroyed 95 percent of human cancer cells of the liver and colon; extracts of sweet onions killed only 10 percent. Sweet onions are also less effective at thinning the blood, so they are less able to lower the risk of heart attack and stroke.

Increasing the size of the onions was another nutritional misstep. The smaller the onion, food chemists have discovered, the less water it contains and therefore the greater its concentration of phytonutrients. Two small onions give you twice as many antioxidants as one large onion of the same variety. The mildness, high sugar and water content, and large size of the supersweet onions work together to lower their antioxidant content, as you can see in the graph below. Western Yellow onions, on the left side of the graph, have eight times more antioxidant punch than the Vidalias on the far right.

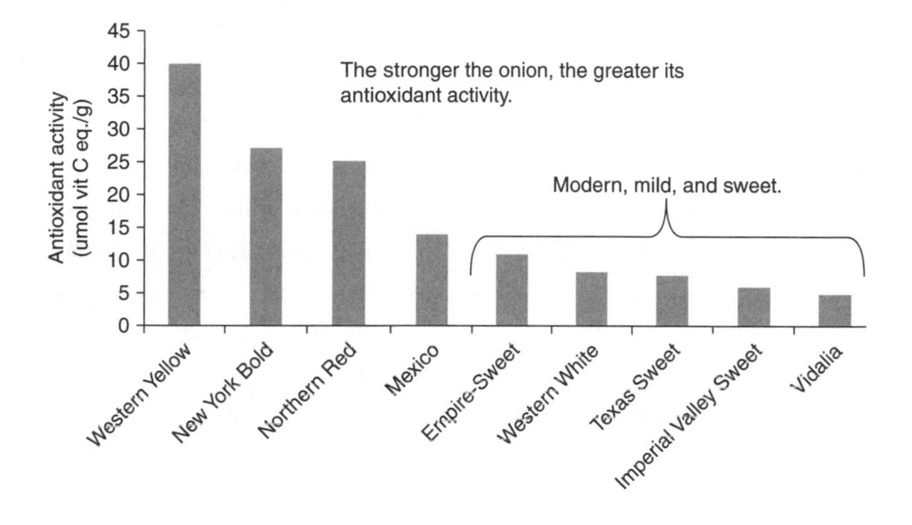

CHOOSING THE MOST NUTRITIOUS ONIONS IN THE SUPERMARKET

You can choose the most nutritious onions in the supermarket if you know what to look for. Scan the produce section and you will see six or more different varieties of onions, including white onions, yellow onions, red onions, pearl onions, boiling onions, and sweet onions. But you can't always distinguish between pungent onions and sweet onions by looks alone. In some stores, the varietal names are displayed, which makes selecting the most nutritious varieties much easier. (You'll find a list of recommended varieties on pages 71–72.) Varieties that are most likely to have their names displayed, however, are the sweet onions, such as Vidalia, Walla Walla, and Texas 101. In other stores, no names are listed, but most of the sweet varieties have the word *sweet* on their stickers.

Although sweet onions are less nutritious than hotter varieties, they are a reasonable choice if you want to eat raw onions. If you were to add slices of a Western Yellow onion to a hamburger, for example, all the other flavors would run and hide. The Empire-Sweet cultivar, a yellow onion popular in New York and its surrounding states, has more phytonutrients than other sweet varieties. (See the above chart.)

Some red onions are very pungent, but others are mild and sweet. This is an instance in which you can differentiate onions by shape. Mild red onions, sometimes called hamburger onions or sandwich onions, are wide and flat. Hot red onions are round or oblong and are much higher in antioxidants. The hot varieties are the ones that bring tears to your eyes; when you are struggling to see through a veil of tears, you know you've made a nutritionally sound choice. But there are ways to lessen your agony. Chopping or slicing onions under running water keeps the irritating fumes to a minimum. Some people swear by "onion goggles," close-fitting goggles that keep the fumes from reaching your eyes. (They're available on the Internet.) You can also pour a tablespoon or two of vinegar on the surface of the cutting board before you start to chop. If you turn the sliced or diced onions to coat them with vinegar, your discomfort will be reduced.

After you've decided which onions to buy, examine them carefully. Look for firm onions with an intact outer skin. The papery outer skin preserves the juiciness of the onions. It also contains natural compounds that protect the vegetable from fungal infections and mold. If the outer skin is flaking off or has been removed by an overzealous produce manager, the onion has less overall protection and will not keep as long.

Interestingly, the high concentration of bionutrients in onion skins makes them the most nutritious part of the vegetable. Although eating the skins would be unpleasant, you can save them and add them to soup stocks, which will enrich the broth with flavor and bionutrients. The skin of yellow onions gives the broth a golden color. You can also crunch the skins and wrap them in cheesecloth or put them in a netted bag or a large tea ball and add them to soups, stews, or pot roasts. It will be easy to remove the skins before serving.

BEYOND THE SUPERMARKET

When you shop for onions at a farmers market or buy seeds for a garden, you can choose from many more varieties than are available at the supermarket. Typically, market vendors display the varietal names of their onions. Look for Red Walking onions, which form a tight cluster of small, dark red bulbs; Red Baron onions, which look like overgrown scallions dipped in red dye; and the heirloom Red Wethersfield onion, a large flattened globe with purple-red skin. Varieties of yellow onions to look for include New York Bold and Western Yellow. You'll find other worthy varieties in the chart at the end of this chapter.

STORING ONIONS

Sweet onions do not keep well because they are high in moisture and their skins are thinner and less protective than the skins of other onions. Store them on a refrigerator shelf and eat them within a week or two. Other onions can be kept a month or longer. To store onions for more than two weeks, put them in a net bag or open paper bag and store in a cool, dark, moderately humid location, such as a basement cabinet or an unheated room. You can also store them in an unheated garage as long as the temperature stays above freezing. If you have only a few onions, store them on a refrigerator shelf. The crisper drawer is too humid.

PREPARING AND COOKING ONIONS

Unlike garlic, onions can be exposed to heat as soon as you slice or chop them without losing any of their health benefits. (Allicin is not an essential part of their nutritional content, so there is no need to protect the heat-sensitive enzyme that triggers its formation.) One of the most beneficial phytonutrients in onions is quercetin, a compound that is being investigated for its antiviral, antibacterial, and anticancer properties. Studies show that baking, sautéing, roasting, or frying onions *increases* their quercetin content. Boiling is the only cooking method that reduces it. By the time onions are fully cooked, 30 percent of their quercetin has been transferred to the cooking water. If you use the cooking liquid, however, you can recoup the loss.

Cooking pungent red and yellow varieties has another effect—it tames their heat. Sauté the hottest yellow onion for five minutes and it will become mild and sweet. The sweetness was there all along, but it was overpowered by more assertive flavors. For the most health benefits, use pungent varieties whenever you cook. You can also sauté or grill spicy varieties, let them cool, and add them to salads and sandwiches. The onions will become as mild-mannered as Vidalias, but will give you twice as much antioxidant protection. Another option is to slice raw, pungent onions so thinly that they are translucent. (You should be able to see the shadow of the knife blade through the slice as you cut it.) Add these wisps of onions to a salad or sandwich and their pungency will be much less apparent.

But I Can't Eat Onions!

Some people can eat cooked onions and garlic without gastric distress, but when they eat them raw, they are plagued with stomach pains, bloating, cramping, or intestinal gas. Other people have these reactions whether the alliums are cooked or raw.

Allicin is the source of discomfort for many people. It stimulates the valve that connects the esophagus and the stomach. After a meal that contains onions, scallions, or garlic, the valve opens and closes more frequently, which allows some of the stomach contents to flow up into the esophagus. The result is heartburn, or gastric reflux. Sweet onions are lower in allicin and are less likely to cause this problem.

The source of misery and embarrassment for others is a condition called complex carbohydrate intolerance, or CCI, which is an inability to digest certain types of carbohydrates. Normally, the body breaks down complex carbohydrates into simple sugars. People with CCI lack sufficient quantities of an enzyme called alpha-galactosidase, which is necessary for complete digestion. This deficiency runs in families. The undigested sugars reach the large intestine, where they ferment and produce gas, pain, and bloating. Some people get relief by taking over-the-counter preparations such as Beano, which supply the missing enzyme.

SHALLOTS

Shallots (*Allium cepa* var. *aggregatum*) look like big bulbs of garlic, each of which has between two and four large cloves. Unlike garlic, the bulbs are cloaked in colorful skins of mahogany, rose, gray, or amber. Julia Child was initiated into the cult of the shallot during her training at Le Cordon Bleu, France's celebrated cooking school. When she wrote *Mastering the Art of French Cooking,* first published in 1961, she could not find shallots in American supermarkets, so she had to substitute scallions in all her recipes. *Sacre bleu!*

In this country, shallots have remained the province of chefs and the most devoted cooks and gourmands. It's time they became better known. Shallots are now available in most large supermarkets. Their mild but complex flavor makes them an excellent addition to egg dishes, cream soups, sauces, and stir-frys. Sauté them in olive oil and serve over fresh salmon, halibut, or tuna.

A little-known fact is that shallots are superstars of nutrition. Ounce for ounce, they have six times more phytonutrients than the typical onion. They are second only to garlic in their ability to destroy cancer cells. Pliny the Elder, a gifted naturalist who lived in the first century AD, described the healing properties of six different kinds of alliums and pronounced that shallots were the best of them all. Two thousand years later, food scientists are coming to the same conclusion.

Shallots are relatively expensive, which is one reason they are not used more often. If you shop in Asian produce markets, however, shallots sell for about the same price as onions. Wherever you buy them, look for firm shallots with tight outer skins. If you store them in a cool, dark location with good air circulation or on a shelf in the refrigerator, they will last for about a month.

Shallots are an excellent vegetable for the home garden. They take up little space and are easy to grow. For a culinary adventure, grow French Gray shallots (*Allium oschaninii*). They are rare and exquisite—the truffles of the allium world. They have a more complex and less "oniony" flavor than other shallots, making them de rigueur for many European and top-ranked American chefs. They are the antithesis of the mass-market vegetable. First of all, they do not store well. They are also relatively small, have a paltry yield per acre, and take longer to grow than other shallots. To top it off, they are ugly. French Gray shallots have a tough, wrinkled, gray outer skin. They are not your cosmetically perfect vegetable.

The reason for the dowdiness of the gray shallot is that it has not been given a human makeover. Shallots that are genetically identical to the ones you find in the supermarket grow in wilderness areas from central to southwest Asia. Many people continue to harvest them. The ones now being cultivated are as close to wild as one can get, and they have the nutritional bounty to prove it. Think of them as an heirloom vegetable with roots that go back thousands of years, not just a century or two. Ounce for ounce, shallots have twice as much quercetin as their cultivated allium cousins. I give them a

10—5 points for exceptional flavor and another 5 for their unsurpassed native nutritional value. You can order shallot bulbs on the Internet or from select seed companies. (They sell out early in the season.) An age-old French tradition is to plant them on the winter solstice and harvest them on the summer solstice. If you don't live in a Mediterranean climate, plant them in the spring instead.

LEEKS

Leeks (*Allium ampeloprasum* var. *porrum*) are tall, mild-flavored alliums that have one slender bulb at the end of a long stalk. They look like scallions on growth hormones. Despite their mild flavor, they are rich in beneficial phytonutrients. The nutrients are most concentrated in the leaves and the green portions of the stalk—the parts that most people discard. If you want to use the leaves, buy the smallest leeks you can find, because their leaves will be more tender. To use the greens in a stir-fry or other sautéed dish, cut them into eighth-inch slices and sauté for a few minutes before adding the white part of the leek. Unlike onions and garlic, leeks lose most of their antioxidant benefits after spending just a few days in your refrigerator. Cook them as soon as you buy or harvest them.

Many people don't know what to do with leeks once they get them home. Apart from one classic dish—leek and potato soup—they draw a blank. The following quick and easy recipe provides a tasty alternative. It uses a portion of the greens as well as the bulb. You can serve the sautéed leeks as a side dish, add them to soups and pot roasts, or pile them on sandwiches or hamburgers. Use them in omelets, frittatas, and poultry stuffing, or serve over fish, beef, pork, poultry, or lamb. I make a large quantity and freeze some in pint-size freezer bags so I can have them readily at hand.

SAUTÉED LEEKS WITH MUSTARD AND CUMIN

PREP TIME: 10–15 MINUTES
COOKING TIME: 10 MINUTES
TOTAL TIME: 20–25 MINUTES
YIELD: 2 CUPS

2 medium-size leeks
¼ cup extra virgin olive oil, preferably unfiltered
1 teaspoon cumin seeds
2 tablespoons prepared mustard
1 teaspoon honey

Trim the bulb ends of the leeks to remove their tiny rootlets. Trim the tops of the leaves, leaving three inches of dark green above the white. Cut the leeks into quarters lengthwise, then rinse well to remove any dirt. Beginning at the root end, slice the white part of the leeks crosswise into ¼-inch slices, then slice the green portion into narrower, ⅛-inch slices.

Combine the oil, cumin seeds, and green portions of the leeks in a medium frying pan. Sauté over medium-low heat for 2 minutes, then add the white portions of the leeks and cook for another 8 minutes. Stir frequently. Add the mustard and honey and sauté over low heat for another 2 minutes. Serve hot, cold, or at room temperature.

ONION CHIVES AND GARLIC CHIVES

There are two types of chives—onion chives (*Allium schoenoprasum*) and garlic chives (*Allium tuberosum*). They are the smallest of the alliums and the only ones that are native to both the Old World and the New World. They are a boon to gardeners because their violet flowers attract bees but their roots and stems repel less desirable insects.

In the United States, we are most familiar with the onion variety of chives. Onion chives have long, thin, tubelike leaves and taste like mild onions. They are a perfect complement to omelets and quiches, and they make a bright green garnish for soups. Baked potatoes with sour cream and chives is an American classic. Go heavy on the chives. To make the traditional French seasoning known as fines herbes, combine equal portions of minced fresh onion chives, tarragon, parsley, and chervil.

Garlic chives have flat, straplike leaves. They are more popular in Asia than in the West, which is why they are often referred to as Chinese chives or Asian chives. Typically, onion chives are eaten raw, but garlic chives are sautéed. Garlic chives are a prime ingredient in spring rolls, stir-frys, hot-and-sour soup, and many meat and seafood recipes. The Japanese call garlic chives nira. A popular Japanese dish is stir-fried liver and nira. Nira is also a common ingredient in gyoza (pot stickers), a dish that appeals to American tastes. Shop in Asian markets for the freshest supply at the lowest price.

Ounce for ounce, garlic chives have more antioxidants than the hottest red onions. The reason they are so potent is that they are all greens and no bulb. Practitioners of Chinese medicine have long used garlic chives to treat a variety of maladies, including fatigue and disorders of the kidney, liver, and digestive tract. Their seeds have also been prescribed as an aphrodisiac.

Do their aphrodisiac properties stand up to the rigors of science? The Shanghai Municipal Education Commission decided to find out. In a 2009 study, male lab rats were fed the seeds of garlic chives for forty days. Every ten days, the rats were introduced to receptive female rats. By the end of the study, the chive-fed males were mounting the females twice as often as they had before being given the herb. Males that were not given the chives maintained their original level of interest. The commission has funded a new study to see if female rats become equally inspired. No such human studies have been conducted to date.

Once you purchase or harvest chives, it's best to eat them right away. If you plan to store them for a few days, put them in a micro-perforated bag and store in the crisper drawer of the refrigerator. Some grocery stores sell onion chives as living plants. (Make sure you are buying chives and not wheatgrass; they look similar.) Take them home and you can enjoy their fresh-picked flavor for days. Growing your own chives is even better. When you harvest them, clip them back to about four inches and they will grow back very quickly. You can clip them several times over the course of a single summer. As is true for all herbs, the closer you plant chives to your kitchen, the more often you will use them.

SCALLIONS

Scallions (*Allium fistulosum*) go by many names, including green onions, spring onions, and salad onions. They have slim white bulbs, dark green tubular leaves, and a tassel of roots. Scallions, like chives, should be eaten soon after you purchase or harvest them. If you're going to keep them for a few days, place them in a plastic bag that you have perforated with pinpricks.

Despite appearances, scallions are not miniature onions (*Allium cepa*) but a species unto themselves. New studies show that they have an incredible 140 times more phytonutrients than common white onions. The green portions are a more concentrated source of phyto-nutrients than the bulbs. This highly nutritious allium shows promise in reducing the risk of cancer. According to a 2002 survey, men who consumed at least a third of an ounce (ten grams) of scallions per day had a 50 percent lower risk of prostate cancer than those who went without scallions. Interestingly, scallions come closest to wild onions in appearance *and* nutrition. It is often the case that the most phytonutrient-rich varieties of fruits and vegetables closely resemble their wild ancestors; in nature, function follows form.

You can use scallions in place of onions in most dishes. Add chopped scallions to raw hamburger before you form the patties. Add them to pasta dishes, soups, egg dishes, pizza toppings, salsa, sandwiches, and dips. If you add them to cooked dishes at the last minute, they add a pleasing crunch.

RECOMMENDED VARIETIES OF GARLIC

IN THE SUPERMARKET	
TYPE	COMMENTS
All types	All varieties of garlic available in supermarkets offer important health benefits. Choose the ones that have the most pleasing flavor to you. The most common variety you'll see, the California Silverskin, is a softneck variety that is rich in allicin. It keeps well, but can become quite pungent when stored.

FARMERS MARKETS, SPECIALTY STORES, U-PICK FARMS, AND SEED CATALOGS			
VARIETY	TYPE	DESCRIPTION	INFORMATION FOR GARDENERS
Chilean Silver	Softneck	Balanced but spicy flavor. A luminous pure white. High in allicin. Contains 15–18 cloves per bulb. Stores well.	You can plant large quantities because it keeps for up to a year. Good for braiding.

VARIETY	TYPE	DESCRIPTION	INFORMATION FOR GARDENERS
Inchelium Red	Softneck	The winner of a number of taste tests. Hot but not overpowering. Large bulbs up to 3 inches across contain 9–20 cloves. Thick skins enable long storage after harvest, up to 7 months.	Ready to harvest in midseason.
Music	Hardneck	Very large cloves, 4–6 per bulb. Rich, pungent flavor. Stores for up to 9 months.	Ready to harvest in midseason. High yields. Vigorous and cold-tolerant. Overwinters without heaving out of the soil.
Persian Star	Hardneck	Magenta-striped skins. Robust flavor. Has 10–12 easy-peel cloves. Stores for up to 6 months.	Winter-hardy.
Pink Music	Hardneck	Similar to Music but has pink-skinned cloves. Rich and pungent flavor. The large cloves, 4–6 per bulb, are easy to peel. Stores for up to 9 months.	Ready to harvest in midseason. High yields. Very cold-tolerant.
Romanian Red	Hardneck	Pungent and hot when eaten raw. Large, plump cloves, only 4–5 to a bulb. Very high in allicin. Stores very well.	Vigorous and cold-tolerant.
Spanish Roja	Hardneck	Taste-test winner. Medium heat. Beautiful, shiny, purple-streaked skin. Good raw or roasted. Has 8–10 large cloves per bulb. Easy to peel. Stores for 2–3 months.	Vigorous grower. Does best in areas with cold winters.

RECOMMENDED VARIETIES OF ONIONS

IN THE SUPERMARKET	
TYPE OR VARIETY	COMMENTS
Red and pungent	All varieties of red, pungent onions are rich in antioxidant value. Their flavor mellows dramatically when cooked.
Yellow and pungent	All varieties of yellow, pungent onions are rich in antioxidant value. Their flavor mellows dramatically when cooked.
Western Yellow	This particular variety of yellow pungent onion is very high in catechins, an important family of phytonutrients. Strong-tasting when raw but mellows when cooked.
Empire-Sweet	Highest in antioxidant value of the common sweet onion varieties, but lower than all the pungent ones. Mild-flavored.
New York Bold	A yellow pungent onion, it is one of the richest in antioxidant activity. Strong-tasting when raw but mellows when cooked.
Scallions, all varieties	One of the most nutritious of all the different species of onions.

FARMERS MARKETS, SPECIALTY STORES, U-PICK FARMS, AND SEED CATALOGS		
VARIETY	DESCRIPTION	INFORMATION FOR GARDENERS
Karmen (also called Red Karmen)	Medium-size flattened globes that look as though they've been dipped in red lacquer. Medium-sweet flavor. Good raw or grilled. Lose some of their color when cooked. High in quercetin. Stores well.	Matures in 65–70 days. Northern long-day onion. ("Long-day" onions require a specific number of daylight hours per day to flower and mature, typically more than 12. For this reason, they are best suited for northern states.)

VARIETY	DESCRIPTION	INFORMATION FOR GARDENERS
Purplette	Small bunching onions with purple skins. Bulbs are 1–2 inches in diameter. Mild, delicate flavor.	Matures in 60–65 days. Can be harvested at the scallion stage.
Red Baron	Small, mild-flavored onions with vibrant burgundy bulbs that keep their color throughout the growing cycle. Extra-high in phytonutrients. Stores well.	Matures in 60 days. Northern long-day onion. Can be harvested in midsummer as a green onion or overwintered to form 3–4-inch bulbs the following spring.
Red Wethersfield (also called Dark Red Beauty or Red Beauty)	Mildly pungent. A large flattened bulb with purple-red skin. Red concentric circles. Stores well.	Matures in 100 days. Northern long-day onion.
Red Wing (also called Redwing)	Red-skinned medium-size onion. Pungent. Alternating red and white rings. Good raw, grilled, or sautéed. High in antioxidant activity.	Matures in 100–120 days. Northern long-day onion.

ALLIUMS: POINTS TO REMEMBER

1. ***Garlic is rich in nutrients and has a number of promising health benefits.***
   Look for garlic with plump, firm cloves enclosed in a tight, intact outer wrapper. To get maximum amounts of allicin, slice, mince, or press the garlic and then let it rest for ten minutes before exposing it to heat. For the best selection, shop for garlic in farmers markets and specialty stores, where you can often find hardneck varieties in a wide range of flavors and degrees of pungency.

2. ***Strongly flavored onions are best for your health.***
   The more pungent the onion, the better it is for you. Bold-tasting red and yellow onions offer the most health benefits. Cooking tames their fire, brings out their sweetness, and increases their nutritional content. Small onions have more nutrients per pound than larger onions. Sweet, mild, and extra-large onions are less

nutritious than bolder varieties. Boiling onions transfers many of their nutrients to the cooking liquid.

3. ***Shallots are mild but nutritionally potent.***
   Shallots are more nutritious than most varieties of onions. Their milder flavor makes them good additions to egg dishes, creamy soups, and sauces. Shop in Asian markets for the lowest price, or grow your own. They take little room in the garden and are easy to grow.

4. ***When cooking with leeks, use the bulbs* and *the greens.***
   The green portions of leeks have more bionutrients than the white portions. Leeks lose their antioxidants very rapidly, so eat them within a few days of purchase.

5. ***Eat plenty of onion and garlic chives.***
   Onion chives have tubular leaves and are sold in most supermarkets. Garlic chives have flat, straplike leaves and are less common. Shop for garlic chives in Asian markets for the greatest selection and lowest price. Eat them within a few days, or store them in a sealed plastic bag perforated with tiny holes.

6. ***Scallions (green onions) are more nutritious than most other alliums.***
   Scallions are closest to wild onions in appearance and nutrition. The green leaves have a greater concentration of nutrients than the slim white bulbs. Store them as you would chives.

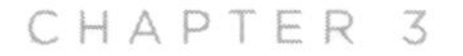

CHAPTER 3

CORN ON THE COB

HOW SUPERSWEET IT IS!

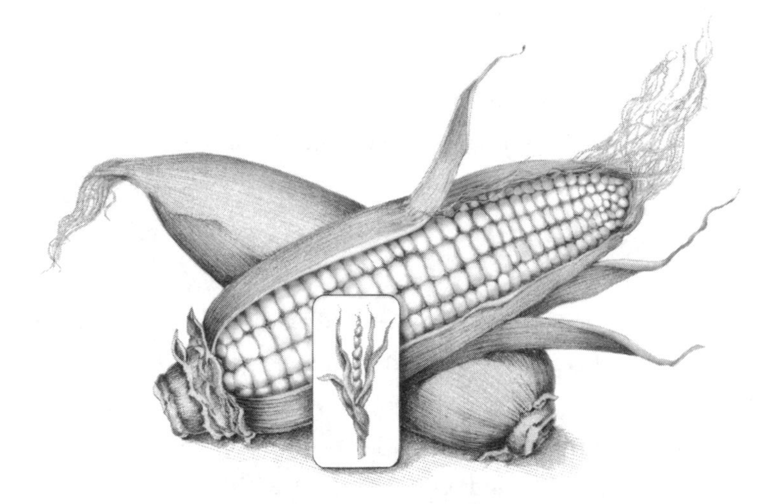

Teosinte and modern corn

The corn we eat today looks nothing like its wild ancestor, teosinte. Teosinte (*Zea mexicana*) is a bushy grass plant native to central Mexico. Each "ear" is a scant five inches long and has only between five and twelve kernels, lined up single file. Each triangular kernel is enclosed in a stony case that is as hard as an acorn shell. Crack one open and you will find a tidbit of dry, starchy food. You would not toss teosinte onto the barbecue or boil it for a summer picnic. The hunter-gatherers who went to the trouble to harvest the seeds did get a nutritional reward, however: teosinte has twice as much protein as our modern corn and significantly less starch.

It took seven thousand years to transform teosinte into our gargantuan modern corn, with its hundreds of succulent, shell-free, ultrasweet kernels. The transformation involved several spontaneous mutations, hundreds of generations of human selection, and, most recently, genetic manipulation. As a result of all these changes, our modern corn differs from its native ancestor more than any other edible plant. It has also become so tasty and productive that it now supplies 25 percent of the calories consumed by the world's population.

In our zeal to create bigger, sweeter, softer, and juicier corn, however, we may have gone a bit too far. Our modern supersweet varieties can contain up to 40 percent sugar, bringing new meaning to the words *candy corn*. There's another concern. Modern corn varieties are much lower in phytonutrients than the varieties raised by the earliest farmers. Blue corn, which has been sacred to the Hopi and other southwestern American Indian nations for several thousand years, is extremely high in anthocyanins, giving it thirty times more antioxidant value than our modern white corn. Multicolored "Indian" corn also contains significant amounts of these compounds.

One of the anthocyanins in blue corn, a compound known as cyanidin-3-glucoside (CG3), promises to have remarkable health benefits. In animal studies, CG3 has slowed the growth of colon cancer, blocked inflammation, lowered cholesterol and blood sugar, and even reduced weight gain caused by a high-fat diet. White and yellow corn varieties, on the other hand, have no anthocyanins and no CG3. In this country, most of the highly pigmented corn is now being produced for seasonal decorations, not human consumption.

People in some South American countries continue to eat great quantities of purple corn, which they call maíz morado. They also use it in a traditional brew called chicha morada, a nonalcoholic beverage made from purple corn, pineapple skins, and cinnamon. This deep purple drink offers more resveratrol than red wine. (Resveratrol is a phytonutrient that thins the blood, calms inflammation, and inhibits the growth of tumor cells.) It also has several times more anthocyanins than most blueberries. News of the possible health benefits of this South American superfood has created a demand for the drink in the United States. You can buy chicha morada at health food stores for about ten dollars a bottle. But do read the label before you buy. Sugar is the number one ingredient in some of the brands. Traditional chicha morada has none.

FROM NATURE'S MUTATIONS TO THE ATOMIC BOMB

We wouldn't be eating any corn today if it hadn't undergone a series of random mutations, nature's way of creating new varieties. DNA experts tell us that teosinte underwent four or five key mutations over the span of several thousand years. Each mutation involved a single gene. These seemingly minor alterations combined to produce spectacular changes. A short bushy plant with multiple stalks, small ears, and cobs containing only a dozen kernels was transformed into a tall plant with one or two stalks, much larger ears, and a hundred or more kernels per cob—all without human intervention.

The earliest farmers were quick to detect and take advantage of nature's changes and began growing corn in large quantities. By about five thousand years ago, farmers in south central Mexico were growing so much corn that it had become their staple crop. It took the place of many of the nuts, roots, greens, and even wild game that had been an essential part of their hunter-gatherer diet.

Corn spread north and south of Mexico over a several-thousand-year span, and eventually became a staple crop throughout the Americas. Christopher Columbus was one of the first Europeans to encounter the New World grain. When he arrived in Cuba, the native people gave him a flat bread made from cornmeal. Columbus noted in his 1492 journal that the grain was "well tasted when baked and dried and made into flour." The tens of millions of people who now eat corn tortillas every day would agree.

When English colonists arrived on the eastern shore of North America in the late 1500s and early 1600s, they encountered a native population that was growing large quantities of corn, a grain that was unknown to them. John Winthrop, the first governor of the Massachusetts Bay Colony, wrote in his journal that the Massachusett, Nauset, and Wampanoag tribes were growing very colorful corn: "Nature hath delighted itself to beautify this Corne with a great variety of colours. . . . They grow white Corne, black Corne, cherry red Corne, yellow, blue, straw-colored, greenish and speckled."

Corn was critical to the survival of the first colonists. All the earliest settlers in the New World faced extreme hardship during their first few years. Hundreds of people died, and entire colonies disappeared. The Pilgrims in the Plymouth Colony fared better, largely because of the corn they obtained from the local tribes. Some of the corn was given to them, some was bartered, and the rest they stole. A little-known fact is that the colony might not have survived if a group of starving Pilgrims had not carted away a cache of corn and bean seeds that they discovered in a Wampanoag dwelling. William Bradford, first governor of the Plymouth Colony, discussed the importance of this event in his book *Of Plimouth Plantation:* "And here is to be noted a spetiall providence of God, and a great mercie to this poore people, that here they gott seed to plant them corne in the next year, or else they might have starved, for they had none, nor any likely to get any till the season had beene past." Without the purloined seeds, the Plymouth Colony might have been a footnote in history, like several of the other early colonies.

Eventually, the Pilgrims mastered the art of growing corn, thanks to the guidance of a Native American named Tisquantum, better known as Squanto. Squanto told the colonists when and how to plant the seeds. He also told them to bury a dead fish at the bottom of each hill of corn. Without the fish, he told them, the corn would "come to nothing." Colonists who tried to grow corn without this natural fertilizer found this to be true. Once the colonists began to grow large amounts of their own corn, they no longer feared starvation and could reduce their dependence on the local tribes. They were overjoyed with their success. Corn produced twice as much food per acre as any of the grains that were growing in Europe. It was also easier to grow than other grains because the fields did not have to be plowed before seeding. In their eyes, and eventually in the eyes of the world, corn was a miracle plant.

THE FIRST SWEET CORN

At some point in corn's evolution, perhaps as long as two thousand years ago, another spontaneous mutation took place that made corn even more pleasing to the human palate. A caprice of nature altered the gene that controls the amount of sugar and starch in the kernels. In a normal ear of corn, a gene called the sugary gene converts sugar into starch as the ear matures. The starch provides the type of energy the kernels need to germinate and grow their first set of leaves. Corn with the mutant sugary gene had less starch and more sugar, making it sweeter to the taste, yet it still had enough starch for the plants to survive. Many of the tribes of the Iroquois Nation were growing this sweet treat before the colonists arrived.

The Iroquois sweet corn did not look like our present-day sweet corn. The ears had only eight rows of kernels—not the fourteen to sixteen rows found in our modern corn—and the cob itself was scarlet red. The Iroquois called it papoon, or "corn for babies," because it was so sweet and soft that they used it to make porridge for their children.

The European settlers were unaware of this novel corn until the Revolutionary War. Then, in 1779, George Washington ordered General John Sullivan to wage an aggressive campaign against the Iroquois to punish them for joining sides with the British. The soldiers destroyed the Indians' settlements and burned their cornfields and storehouses. The story goes that one soldier stopped long enough to taste some of the papoon and was so taken by its sweetness that he brought seeds back with him to Plymouth, Massachusetts. Forty years later, papoon was featured in the seed catalog of G. Thorburn & Sons and was being sold to growers up and down the East Coast. Sweet corn had arrived.

Americans were not satisfied with papoon for long, however. They wanted new and improved varieties. The first documented corn breeding program was launched in the 1830s by Noyes Darling, the mayor of New Haven, Connecticut, and a gentleman farmer. His wish list was short and to the point. He wanted to create "a new white, sweet corn that was fit for boiling by the 18th of July." He was not satisfied with corn that was knee high by the Fourth of July, as the old adage goes—he wanted a variety that was ready to eat just two weeks later!

After six years of painstaking crossbreeding, Darling achieved his goal of developing a pure white, extra-early corn. He took special pride in the fact that he had rid the corn of the "disadvantage of being yellow." Unbeknownst to him, when he bred out the yellow color, he was also stripping away the beta-carotene. Nutritionists would not know until one hundred years later that the "disadvantage of being yellow" had instead been a considerable advantage for human health.

By the late 1880s, most of the corn being grown in the United States was either white or yellow, and Darling's sweet mutant variety was the most popular corn in the country. The original, low-sugar corn was demoted to the status of "field corn" and fed to animals. According to a book on corn written in 1915, "About every American family demands in the planning for a home garden the inclusion of several varieties of this choice garden vegetable. In fact, they never consider the garden complete unless it contains sweet corn."

GENETIC BLUDGEONING

In the 1930s, scientists in the brave new field of plant genetics began to experiment with manipulating corn genes. Their purpose was to learn more about basic genetics, not to develop new varieties of corn.

At the beginning of the genetic experiments, the researchers collected thousands of wild and domesticated corn plants to study their genes. They were especially interested in corn plants that had undergone a spontaneous mutation, because these unusual plants had a novel arrangement of genes that the others lacked. Studying them might provide more insight into the basic function and the normal sequence of key genes.

Over time, the geneticists became more ambitious. In addition to gathering mother nature's mutants, they began to create their own. To do this, they collected normal corn seeds and exposed them to X-rays, UV light, toxic chemicals, and cobalt radiation. The scientists would then plant the mutated seeds to see what they had wrought. Many of the plants were so altered that they no longer looked like corn. Some plants were dwarfed, spindly, or had split leaves. Some had stiff tassels that branched out like a Christmas tree. A few had cobs that hung in clumps, like bananas. No matter how the corn looked or how well it grew, however, it was of interest to the geneticists.

Then, in 1946, the genetic researchers seized upon an even more surefire way to mutate corn seeds—blast them with an atomic bomb, an explosive chapter in the saga of "king corn" that has been untold until now. This bizarre series of experiments took place on the Bikini Atoll in the Marshall Islands as a part of Operation Crossroads, a military research project investigating whether large military ships could survive atomic warfare. A secondary goal was to study the effects of intense radiation on plants and animals. This was more than an academic exercise. The detonation of atomic bombs over Hiroshima and Nagasaki at the end of World War II had ushered in an era of atomic warfare and all its unknown consequences. In the week before the first detonation, biologists ferried goats, pigs, and sacks of corn seeds to a few of the ships that were anchored far enough away from ground zero to stay afloat but close enough to be bombarded with radiation.

The results of the experiment are spelled out in government document AD473888, entitled "Effects of an Atomic Bomb Explosion on Corn Seeds." Although the report was written in 1951, it was not declassified until 1997. According to this document, the military retrieved the irradiated seeds as soon as it was safe to board the ships and planted them in a secure government facility near Washington, D.C. As was true in earlier radiation experiments, most of the corn seeds grew into plants that were freakish and short-lived. Nonetheless, samples of all the viable kernels were collected and sent to a central seed bank called the Maize Genetics Cooperation Stock Center for future research. Geneticists and plant breeders could examine samples from this fast-growing storehouse of mutants as easily as they could check out a book from a library. The vast majority of the seeds were from the atomic bomb experiments.

JOHN LAUGHNAN'S SHRIVELED CORN

Our modern supersweet corn came out of this collection of misbegotten seeds. One day in 1959, a geneticist named John Laughnan was shelling an ear of mutant corn grown from seeds he had ordered from the Maize Genetics center. This particular strain produced corn with shriveled and shrunken kernels that had been given the code name shrunken-2, or sh2. Laughnan absentmindedly popped a few kernels into his mouth and was startled by their extraordinary sweetness. The sh2 mutation had turned a normal corn gene into a sugar factory! Lab tests showed that the strange-lookingkernels were ten times sweeter than the so-called sweet corn of his day.

Laughnan was a geneticist, not a plant breeder, but he changed overnight into an avid entrepreneur. He knew at once that he had stumbled upon a gold mine. As soon as possible, he planted the sh2 corn to study its growth and palatability. When he harvested the first planting, his excitement intensified. The kernels were not only extra-sweet, they stayed sweet for a remarkable amount of time. The sugar in ordinary sweet corn begins to convert to starch just a few hours after picking; half the sugar is gone in eight hours. To maintain its flavor, people cook it within a few hours of harvest. Zealots put the water on to boil *before* they pick the corn. Laughnan realized that his sh2 corn would get rid of all this fuss and bother. When properly chilled, the corn stayed sweet for ten days! Sh2 would revolutionize the corn industry. For the very first time, corn could be grown in the Midwest and still be lip-smacking sweet when it arrived in grocery stores in Maine or Los Angeles. The ability to grow corn on megafarms in central locations and ship the ears long distances would make corn production more profitable than ever before.

Before Laughnan could put sh2 corn on the market, however, he had to find some way to make the seeds easier to sprout. They were so unnaturally high in sugar and deficient in starch that they had difficulty germinating. They also struggled to grow during the first critical weeks. Without more intervention, his mutant corn would never thrive. Laughnan spent years fixing this flaw. He finally succeeded by crossing sh2 with several old-fashioned cultivars of sweet corn. Although these new hybrids were not as sweet as sh2, they were still many times sweeter than any corn on the market.

In 1961, Laughnan began to market the first of his supersweet corn varieties—Illini Xtra-Sweet, along with an extra-sweet version of the popular Golden Cross Bantam. Consumers fell head over heels for the sugary corn. In 1962, the Florida State Horticultural Society helped promote the new corn by giving three ears of Illini Xtra-Sweet to each of two thousand consumers in Gainesville, Florida. Even though the corn had been picked at least five days earlier, people said that it was the best corn they'd ever eaten and begged to know where they could get more. Old-fashioned sweet corn, the beloved corn of our parents' and grandparents' generations, was about to be pushed off the market.

FOR OUR NEXT TRICK—DOUBLE AND TRIPLE MUTATIONS

Laughnan was not the only geneticist to stumble upon a supersweet strain of corn. In the late 1960s, a professor from the University of Illinois named Ashby M. Rhodes identified another extra-sweet mutant. This corn did the sh2 one better. It was not only extra-sweet, it was extra-tender as well. This new mutant strain was named the sugar-enhanced or se, corn. The first of many se cultivars began to arrive on the market in the 1980s.

More recently, plant breeders have been using advanced breeding techniques to "stack" multiple mutations onto a single variety of corn, creating a new phenomenon called augmented supersweet corn. Augmented supersweet varieties have all the bells and whistles: they are extra-sweet, extra-tender, extra-creamy, and they retain their sweetness for days. To most consumers, this is the ultimate corn on the cob.

In just sixty years, the new science of plant genetics had transformed the entire sweet corn industry. Ninety-five percent of the sweet corn being grown today has Laughnan's sh2 mutation, the se mutation, or some artful combination of the two. We Americans love these man-made creations so much that we are now eating 30 percent more fresh corn than we did just a few decades ago. Build a sweeter vegetable—by any means—and consumers will come.

It is important to note that out of the thousands of mutant corn seeds sequestered in the Maize Genetics Cooperation Stock Center, the only varieties that have made it to our tables are the ones that are extra-sweet, soft, and either yellow or white in color, despite the fact that the center's collection includes kernels that are unusually high in protein, anthocyanins, or beta-carotene. But all these more nutritious varieties have been passed over in favor of sweeter, milder-flavored corn.

Why We Love Sweets

Our love of sugar is not caused by a sweet tooth, but by reward centers embedded deep within our brains. When we taste something sweet, receptors on the tongue and the lining of the mouth send instant messages to those centers, triggering the release of feel-good chemicals, including dopamine and endorphins. These are the same chemicals that people experience when they take first prize in a competition, win at gambling, go on a shopping spree, or engage in sexual activity. Whenever this part of the brain is activated, people feel so good about what they are doing that they are highly motivated to do it again.

Using advanced technology called functional magnetic resonance imaging (fMRI), neuroscientists can now monitor brain activity without invasive procedures. When volunteers eat sweet foods while undergoing a scan, the pleasure centers of their brains become much more active. On the imaging screen, those areas show up in brighter colors. Of all the types of food tested to date, sugar has caused the biggest light show. Even *thinking* about a favorite dessert can light up the screen.

Interestingly, other scans have shown that our brains can tell the difference between sugar and artificial sweeteners, even when our taste buds are fooled. In one study, healthy volunteers were given fMRI scans while tasting either sugar or the noncaloric sweetener sucralose. Even though the volunteers had difficulty distinguishing between the tastes of the two compounds, their brains knew the difference. When they tasted sugar, ten areas of their brains lit up in bright colors. When they tasted sucralose, only three regions were activated, leaving the seven other pleasure centers in the dark.

Why are we hardwired to want sweet flavors? As hunter-gatherers, we were so active that we needed to eat food with high concentrations of fat, starch, and sugar in order to survive. This type of food was so scarce in the wilderness environment that we had to search high and low for it. Nature gave us the chemical rewards we needed to stay on task. Even though we are now inundated with rich food, our archaic brains still reward us with dopamine whenever we indulge. Although we've succeeded in turning our food supply upside down, we have yet to rewire our sugar-hungry brains.

CHOOSING THE MOST NUTRITIOUS CORN IN THE SUPERMARKET

After many decades of selecting low-nutrient, extra-sweet corn, it's time we turned away from sugar and went in a healthier direction. A good first step is to choose the most colorful varieties of corn available. You won't see red, blue, or purple corn in conventional supermarkets, but you can choose the ears with the deepest yellow kernels. Deep yellow varieties have up to fifty-eight times more beta-carotene and the related compounds lutein and zeaxanthin than white corn. Lutein and zeaxanthin reduce the risk of two common eye diseases, macular degeneration and cataracts. If you prefer the taste of white corn to yellow corn, try sampling more varieties of yellow corn. There are dozens of cultivars, each with its own flavor and texture. You're likely to find more than one that pleases your palate.

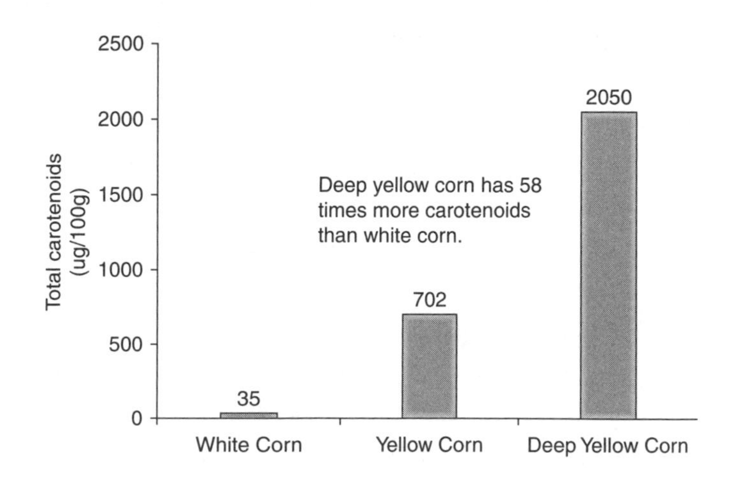

ORGANIC CORN

Regular sweet corn has relatively low levels of pesticide residues. In fact, in 2012, sweet corn was ranked number two on the Environmental Working Group's "Clean 15" list. Supersweet corn is another matter. Consumers want the ultrasugary varieties to be sweet, tender, creamy, and *flawless.* According to the USDA's Agricultural Research Service, this desire for perfection is causing corn growers to use more chemicals more often. "Because of the consumer's zero tolerance for sweet corn ear damage in US markets," the USDA stated in a recent bulletin, "growers in the southern United States spray insecticides as many as twenty-five to forty times per season. This extensive use of synthetic insecticides in agriculture is of concern because of worker and consumer safety and environmental contamination." Buying organically raised corn eliminates all these problems. Does organic corn have more nutrients than conventional corn? A few, but not all, studies say this is so. In a 2003 survey, organic corn was found to have 50 percent more phytonutrients than conventionally raised corn. More testing is under way.

BEYOND THE SUPERMARKET

Blue, purple, orange, black, and red corn varieties are extra-nutritious, but they are very hard to find, even in farmers markets. One advantage of shopping for corn in a farmers market, however, is that you will be able to buy heirloom varieties of yellow corn. Created before the 1960s, these varieties are free from genetic manipulation. Some heirlooms have deep yellow kernels and are sweet enough to be tasty but not so sweet that they wreak havoc with your blood sugar. They also have a "cornier" taste and creamier kernels than the supersweet cultivars. (Regular sweet corn is high in a starch called phytoglycogen, which has a smooth texture. In most supersweet cultivars, the phytoglycogen has been converted to sugar, robbing the corn of its creaminess.) In fact, some fans of heirloom varieties refer to supersweet corn as "sweet mush on a cob." When you're shopping at a farmers market, the vendors can tell you the varietal names of the corn they sell and whether these varieties fall into the category of ordinary sweet corn or the extra-sweet category.

GROWING CORN

When you grow your own corn, you have the most choices. The majority of the varieties available in conventional seed catalogs, however, are extra-sweet varieties. Their names are a dead giveaway: Sugar Buns, Honey, TripleSweet, Kandy Korn, and How Sweet It Is. To find varieties that are not extra-sweet, look for those labeled "old-fashioned," "heritage," or "heirloom," or look in a specialty seed catalog that features heirloom plants such as those published by the Seed Savers Exchange or the Southern Exposure Seed Exchange.

In some seed catalogs, you can also choose corn varieties based on the exact nature of their genetic mutations, spelled out in a code printed beside each variety. If you understand the code, you can glean a great deal of information. The sweetest varieties of all are called supersweets and are labeled "sh2." (This is the variety discovered by Laughnan.) Sh2s can be four to ten times sweeter than old-fashioned sweet corn. Sugar-enhanced, or se, corn is very sweet, but not as sweet as sh2. Old-fashioned sweet corn is labeled "su," for "sugary." The chart on page 92, entitled Cracking the Corn Code, provides more details.

When you grow old-fashioned varieties, harvest them from a U-pick farm, or grow them in your own garden, chill the ears as soon as you pick them, then eat them that day. (Bring along a cooler filled with ice when you harvest corn at a farm.) If you wait until the next day to eat the corn, much of the sugar will have been converted to starch.

HOW TO COOK CORN ON THE COB

The most common way to cook corn on the cob is to rip off the husks, strip off the silk, and plunge the naked ears into a big pot of boiling water. This brutality has got to stop. Boiling corn and other vegetables dissolves most of their water-soluble nutrients into the cooking water. The less contact corn has with water, the more nutrients stay in the kernels.

You can steam corn on the stove top or in the microwave. If you microwave corn in its husks, no water comes in contact with the corn, so all its nutrients are retained. To prepare the corn, cut off the silks that extend outside the husks, because they burn easily. Do not cut or open the husks themselves. Arrange the corn evenly in the microwave and cook on high. Microwaves have different wattages, so cooking times will vary. As a rough guide, allow three to four minutes for a single ear of corn, five to six minutes for two ears, and an added one to two minutes per ear for larger quantities. To check for doneness, carefully peel back the top portion of the husk of one ear of corn. If the corn is not done, close the husk and cook a minute or two longer. Let the corn cool down for five minutes before husking and removing the silk. You'll be delighted by the intense corn flavor. You can grill corn in its husks as well. Cut off the silks that stick out of the husks. Grill the corn in its husks for five minutes, turning several times. Remove the husks and silk, then put the ears back on the grill. Turn the corn until it is lightly grilled on all sides. (The amount of time will depend on the heat of your grill.) Eat the corn as is or add butter and salt. For more pizzazz, drizzle with lime juice and flavor with chili powder or hot pepper sauce.

COLORFUL CORNMEAL

As a nation, we consume more cornmeal, grits, polenta, tortillas, and corn chips than we do fresh corn. Most of these corn-based products are made from yellow or white field corn. The corn is dried, ground, and then refined, or, as one label states: "Dehulled and degermed to reduce susceptibility to rancidity." A more truthful label would read: "In order to extend the shelf life of the cornmeal, we have removed the germ (which is rich in vitamin E) and the hulls (which are high in fiber and antioxidants). During the processing, a significant loss of flavor and nutrients has occurred."

Fortunately, although colorful corn on the cob is very rare, colorful cornmeal is much easier to find; it's a great way to bring back some of the phytonutrients we've lost over the past several hundred years. Choose whole-grain yellow cornmeal, available in some large supermarkets and most natural-food stores, whenever possible. You will be getting more fiber, antioxidants, magnesium, phosphorus, potassium, choline, and more of a beneficial phytonutrient called betaine. Because whole-grain cornmeal includes the oily germ, it becomes rancid more quickly than refined cornmeal. Buy only the amount you will use in a month or so, seal it in a container or plastic bag, and store it in the freezer or refrigerator. This preserves the nutrients and prevents bug infestation as well.

Cornmeal made from blue, red, and purple corn provides many more bionutrients than yellow or white cornmeal. Look for these products in large supermarkets, ethnic markets, natural-food stores, or order them on the Internet. If you shop around, you will also find prepared mixes for blue cornmeal pancakes and muffins.

Order dishes made from colorful corn when you eat away from home. Recipes that feature blue corn or blue cornmeal are now showing up on restaurant menus around the country, not just in New Mexico, Texas, and Arizona. You can buy blue corn tortilla chicken taquitos in Chicago, blue corn buttermilk waffles in Manhattan, blue corn enchiladas in Portland, Oregon, and blue corn–encrusted cod in Alaska.

The following recipe for blue or purple cornbread is a welcome change from conventional cornbread. Honey is the only sweetener, and the cornbread is colorful and moist. Consider making a double batch and freezing some for later use. (You can make the cornbread from whole-grain yellow cornmeal as well.)

COLORFUL CORNBREAD

PREP TIME: 15–20 MINUTES
COOKING TIME: 20–25 MINUTES
TOTAL TIME: 35–45 MINUTES YIELD: 6 SERVINGS

1 cup purple, red, or blue whole-grain cornmeal
1 cup all-purpose flour
2 teaspoons baking powder
½ teaspoon baking soda
½ teaspoon salt
2 large eggs
⅓ cup honey
3 tablespoons melted unsalted butter
⅔ cup plain nonfat, low-fat, or full-fat yogurt
⅔ cup skim, low-fat, or whole milk

Preheat the oven to 425°F. Grease an 8-inch or 9-inch square baking pan.

Combine the dry ingredients in a medium mixing bowl. Using a spoon, make a well in the center.

In a small mixing bowl, whisk together the remaining ingredients until thoroughly combined. Pour the liquid ingredients into the well in the dry ingredients and stir briefly, until just combined. Pour the batter into the prepared pan and put it on the middle shelf in the oven.

Bake 20–25 minutes, or until the top is golden brown and the cornbread springs back when you touch it in the middle. Cool slightly and cut into 6 to 8 squares. Serve warm or at room temperature.

CANNED AND FROZEN CORN

Most people assume that canned fruits and vegetables are less nutritious than fresh produce. This makes sense, given the fact that high canning temperatures can destroy vitamin C and other heat-sensitive vitamins. New findings from food science labs, however, are revising this notion. It is now clear that vitamin C provides only a fraction of the antioxidant power in most fruits and vegetables. The majority comes from their phytonutrients. Unlike vitamin C, many phytonutrients maintain their antioxidant properties when they are heated. Some even become more potent, because the heat transforms them into more active forms or makes them easier to absorb. This explains why canned corn is even *higher* in carotenoids than fresh corn. Canned corn does not taste like fresh corn, of course, but it can be as good for you or better. If you're in a hurry, reach for a can. You'll find canned white and yellow corn on the grocery shelves. The yellow corn is much more nutritious.

In the past, most producers added sugar to canned corn to appeal to consumers. The invention of supersweet corn has made this unnecessary because the corn itself is so sugary. Food companies have been quick to slap "no sugar added" labels onto their canned supersweet corn to attract people who are trying to cut down on sugar. Consumers read those words and assume that the corn is a more healthful product, but it has just as much sugar as the sugar-added corn of earlier decades. The only difference is that the sugar is in the corn, not in the canning liquid.

Frozen yellow corn has the same nutritional content as fresh yellow corn. Most of the frozen corn on the market is made from supersweet varieties, however, so it has a relatively high glycemic index. Steam frozen corn without thawing to retain the most nutritional value. Boiling leaches out water-soluble nutrients.

CRACKING THE CORN CODE

TYPE AND CODE	DESCRIPTION	INFORMATION FOR GARDENERS
Old-fashioned sweet corn Code: su	Sweeter than field corn, but not as sweet as most modern varieties, which can be up to 44 percent sugar. Very creamy, with traditional "corny" flavor. The sugar changes to starch within 1–2 days. Cook within hours of harvest.	Plant at least 250 feet away from sh2 varieties. You can save the seeds of su corn because, unlike the seeds of hybrid corn, they produce corn nearly identical to the original plant. Old-fashioned sweet corn is better suited for cool climates than supersweet varieties.
Sugar-enhanced corn Code: se	Sweeter and more tender than old-fashioned sweet corn, which is 14–25 percent sugar. Stays sweet for 2–3 days after harvest with prompt refrigeration.	Plant at least 250 feet away from sh2 varieties. Less hardy than su corn. Requires extra moisture to germinate.
Supersweet corn Code: sh2	The mutant discovered by geneticist John Laughnan. Some varieties are 10 times sweeter than su corn, and are as high as 28–44 percent sugar. With proper handling, it can be stored up to 10 days without losing its sugar.	Plant 250 feet from all other varieties to prevent cross-pollination, which will turn the corn starchy. Plant when soil temperatures are at least 60–65 degrees and the soil is moist but not saturated. Do not plant as deep as other types. Yields are relatively low.
Augmented sweet corn Code: au	The sh2 type with additional mutations that make the kernels extra-tender. Sugar content varies greatly.	Plant when soil temperatures are at least 60–65 degrees and the soil is moist but not saturated. Do not plant as deep as other types.
Synergistic corn Code: se/sh2 or sy	Synergistic corn is a hybrid of se and sh2 corns. (It is up to 40 percent sugar.) On a single ear of corn, some kernels are se and others are sh2. The tastes and textures blend together when you eat them. Most bicolored corn is synergistic corn.	Isolate from sh2 corn and au corn. Does not need to be isolated from se or su corn. Tolerates cold better than other high-sugar varieties. Sow 7–10 days later than other early varieties.

RECOMMENDED VARIETIES AND TYPES OF CORN

IN THE SUPERMARKET	
TYPE OR VARIETY	COMMENTS
Yellow corn	All varieties with yellow or deep yellow kernels are higher in beta-carotene than varieties with white or pale yellow kernels. Most of the varieties of yellow corn in the supermarket are supersweets and very high in sugar, however.

FARMERS MARKETS, SPECIALTY STORES, U-PICK FARMS, AND SEED CATALOGS			
VARIETY	TYPE	DESCRIPTION	INFORMATION FOR GARDENERS
Blue Jade	Sugary corn (su)	Old-fashioned sweet corn. Small ears; silvery blue kernels. Seeds may be difficult to find.	Matures in 70–80 days (extra-early). Short stalks, 3–4 feet tall. Good for cool climates.
Double Red Sweet	Sugary corn (su)	Intensely red or purple kernels. Sweet when harvested before fully ripe and cooked within a few hours of picking. Also makes good cornmeal when harvested at maturity. High in anthocyanins. Rare.	Matures in 85–100 days. Grows 6–7 feet tall.
Floriani Red	Flint corn (nonsugary)	Dark red kernels with yellow interior. Makes flavorful cornbread, polenta, and grits. Rare. (Flint corn is also called Indian corn.)	Matures in 100 days. Grows 7–10 feet tall.

VARIETY	TYPE	DESCRIPTION	INFORMATION FOR GARDENERS
Golden Bantam	Sugary corn (su)	Old-fashioned sweet corn with deep yellow kernels. Traditional corn flavor. Freezes well on the cob and good for roasting.	Matures in 85 days.
Hopi Blue	Field corn (nonsugary)	Ancient variety. Large (8–10-inch) silvery-blue ears — somewhat sweet when picked young and roasted, but best known for making high-protein corn flour and cornmeal.	Matures in 75–110 days. Grows to 5 feet tall with 2 ears per stalk.
Indian Summer	Supersweet (sh2)	Large ears; yellow, white, red, and purple kernels. Color intensifies when cooked. Good for eating fresh. Steam or microwave to cook (red kernels turn brown when boiled). One of the few supersweet varieties with colorful kernels.	Matures in 79 days. Plant 500 feet away from other varieties, or plant so that it will mature 2 weeks earlier or later than others, to prevent cross-pollination.
Ruby Queen	Sugar-enhanced (se)	Red kernels with old-fashioned flavor. Has decorative red tassels and stalks. Steaming or microwaving enhances color. Pick young for maximum sweetness. Rare.	Matures in 75 days. Does best with another se variety for cross-pollination.
Seneca Red Stalker	Field corn (nonsugary)	Large (8–9-inch) ears; white, yellow, red, blue, and black kernels. Highly ornamental purple-red stalks. Originally grown by the Seneca Nation. Rare.	Matures in 100 days. Ancient variety.
White Eagle (also called Cherokee White Eagle)	Field corn (nonsugary)	Large ears; white and blue (and sometimes all blue) kernels on a red cob. Good for cornmeal, or for roasting when harvested young. Ancient variety grown by the Cherokee Nation.	Matures in 110 days.

CORN: POINTS TO REMEMBER

1. ***Choose colorful corn.***
   Varieties that are deep yellow, red, blue, black, or purple—or any combination thereof—give you more phytonutrients than pale yellow or white corn.
2. ***Choose old-fashioned or moderately sweet corn.***
   Select old-fashioned sweet corn or one of the moderately sweet varieties to help maintain optimum blood sugar levels. For maximum freshness, buy corn at a farmers market or U-pick farm.
3. ***Steam, grill, or microwave corn; do not boil it.***
   When you boil corn, valuable nutrients leach into the cooking water. Steaming, grilling, or microwaving will preserve those nutrients. Corn cooked in its husk retains the most nutrients of all.
4. ***Canned and frozen corn can be as nutritious as fresh corn.***
   Canning corn reduces its vitamin C content, but does not destroy its phytonutrients. Freezing corn has a minimal effect on its nutritional profile. Frozen and canned supersweet corn, however, have a relatively high glycemic index.
5. ***Cook with whole-grain cornmeal.***
   Buy whole-grain yellow cornmeal so you can benefit from the nutrients in the bran and the germ. Keep cornmeal refrigerated. For added nutrition and variety, cook with red, blue, or purple whole-grain cornmeal.
6. ***Buy organic corn to reduce your exposure to pesticides.***
   Supersweet varieties of corn grown in some areas of the country are heavily sprayed with pesticides. You can find organic sweet and supersweet corn in natural-food stores and farmers markets.
7. ***Grow your own corn.***
   Choose the most colorful supersweet cultivars, or grow old-fashioned sweet corn. If you choose the latter, cook the corn within a few hours of harvesting to keep the sugar from converting to starch.

CHAPTER 4

POTATOES

FROM WILD TO FRIES

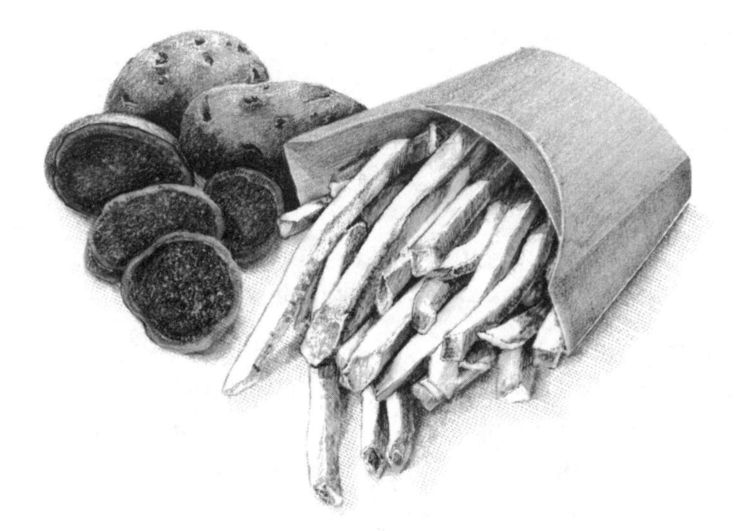

Wild potatoes and modern fries

The Mall of America, or MOA, as fans call it, is a gargantuan shopping center in Bloomington, Minnesota, which sprawls over 4.2 million square feet of land. Forty million people shop there every year. As you might expect, shoppers do not go hungry in the Mall of America. MOA boasts more than twenty-five fast-food chains and dozens of independent eateries. Potatoes are one of the most popular foods in the mall. Shoppers can treat themselves to french fries, cheese fries, potato chips, jojos, fish and chips, hash browns, garlic mashed potatoes, potato salad, fried potato skins, and baked potatoes with a dozen different toppings.

Outside the mall, potatoes are just as popular. On average, each of us eats 130 pounds of potatoes a year—twice as much as we did in the 1960s. This surge in consumption was sparked by the rapid proliferation of fast-food chains in the 1970s, which got America hooked on fries. We eat 7.5 billion pounds of french fries a year—that's thirty pounds of the deep-fried snacks per person per year. We consume eighteen million pounds of potato chips on Super Bowl Sunday alone. One-third of the vegetables consumed by teenagers comes in the form of french fries. In their many manifestations, white potatoes account for 32 percent of all the vegetables consumed by adults. Our intake of dark green and cruciferous vegetables, by contrast, is less than 1 percent of the recommended daily allowance. Starch rules.

Four hundred years before the Mall of America opened its doors, the land it occupies belonged to the Sioux Nation. The Sioux scouted the area for deer, elk, and caribou, and they foraged for wild fruits and vegetables. Their favorite root crop was the apio (*Apios americana*), a wild vegetable that has many common names, including Indian potato and potato pea. The tubers range from pea size to grapefruit-size, and they are strung along their thin roots like chunky beads on a necklace. The clever Sioux discovered a lazy way to gather them: they raided the burrows of field mice, who stuff their hideaways with up to half a bushel of apios.

Hundreds of years after apios disappeared from the menu, scientists have become curious about what they might have to offer us in terms of nutrition. Apios, they've discovered, have three times more protein than our modern potatoes. Like soybeans, also a member of the pea family, they are a rich source of the phytonutrient genistein. Genistein has been linked with a lowered risk of breast and prostate cancer. (Interestingly, the Sioux made a paste out of apios and applied it directly to skin tumors.) Apios may prove beneficial to the cardiovascular system as well. In an animal study, this forgotten root reduced the blood pressure of hypertensive rats by 10 percent. Despite these benefits, apios will never be served in the Mall of America. First of all, they grow too slowly: it takes three years before they produce tubers large enough to appeal to present-day consumers. More important, apios would make lousy french fries and potato chips. No slicing machine could ever cope with their irregular sizes and shapes. Lacking commercial appeal, apios are now classified as an invasive and noxious weed.

The large, sliceable, quick-growing tubers we eat today, *Solanum tuberosum,* commonly known as Irish potatoes, are native to Chile and Peru, not Ireland or the United States. Their native territory is twelve thousand feet above sea level, in mountainous regions of the Andes known as the altiplano, or high plateau. As they have for tens of thousands of years, the wild tubers survive and thrive despite poor soil, strong winds, and temperatures that can reach twenty degrees below zero.

There are as many as five thousand varieties of wild potatoes, which range from marble-size to football-size. In addition to white potatoes, there are black, tan, red, purple, blue, brown, yellow, orange, and green varieties. Place these exotic tubers next to our uniform, buff-colored russets and they would look gnarly and garish.

About eight thousand years ago, the first farmers in Peru began growing wild potatoes in their terraced, irrigated gardens, which were midway up the flanks of the Andes. The Peruvians selected the sweetest, largest, least bitter, and least fibrous potatoes to cultivate. Choosing mild-tasting potatoes was more than a matter of pleasing their taste buds, however. It was also a matter of survival. Potatoes and other members of the nightshade family have bitter compounds called glycoalkaloids that can be as deadly as strychnine.

Unlike most present-day potato farmers, the Peruvians did not grow just one or two varieties—they grew dozens. Even today, some high-altitude farmers grow as many as forty-five different varieties in a single year. A common practice is to plant five different varieties in a single hole. Planting a multitude of varieties, they have learned over millennia, insures that some potatoes will survive even the most unfavorable conditions. Genetic variation is their crop insurance.

Over the ages, Andean farmers invented a multitude of ways to prepare and store the tubers. People in remote villages still follow some of these traditions. To store potatoes for long periods of time, for example, they dig up mature potatoes and spread them out on the ground. The potatoes freeze during the cold nights and dry out in the daytime sun. This freezing and drying process goes on for weeks. Eventually, the potatoes become so dry that they are as brittle as chalk. Some of these "freeze-dried" potatoes are stored whole and others are turned into flakes called chuñu. To make chuñu, they heap the dried potatoes into piles and stomp on them. If the chuñu is kept in a cold, dry place, it remains perfectly preserved for as long as ten years. To reconstitute the flakes, they add water, just as we add water to dried potatoes to make instant mashed potatoes.

During the Korean War, food specialists from the US military visited Andean farmers to observe this simple but ingenious storage technique. Suitably impressed, the scientists went home and adapted the ancient method to create an instant potato product to add to the K rations for combat troops.

IMPROVING THE POTATO

New and improved cultivars of potatoes now grow in hundreds of countries around the world. All the "defects" of their wild ancestors have been remedied. Most potatoes are now medium to large in size and have a machinelike uniformity. A high percentage of their glycoalkaloids have been bred out of them, so you no longer have to worry about dying from eating a toxic potato. The greatest success story, however, has been a stunning increase in productivity. The yield per acre has increased sixfold in just the last eighty years. If you were to plow a football field, douse it with ammonium sulfate, dig in some seed potatoes, water as needed, and then wait four months, you would harvest up to forty-five thousand pounds of potatoes. Potatoes have become one of the most productive crops in the world.

In terms of food value, however, potatoes have been on a downhill slide for hundreds of years. Somewhere between the high plateaus of the Andes and the flat potato fields of Idaho and Washington, a great many nutrients have disappeared. The loss of color is the major reason for this decline. The Purple Peruvian potato (*Solanum tuberosum* subsp. *andigena*) is a small knobby potato that has been cultivated for several thousand years. To call it an heirloom is like calling Methuselah a senior citizen. Its abundance of anthocyanins makes it one of the most nutritious of all varieties. On an ounce-per-ounce basis, it has twenty-eight times more bionutrients than our most popular potato, the Russet Burbank, and 166 times more than the Kennebec white potato.

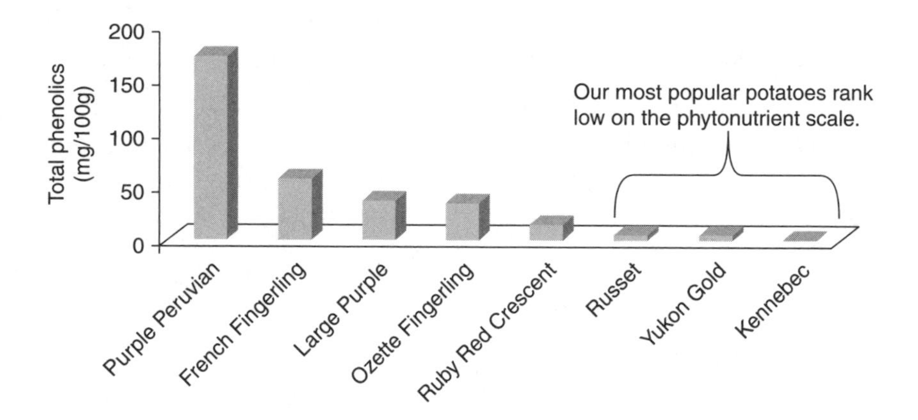

Wild potatoes are also lower in sugar and rapidly digested starch than the ones we eat today. Most of our modern varieties are high-glycemic, which means that we digest their sugars so rapidly that they give us a sharp rise in blood glucose. Our bodies are poorly equipped to handle this rapid infusion of sugar. People who consume a high-glycemic diet over a long period of time—which many Americans do—have a higher risk of prediabetes, also known as metabolic syndrome, which can lead to type 2 diabetes. (See boxed text below.) Type 2 diabetes is our leading cause of blindness, amputation, neuropathy, and cardiovascular disease. People who are diabetic or have the early signs of the disease are advised to limit their consumption of potatoes.

How Starch and Sugar Disrupt Your Metabolism

When you eat refined sugars and carbohydrates, your digestive system breaks them down into a simple sugar called glucose that is released into your bloodstream. Glucose is essential for your survival. It is the primary source of energy for all of the cells in the body and the *only s*ource of energy for your brain.

Your body functions best when you eat low-glycemic foods that release their sugar over a span of a few hours rather than in a short burst. As the glucose trickles into your bloodstream, your pancreas releases measured amounts of the hormone insulin. Insulin attaches to receptors on your fat and muscle cells, which prompts them to open up and receive the sugar and either burn it as fuel or store it for later use. Glucose cannot be cleared from your bloodstream without adequate amounts of insulin; it's a tightly choreographed dance.

High-glycemic foods have large amounts of rapidly digested carbohydrates and sugars. If you eat a high-glycemic meal, you experience a sudden surge in blood sugar, which must be countered by an equal surge in insulin. If all goes well, the extra infusion of insulin will drive the sugar out of your blood, restoring normal levels.

If you make a habit of eating high-glycemic food — as most Americans do — your fat and muscle cells are likely to stop reacting to the insulin. In medical terms, they will become insulin resistant. Because of this abnormal response, high levels of glucose linger in your bloodstream, resulting in chronic high blood sugar.

At some point, your pancreas may no longer be able to keep up with the incessant demand for insulin. As a result, even more glucose accumulates in your blood. If your fasting blood sugar climbs above 126 mg/dL (milligrams per deciliter) for two consecutive blood tests, you meet the criteria for type 2 diabetes. Our highly refined, starchy, high-sugar Western diet is pushing tens of millions of adults and teenagers into this deadly zone.

Our native diet was low-glycemic. When we choose to eat more low-glycemic meals, we are giving our bodies the types of food they are designed to handle. As a result, we have a lower risk of obesity and diabetes and their many negative consequences.

HIDDEN PESTICIDES

Year after year, potatoes make it to the "Dirty Dozen," the Environmental Working Group's annual list of the most contaminated foods in the US food supply. Potatoes are sprayed with fungicides and insecticides while they are growing in the field, and then are treated with sprout inhibitors while they are in storage. Some of these chemicals are highly soluble and penetrate beneath the skin of the potato. Scrubbing the potatoes removes only 25 percent of these hidden compounds. Peeling gets rid of up to 70 percent, but the rest remains inside the potato—unwelcome ingredients in your baked potatoes and potato salad.

Although peeling potatoes gets rid of many of the contaminants, the peels are the most nutritious part of the vegetable. Remove the skins and you lose 50 percent of the total antioxidants in the potato. You will also lose fiber, which slows the release of glucose into your bloodstream. The way out of this conundrum is to buy organic potatoes and eat the skins. Shop around and you will find organic potatoes that are only twenty to thirty cents more per pound than conventionally raised potatoes.

As you will discover in the following pages, there are other ways to make potatoes a more healthful part of your diet. Choosing highly nutritious varieties is one of the most effective. You'll find at least one of the varieties recommended on pages 108–9 in your local supermarket and many more at farmers markets. If you're a gardener, you can plant varieties that give you almost the same benefits as wild potatoes. Once you've chosen your potatoes, you can prepare and cook them in ways that preserve their nutrients and further lower their adverse effect on your blood sugar. Even if you are diabetic, overweight, or have metabolic syndrome, potatoes can become a nutritious part of your diet.

SHOPPING FOR POTATOES IN THE SUPERMARKET

The typical supermarket carries a number of varieties of potatoes. The most common are the buff-colored Russet Burbanks, red and white new potatoes, boiling potatoes, white baking potatoes, and Yukon Golds. Surprisingly, our most popular potato, the Russet Burbank, has the most phytonutrients. It is also a great source of potassium, a good source of vitamin C, and is unusually high in vitamins B2, B3, and folic acid. Its main failing is that it also has a very high glycemic index.

New potatoes are potatoes that are harvested early in the season and sold soon thereafter. They have a waxy, creamy flesh that makes them ideal for potato salads and casseroles. Common varieties of new potatoes include small red or white potatoes and boiling potatoes. Old potatoes are potatoes that are harvested when fully mature and then stored at least a few weeks before making their way to the market. (In earlier days, they were referred to as storage potatoes.) Old potatoes, such as the russet, have a thicker skin than new potatoes and a fluffier, drier texture. Most people use old potatoes for baking, frying, mashing, and making french fries.

New potatoes cause a lower rise in blood sugar than old potatoes—in some cases half as much. They also have thinner skins, making it more likely that people will eat them. Europeans eat more new potatoes than old ones, the reverse of our eating habits. We would do well to emulate them.

Some large supermarkets have begun to sell more colorful potatoes, primarily for the sake of novelty. Many of these potatoes are far more nutritious than people realize. The potatoes with red, blue, or black skins and deeply colored flesh approach the phytonutrient content of their wild ancestors. If you don't know the color of the flesh, ask the produce manager to cut one open for you. A potato can be blue-skinned but stark white inside. Some stores sell bags of assorted varieties, which is a good way to find out which ones you like best.

BEYOND THE SUPERMARKET

You'll have the most choices when you shop for potatoes in a farmers market or buy seed potatoes for a garden. The list of recommended varieties at the end of this chapter will help guide your choices. Most farmers display the names of their varieties or can identify them for you. Three potatoes on the list—Mountain Rose, Purple Majesty, and All Blue—were bred specifically to increase their nutritional content. The developers used traditional breeding techniques, not genetic modification, to create these high-nutrient cultivars. In an animal study, Mountain Rose was found to be highly effective in inhibiting human breast cancer cells that had been implanted in rats. Purple Majesty contains at least 235 milligrams of anthocyanins per serving. According to its developers, this is "twice the amount found in any other fruit or vegetable." A 2012 study determined that eating Purple Majesty potatoes can lower the blood pressure of people with hypertension. The reduction was enough to lower the risk of stroke by 34 percent and the risk of heart attack by 21 percent. Despite the fact that the volunteers added the potatoes to their normal diet, they did not gain weight.

The Red French Fingerling, or French Fingerling, is one of my all-time favorite varieties. This heirloom potato has rose-colored skin and creamy yellow flesh that is similar to the flesh of Yukon Gold, but it has ten times more antioxidants. The skin is thin enough that you won't be tempted to peel it. I grow it every year, and it has become a favorite of family and friends. It makes a beautiful potato salad.

STORING POTATOES

New potatoes do not store well because their thin skins offer little protection against moisture loss, mold, and disease. Store them in the refrigerator and eat within a week of purchase. Old potatoes have a low rate of respiration and can be stored for several months without losing any of their nutritional value. Their thick skins also prevent rapid moisture loss.

Do not store old potatoes in the refrigerator for more than a week or two. The cold temperatures increase their already high sugar content and make them discolor when cooked. The potatoes also release ethylene gas, which reduces the storage life of other vegetables. Ideally, store them in a cool, dark location with good ventilation. The ideal storage temperature is between forty-five and fifty degrees. These conditions were easy to come by in the days when most people had a root cellar, but not so today: the refrigerator is too cold and heated spaces are too warm. A workable compromise is to put potatoes in a netted bag, open paper bag, or a box with a few nickel-size holes for ventilation. Store them in an unheated basement or garage. If you don't have a basement or garage, buy them at the store as you need them.

HOW TO MAXIMIZE THE FLAVOR AND HEALTH BENEFITS OF POTATOES

There is a slick trick you can use to tame the sugar rush of high-glycemic potatoes. If you cook potatoes and then *chill them for about twenty-four hours before you eat them,* they are magically transformed into a low- or moderate-glycemic vegetable. The cool temperature converts the potatoes' rapidly digested starch into a more "resistant" starch that is broken down more slowly. All cold potato dishes, from the humble potato salad to the urbane salade niçoise, are moderate-glycemic foods—provided you chill them overnight before you eat them.

Once you cook potatoes and chill them overnight, you can reheat them and they will retain their lower glycemic status. Bake potatoes today, chill them tonight, and then reheat them for dinner tomorrow. Your blood sugar response will be reduced by as much as 25 percent. If you or someone in your household is overweight or struggling with high blood sugar, prediabetes, or diabetes, it is worth your while to take this extra step. In just one day of chilling, you can reverse thousands of years of human intervention that have turned a low-glycemic tuber into a contributing cause of obesity, diabetes, and cardiovascular disease.

Adding fat to potatoes or cooking them in fat also slows down the digestive process. For this reason, french fries produce a smaller increase in blood sugar than baked or steamed potatoes. Sprinkling fries with vinegar, an English tradition, slows down digestion even more.

The following recipe for potato salad uses all these tricks. The potatoes are cooked in their skins and then chilled overnight, and the dressing contains both oil and vinegar. It's a delicious salad that will please everyone, not just those concerned about high blood sugar. For the most health benefits, use blue, red, or purple potatoes, but conventional varieties can be used as well.

POTATO SALAD WITH SUN-DRIED TOMATOES AND KALAMATA OLIVES

PREP TIME: 15 MINUTES
COOKING TIME: 20–45 MINUTES, DEPENDING ON METHOD
CHILLING TIME: 24 HOURS YIELD: 5 CUPS (ABOUT 4–5 SERVINGS)

2 pounds unpeeled new potatoes or unpeeled baking potatoes, preferably with red, blue, or purple flesh
½ cup oil-packed sun-dried tomatoes, drained and chopped or julienned
½ cup thinly sliced red onions or chopped scallions (including white and green parts)
⅓ cup extra virgin olive oil, preferably unfiltered
3 tablespoons red or white wine vinegar
1 tablespoon sugar
1–2 garlic cloves, pushed through a garlic press
½ teaspoon powdered mustard or 1 teaspoon prepared mustard
½ cup pitted and chopped kalamata olives
⅓ cup chopped prosciutto or diced cooked bacon (optional)

Steam or microwave the potatoes in their skins until they are tender. Cool and store in the refrigerator for 24 hours. Quarter the chilled potatoes, then cut into ¼-inch slices and place in a large mixing bowl. Do not remove the skins.

Combine remaining ingredients in a small bowl and pour over the potatoes. Toss to coat evenly. Serve cold or at room temperature.

RECOMMENDED TYPES AND VARIETIES OF POTATOES

IN THE SUPERMARKET	
TYPE OR VARIETY	COMMENTS
All varieties of new potatoes	All new potatoes, or "waxy" potatoes, have a lower impact on your blood sugar than old, or "baking," potatoes.
Russet Burbank	Relatively high in antioxidants. Bake, refrigerate overnight, then reheat to lower the impact on your blood sugar.
Colorful "novelty" potatoes	Potatoes with blue skins *and* flesh are the most nutritious, followed by potatoes with red skins and flesh. (See descriptions of specific varieties below. They are available in some supermarkets.)

FARMERS MARKETS, SPECIALTY STORES, U-PICK FARMS, AND SEED CATALOGS		
VARIETY	DESCRIPTION	INFORMATION FOR GARDENERS
All Blue	Very high in anthocyanins. Medium-size oblong tubers with deep blue skin and nearly purple flesh. Good for baking and oven fries.	Matures in 90 days; a midseason variety.
All Red (also called Cranberry Red)	Medium-to-large potatoes with bright red skin and rose-swirled flesh; they keep their color when cooked. Fine, moist texture good for potato salads. Store well.	Matures in 80–95 days; a midseason variety.
Mountain Rose	Red inside and out. Good for baking, mashing, and potato salads.	Matures in 70–90 days; an early-to-midseason variety.
Nicola	Yellow skin and flesh. Good for mashing, roasting, and salads. Waxy, with a nutty potato taste. Low glycemic index. Uncommon.	Matures in 95 days; a midseason variety.

VARIETY	DESCRIPTION	INFORMATION FOR GARDENERS
Ozette	Pale skin and creamy yellow fingerling potato with a slightly earthy, nutty flavor. Ancient heirloom that originated in South America. Rare.	Matures in 120–130 days; a late-season variety.
Purple Majesty	Uniform; oblong; purple inside and out. Good for frying, baking, and potato salad. Stores well. Very high in anthocyanins.	Matures in 85 days; an early-to-midseason variety.
Purple Peruvian	Deep purple skin and flesh. Small-to-medium tubers with many eyes. An earthy flavor. Good fried or roasted. Very high in anthocyanins. Ancient heirloom from Peru. Rare.	Matures in 100–120 days; a late-season variety.
Ranger Russet	Long, slightly flattened, with russeted (roughened) brown skin and white flesh. Good for roasting, mashing, frying, and baking. Higher in antioxidant activity than the Russet Burbank.	Matures in 120 days; a late-season variety.
Ruby Crescent	Slender fingerling only 2–3 inches long, with thin, rosy-colored skin. Yellow flesh is waxy. Good for potato salads and roasting. Earthy, nutty flavor.	Matures in 120 days; a late-season variety.
Russet Norkotah	Large, oblong tubers with russeted (roughened) skin and white flesh. Higher in phytonutrients than Russet Burbank. Stores well.	Matures in 60–75 days; an early-to-midseason variety.

POTATOES: POINTS TO REMEMBER

1. ***Choose the most colorful potatoes.***
   Choose potatoes with the darkest skins and flesh. Blue, purple, and red potatoes give you more antioxidants than yellow potatoes. Russet Burbank potatoes are higher in phytonutrients than most white potatoes, but they are also high in rapidly digested carbohydrates.

2. ***Eat the skins.***
   The skin contains 50 percent of the antioxidant activity in the entire potato. Its high fiber content slows the digestion of starch and sugar, giving the potato a lower glycemic value.
3. ***Shop beyond the supermarket.***
   When you are choosing potatoes in farmers markets, natural-food stores, and specialty produce stores, look for the recommended varieties listed on pages 108–9. Some of the most nutritious varieties are available only in these markets and in select seed catalogs.
4. ***Buy organic potatoes to reduce your exposure to pesticides.***
   Conventionally grown potatoes are heavily sprayed with pesticides and other chemicals. Scrubbing and peeling them do not remove all the unwanted compounds. Buying organic potatoes will reduce your intake of toxins and is highly recommended if you eat the skins.
5. ***Store potatoes in a cool, dark location with adequate ventilation.***
   New potatoes can be stored in the refrigerator for one or two weeks. Old potatoes are best stored outside the refrigerator in a dark, cool location, ideally between forty-five and fifty degrees. Storing them in a partially closed paper sack or a box perforated with a few nickel-size holes will provide adequate ventilation.
6. ***Tame the sugar rush.***
   New potatoes do not raise your blood sugar as much as mature potatoes do. In addition to eating the skins, you can lower the glycemic index of potatoes by (1) eating them with some type of fat, (2) chilling them for twenty-four hours after they've been cooked, and (3) flavoring them with vinegar.

CHAPTER 5

THE OTHER ROOT CROPS

CARROTS, BEETS, AND SWEET POTATOES

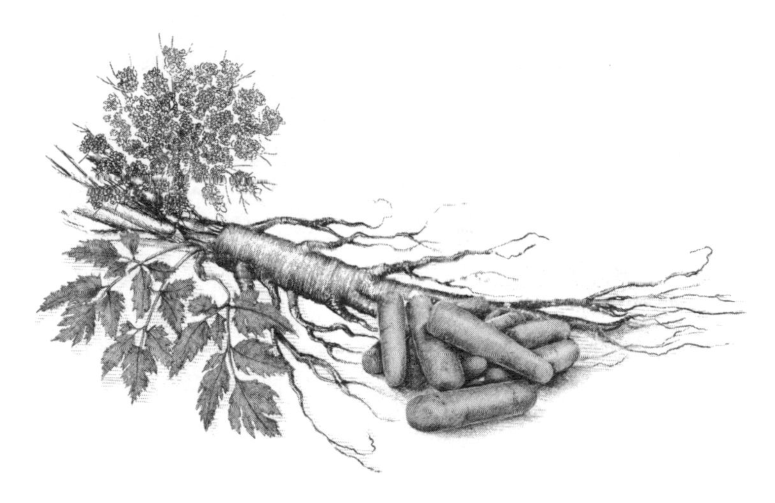

Wild carrots and modern baby carrots

For most hunter-gatherer tribes, the transition from living on wild plants to getting most of their food from their gardens took place over the course of hundreds of years. When a tribe is introduced to a carbohydrate-rich crop, however, the change can take place in one or two generations. This was the case for a tribe of Maku Indians, who live in the northwest corner of the Amazon rain forest. The region is so remote that the tribe had little contact with outsiders until well into the twentieth century. In 1927, they were studied by an anthropologist who observed that the tribe was living on fish, wild plants, insects, and the small game that they captured with their bows and arrows or poison-tipped darts. He saw no traces of agriculture.

In 1972, just forty-five years later, an anthropologist named Peter Silverwood-Cope encountered the same tribe. He was surprised to see they were now growing large quantities of manioc, a starchy root also known as cassava. (Tapioca is made from manioc roots.) The tribe had learned how to grow manioc from a neighboring farming tribe. Even though the Maku had been growing it for only two generations, it was supplying up to 80 percent of their calories. The Maku still remembered how to gather wild plants, Silverwood-Cope reported, and they would talk to him about the time of their grandfathers, when all their food had come from the forest. Once they had found a reliable supply of starch, however, there had been no turning back. In fact, when they ran out of the roots, they would complain loudly that they had "no food," even though they had drying racks piled with meat and forest fruits. In desperation, they would beg manioc from neighboring tribes, or they would walk long distances to a manioc plantation and trade their dried meat and fruit for the starchy roots. The wild plants and game that had sustained the Maku for countless generations had been reduced to mere bargaining chips in their quest for more carbs.

Today, manioc is a staple food for approximately five hundred million people worldwide. The vegetable is low in protein, phytonutrients, and vitamins, but it yields more carbohydrates per acre than all other crops in the world except for sugarcane and sugar beets.

ROOT CROPS IN THE UNITED STATES

The most important root crops in this country—apart from the common potato—are carrots, beets, and sweet potatoes. Unlike manioc, they can be very nutritious. Like all root crops, they were more popular before the days of home canning and freezing because they could be stored in root cellars and brought to the table whenever needed. The vegetable lairs kept the roots from freezing, drying out, rotting, and sprouting. Our modern refrigerators don't do nearly as well.

There is a wide range of nutrients and flavors in our many cultivars of carrots, beets, and sweet potatoes, as there is in all our produce. Knowing which ones to choose and how to prepare them could make a significant difference in your health. Pick the right varieties of beets, for example, and research shows that you might be able to run faster, walk with less effort, and even reduce your risk of a stroke.

CARROTS

In North America, the most common wild carrot is the taproot of a plant known as Queen Anne's lace. You may have seen it growing in an open field. It is a thigh-high weed with an umbrella-shaped canopy of flowers made up of hundreds of smaller flowers. Some varieties have a single dark red flower in the center. People who study insects say that this single red flower is as attractive to insects as rosy lips are to lovers. The root of the plant is spindly and cream-colored and looks nothing like the carrots we eat today. If you crush the root and inhale its scent, however, you will smell the family resemblance; there's no mistaking the aroma of a carrot.

Numerous Native American tribes gathered these wild carrots and stored them for winter use. The Navajo made a vegetable soup of dried wild carrots and celery. The Pacific Northwest Klallam tribe arranged fresh carrots in large pits lined with red-hot rocks that were covered with seaweed. The carrots steamed in their hot, salty sauna for up to two days. More seaweed was heaped on top.

DOMESTICATED CARROTS

The wild ancestor of our present-day orange carrot is a plant with a purple taproot that is native to Afghanistan. It was first cultivated several thousand years ago. By the 1300s, purple carrots were growing in Spain, France, Germany, and the Netherlands. Two mutant varieties—white and yellow carrots—began to be cultivated as well. Sixteenth-century Europeans were growing four colors of carrots—red, yellow, purple, and white.

You might have noticed that orange carrots have yet to be mentioned. In fact, orange carrots did not exist until four hundred years ago, when two plant breeders in the Netherlands crossed a yellow mutant carrot from Africa with a local red carrot. The impetus for this botanical merger is that the men wanted to honor the House of Orange, the princely dynasty that had spearheaded the Netherlands' revolt against Spain in the mid-sixteenth century.

The new designer vegetable was first referred to as "the long orange Dutch carrot." It became so popular that Dutch entrepreneurs began promoting it outside the country, along with their wildly popular tulip bulbs. Over the span of two hundred years, orange carrots became the most common variety in the Western world. Although purple carrots still appear in food markets in Egypt, India, Japan, and China, most stores in the United States carry only the orange varieties.

Too bad for us that the House of Orange was not called the House of Purple. A fit of patriotism hundreds of years ago gave us the short end of the carrot stick. As is the case with most vegetables, the color of carrots is a good indicator of the amount and kinds of bionutrients they contain. Purple carrots are a concentrated source of anthocyanins, which have more antioxidant activity and potentially more health benefits than the beta-carotene in orange carrots. As you will discover later on, we have not only "depurpled" corn and carrots, we have removed the anthocyanins from a number of other fruits and vegetables as well, including broccoli and cauliflower. The green, yellow, orange, and white varieties of produce that predominate in our supermarkets do not come close to the healing properties of their purple-hued and red-hued ancestors.

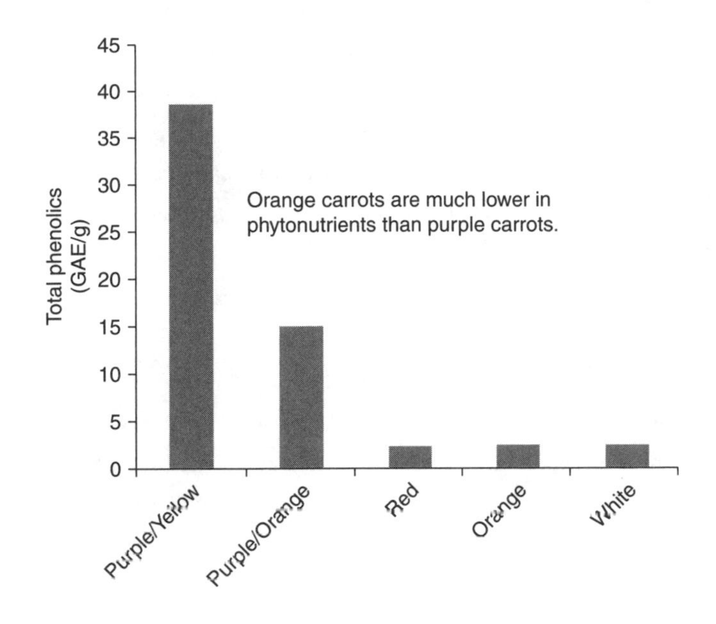

GETTING THE MOST FROM ORANGE CARROTS

Although orange carrots do not have the potentially disease-preventing properties of purple carrots, they are nutritious vegetables nonetheless. The admonition "Eat your carrots" is a good one. Carrots are low in fat, high in fiber, low in calories, and a good source of beta-carotene. Most of their calories come from sugar, but there is not enough sugar in a serving of carrots to wreak havoc with your blood sugar.

With just a few simple changes, however, you can triple the nutrients you get from orange carrots and enhance their flavor at the same time. First of all, think twice before you buy so-called baby carrots. Those convenient little nubbins that come in plastic bags are pretrimmed and scrubbed. You can reach into the bag, grab some carrots, and nosh. In reality, baby carrots are misshapen mature carrots that have been whittled down to a smaller and more uniform size. The outer part that's thrown away, food scientists have learned, is much more nutritious than the inner core that remains. As with most fruits and vegetables, the greatest concentration of nutrients is in the skin and the tissue right below it. This makes sense, because the outer layers of a plant are its first line of defense against UV rays, mold, grazing animals, insects, fungus, and disease. The more phytonutrients in those outermost layers, the better it can defend itself. When you whittle away the outer portion of a carrot, you remove one-third of its phytonutrients. Cutting mature carrots into sticks would make a more nutritious snack.

For the freshest and sweetest flavor, buy carrots with their green tops still attached. They are, at most, a few weeks old; carrots sold without their tops can be several months old, which can give them a bitter, off-putting flavor. (Cut the tops off the carrots before refrigerating to preserve the moisture in the carrot.)

Some vegetables are as nutritious frozen as they are when fresh. Not so carrots. The peeling and processing that carrots undergo before freezing, along with the freezing-and-thawing cycle itself, can destroy half their antioxidant value. Take an extra fifteen minutes to cook fresh carrots. All too often, when we try to speed up meal preparation, we cheat ourselves out of some wholesome nutrients.

Some foods are more nutritious when eaten raw, but carrots are better for you when cooked. The heat breaks down their tough cell walls, making some of their nutrients more bioavailable. A 1998 study determined that volunteers who consumed cooked carrots for a month absorbed three times more beta-carotene than people who consumed the same amount of raw carrots. Practitioners of Chinese medicine intuited this eons ago. They have long advised their patients that cooking carrots increases their medicinal benefits.

It also matters *how* you cook carrots. Boiling them allows many of their water-soluble nutrients to leach into the cooking water. Sautéed or steamed carrots retain more of their food value because the carrots are in contact with less water.

There's another recent discovery you should know about. If you cook carrots whole and then slice or chop them *after* they've been cooked, you get more nutrients than if you cut them *before* you cook them. Whole carrots do take longer to cook than sliced carrots, but more of their nutrients stay in the vegetable. Once the carrots are cooked, you can carve away at them with no nutritional loss.

Eating carrots that have been cooked whole may even reduce your risk of cancer. Carrots contain a cancer-fighting compound called falcarinol. British researchers at Newcastle University discovered that whole-cooked carrots have 25 percent more falcarinol than carrots that have been cut before cooking. As an added bonus, whole-cooked carrots retain more of their natural sweetness. In a blind taste test of one hundred volunteers, 80 percent of them preferred the flavor of whole-cooked carrots, making this a win-win situation.

Finally, carrots are best for you when you eat them with some type of oil or fat. Beta-carotene is a fat-soluble nutrient that needs to be coated in fat for greatest absorption. Combining these four simple steps—(1) choosing whole carrots rather than baby carrots, (2) cooking them whole, (3) steaming or sautéing them rather than boiling them, and (4) serving them along with some oil or fat can give you eight times more beta-carotene than eating raw baby carrots, and at no extra cost.

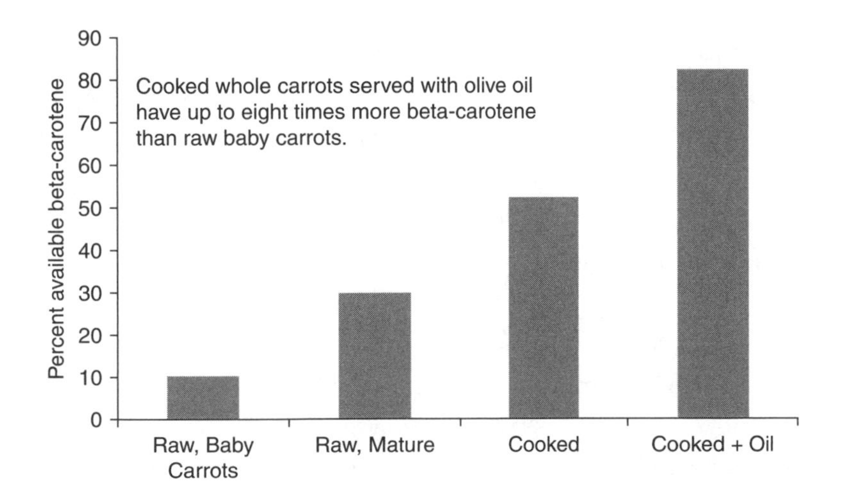

COLORFUL CARROTS MAKE A COMEBACK

At long last, the orange carrot fetish that began in the Netherlands is finally losing its grip. Scout around in farmers markets, natural-food stores, seed catalogs, and some of the larger supermarkets and you'll see yellow, red, and purple carrots for sale alongside their orange cousins. Don't think of them as designer foods or nutraceuticals but rather as a return to our culinary and nutritional heritage.

The purple varieties of carrot are more nutritious than all other colors, as illustrated in the chart on page 115. The purple color comes from anthocyanins. Compared to orange carrots, they are also higher in beta-carotene and a related compound called alpha-carotene, which has been linked with a lowered risk of dying—from any cause—during a fifteen-year period.

A few animal studies have shown that eating purple carrots could be the perfect antidote to the standard American diet, also known as SAD. In an Australian study, a colony of healthy rats was placed on a high-fat, high-carbohydrate diet similar to the diet most Westerners eat today. The researchers left nothing out. They even replaced the rodents' drinking water with a 25-percent fructose solution, which is the percentage of fructose in a Pepsi or a Coke that has been sweetened with high-fructose corn syrup.

After only two months on the unwholesome diet, the rats had the same physical problems many overweight middle-aged Americans do. They had gained weight, especially around the middle. The walls of their hearts had thickened, a sign that their hearts were under increased strain. They had higher blood pressure, and fat had infiltrated their livers, which is the first step in fatty liver disease. On top of that, their cells had become insulin resistant and they had higher levels of triglycerides and cholesterol in their blood. All these symptoms are part of the condition called metabolic syndrome. Doctors treat these symptoms with blood-pressure medications and cholesterol-lowering drugs, and issue stern warnings about the consequences of a "fatty liver" and abnormal liver function.

The scientists kept the beleaguered rodents on this unhealthy diet for another eight weeks. At this point, half the rats were given purple carrot juice to drink in addition to the high-fructose water. In just two months, their heart and liver functions improved. They lost weight and their bellies shrank. They had less chronic inflammation and lower blood pressure, and their cholesterol, glucose response, and triglycerides dropped back to normal. *Remarkably, all these changes took place despite the fact that the rodents were still on the high-fat, high-carbohydrate, high-fructose diet.* The anthocyanins in the purple carrot juice had made all the difference.

If you need more incentive to try purple carrots, you should know that they are sweeter than orange carrots. Professional food tasters say they have less of a "petrol" flavor as well. If you are a gardener, look for the following cultivars of purple carrots: Cosmic Purple, Deep Purple, Purple Haze, and Purple Rain. Deep Purple has the most anthocyanins by far.

STORING CARROTS

Carrots, like most root crops, have a low respiration rate and can be stored for weeks without losing their food value. It's best to keep them away from fruits and vegetables that produce ethylene gas, however. Ethylene gas triggers the formation of bitter compounds in carrots. Ethylene producers include apples, cantaloupe, scallions, tomatoes, plums, potatoes, and dozens of additional fruits and vegetables, many of which are stored in the refrigerator. To protect carrots from ethylene gas, put them in a sealed plastic bag and store them in the crisper drawer of the refrigerator or in another dark, cool, and humid environment. (Their respiration rate is so low that their flavor is not compromised by being stored in a sealed plastic bag.)

How Healthy Were Hunter-Gatherers?

Hunter-gatherers consumed far more phytonutrient-rich food than we do today. How did that influence their health and longevity? Despite their high consumption of phytonutrients and their lack of exposure to high-sugar, high-fat foods, hunter-gatherers did not live nearly as long as we do today. Anthropologists estimate that a baby born into a hunter-gatherer tribe ten thousand years ago had a life expectancy of only twenty-five to thirty-five years; an infant born in the United States in 2012 can expect to live seventy-five or eighty years.

But to what do we owe our greater longevity? Not to an improvement in diet or lifestyle but to dramatic advances in medicine and sanitation that have taken place within the past 250 years. Roll back the clock to the mid-1770s, and many Europeans had an average life span similar to most hunter-gatherers. People living in Sweden in 1750, for example, had a life expectancy of only thirty-four years. Shortly after that time, highly effective vaccines began to be developed that greatly reduced the mortality rate from smallpox and other infectious diseases. Improved sanitation put an end to cholera epidemics that had been claiming countless lives. Penicillin became available in the early 1900s and was followed by other highly effective antibiotics. Today we have all these benefits plus sophisticated diagnostic tools, advanced surgical procedures, a broad array of pharmaceuticals, expert trauma care, and an untold number of other medical advances. Take them away and we might be living no longer than people who lived ten thousand or more years ago.

There's another point to consider. Although we now have an enviable life span, we have a rapidly decreasing "health span." The majority of people in this country are now overweight or obese. Twenty-six million adults have type 2 diabetes, including 30 percent of people age sixty-five and older. An additional seventy-nine million adults have high blood sugar, putting them at risk for developing diabetes. According to the American Heart Association, more than seventy-six million Americans have high blood pressure, which is a contributing cause of heart attack and stroke. Until the late twentieth century, these health problems were restricted to the adult population; now they are being diagnosed in teenagers and younger children as well.

From all available evidence, it appears that hunter-gatherers were relatively free of these afflictions, no matter their age. How do we know this? Although it is not possible to go back in time and give medical exams to people who lived thousands of years ago, anthropologists and medical researchers have done the next best thing: they have studied the health of hunter-gatherers in more than fifty tribes that managed to survive into the nineteenth and twentieth centuries. These tribes lived in such remote areas that they had little or no contact with the outside world; they were living relics of our original lifestyle.

The results of the medical examinations were astounding. The vast majority of the tribal members had blood pressure readings at or below our current gold standard of 120/80. What's more, their blood pressure did not increase with age. People in their seventies had readings as low as 105/60. There was little or no evidence of cancer or cardiovascular disease. Obesity was nonexistent. The body mass index of most adults was below today's ideal of 22. Despite their leanness, the hunter-gatherers were not frail or wasting away. In fact, tests of physical fitness determined that they had the endurance and strength of today's elite athletes.

Now, for the very first time, we can have the best of both worlds. We can reduce our risk of disease by avoiding refined foods and choosing high-phytonutrient, high-fiber fruits and vegetables that can restore a host of lost nutrients to our diet. We can get additional health benefits by ramping up our physical activity so that it comes closer to the levels of our long-ago relatives. We can choose to eat less red meat or switch to the leaner, more nourishing meat of grass-fed animals, which is similar to the meat of wild game. When these lifestyle changes are combined with the best of twenty-first-century medicine, we have the potential to become the healthiest people who have ever walked on the planet.

BEETS

The wild ancestor of our modern beet is the sea beet (*Beta maritima*), which is native to the coastal regions of the Mediterranean. It still grows there, looking more like Swiss chard than our bulbous supermarket beet. In fact, the roots are so small they're not worth eating. Our farming ancestors began to domesticate beets about six thousand years ago, but for several thousand years, people consumed only the leaves, much the same way we eat the leaves of Swiss chard and discard the roots. Beet roots were used primarily for dyes, teas, poultices, and as a treatment for stomach complaints.

By the Roman era, careful selection had created beets with larger and sweeter bulbs, and the bulbs began to be eaten along with the leaves. They continued to be used as a healing food, and were even used to rekindle sexual desire. Evidence for their use as an aphrodisiac comes from the writings of Roman physicians and naturalists of the time, and, more recently, from excavations of the ancient towns that were preserved in volcanic ash from the eruption of Mount Vesuvius in 79 AD. These preserved buildings retained astonishing detail, right down to the brightly colored frescoes on the walls. One of the more titillating discoveries is that *lupanares,* or brothels, were commonplace during this bawdy era.

Archaeologists are able to identify them because their walls are decorated with rows of beet roots.

Beets may indeed have aphrodisiac properties. They are rich in the element boron, which until recently was known only for its bone-building properties. In 1987, a small-scale human study uncovered another effect: boron "markedly elevates" the production of testosterone in both men and women. Higher testosterone levels are linked with greater sexual desire in both sexes. Eating beets also relaxes and widens the blood vessels, allowing greater blood flow throughout the body. Beets show promise of being a veggie Viagra.

As farmers created bigger and sweeter beet roots, the roots eventually became the main course and the leaves became the hors d'oeuvre. Today, we eat only tiny amounts of the greens. Consumers eat more canned beets than fresh ones, and most fresh beets are sold without their tops. But even when beets are sold with their leaves attached, most people chop off the greens as soon as they get home. Once again, it would behoove us to eat the greens. Research shows that the leaves have more antioxidants than the roots themselves. Our ancient ancestors had it right all along.

Beets *without* their greens still rank among the healthiest of all our most commonly eaten vegetables, however. They taste sweet, but they have a surprisingly low impact on your blood sugar. They are also a good source of fiber, folate, and potassium. It wasn't until 1991 that their most remarkable property was discovered: *they have more antioxidant properties than all other common vegetables in the grocery store except for artichokes, red cabbage, kale, and bell peppers.* They have nine times more antioxidant activity than the typical tomato and fifty times more than orange carrots.

Most red-colored fruits and vegetables get their color from either anthocyanins or lycopene. Beets get their red hue from phytonutrients called betalains. Betalains are proving to be good cancer fighters. In a 2009 test-tube experiment, beet juice blocked the proliferation of human cancer cells of the pancreas, stomach, prostate, lungs, and brain by 85 to 100 percent. A dietary survey revealed that people who eat beets on a regular basis have a lower risk of cancer, cardiovascular disease, diabetes, obesity, and diseases of the digestive tract than people who don't eat beets.

Heads up, athletes: the nitrate in beets may enhance your performance in two different ways. (Although the nitrates and nitrites added to processed meats have been linked with an increased risk of cancer, sodium nitrate is a natural ingredient in leafy greens, beets, and a few other vegetables. It can have health-enhancing properties when consumed in its natural, vegetable form.) First, the nitrate can reduce your blood pressure, which increases blood flow to your muscles. Second, it reduces the amount of oxygen required by your muscles during exercise. To test the effects of beets on athletic performance, scientists at England's University of Exeter gave healthy volunteers a glass of beet juice to drink, then asked them to exercise on a treadmill to the point of exhaustion. The volunteers were able to exercise 15 percent longer than they were when given a placebo drink.

Drinking beet juice also gives a boost to sedentary people. In the same study, sedentary volunteers who consumed beet juice required 12 percent less effort to walk a given distance than when they drank a placebo juice. The investigators speculated that this was enough of a difference to improve the daily functioning of older people or people with pulmonary or cardiovascular difficulties.

A 2012 British study determined that fit men and women who had eaten a serving of whole beets daily for several days could run faster than they could when they had eaten a serving of other vegetables. The difference in speed would have been enough to shave off forty-one seconds from a five-kilometer run, which could make the difference between winning and losing. Motivated by these findings, a number of British athletes who competed in the 2012 Summer Olympics drank beet juice rather than Gatorade before their events, including Mohamed (Mo) Farah, who won the gold medal for the men's five- and ten-kilometer races. As of this writing, beets are not considered an illegal performance-enhancing drug. Juice up.

CHOOSING THE MOST NUTRITIOUS BEETS IN THE SUPERMARKET

To get the health benefits of beets, you need to choose the right varieties. Some beets have no betalain, the compound responsible for reducing the risk of cancer and cardiovascular disease. Few supermarkets list the varietal names of beets, however, so you will need to choose them based on color alone. The darkest red varieties are the ones to take home. If the names of the varieties are listed, look for Detroit Dark Red and Red Ace, two of the most popular and nutritious cultivars in the supermarket. White, golden, and the pinwheel-striped Chioggia beets are much lower in red betalains. Yellow beets are a good source of lutein, however, another beneficial phytonutrient. White beets are a mutant variety that has no lutein or betalains. Their only claim to fame is that they don't discolor other vegetables when you cook them together.

Dark red bunch beets are another good choice in the supermarket. Bunch beets are young beets that are sold with their leaves attached. Beet leaves, the only part of the plant that was consumed eons ago, are among the healthiest greens you can buy. They have seven times more antioxidants than romaine lettuce and are on a par with kale in terms of overall nutritive value. Add the greens to salads, substitute beet greens for spinach in recipes, or serve them along with the roots, as in the recipe on pages 127–28.

There's another reason to buy bunch beets—they are likely to be the freshest beets in the store. As beets age, their leaves begin to wilt and turn yellow. As a result, produce managers have to cull them from the display. Beets sold without their leaves can be on display for weeks because the roots are much slower to betray their true age. Bunch beets are a seasonal vegetable in most areas of the country, so make a point to buy them when they're available.

Beets, like corn, do not lose their nutritional value when they are canned. In fact, they become somewhat more nutritious. Canned beets are less flavorful and colorful than fresh-cooked beets, but they provide more antioxidant value.

BEYOND THE SUPERMARKET

When you shop for beets in the farmers market or choose beet seeds for your garden, refer to the list of recommended varieties on pages 133–34. Two of the varieties on the list, Ox Blood and Red Ace, are dark red and extra-nutritious. Ox Blood has been a winner in a number of taste tests because of its sweet and rich flavor. Also, look for extra-leafy varieties so you can get a generous amount of greens. Early Wonder Tall Top and Bull's Blood are good choices. The leaves of the Bull's Blood variety have a deep burgundy hue and give you added betalain. They also complement the bright green color of other salad greens.

STORING AND COOKING BEETS

If you buy bunch beets, store the greens and roots separately. Cut off the greens, rinse them, spin or towel dry, and store in a plastic bag pricked with tiny holes. They spoil rapidly, so eat them within two days. Store the beet roots unwrapped in the crisper drawer of your refrigerator and use them within a week or two.

Beets become more nutritious when you steam, microwave, or roast them. Scrub the beets well and cook them with their skins on. The skin keeps the water-soluble nutrients inside the beets. Once they're cooked, let them cool down and then slip off the skins. If you don't want purple hands, use rubber gloves. Beets stain wooden cutting boards as well.

STEAMED BEETS WITH SAUTÉED GREENS, BLUE CHEESE, AND BALSAMIC VINEGAR

PREP TIME: 10 MINUTES
COOKING TIME: 40–60 MINUTES
TOTAL TIME: 50–70 MINUTES YIELD: 4 SERVINGS

2 bunches red beets (about 8–10 medium), with their greens
2 garlic cloves
¼ cup extra virgin olive oil, preferably unfiltered
¼ cup chopped pungent red or yellow onion
½ cup dark balsamic vinegar
⅔ cup crumbled blue cheese
Grated zest of 1 lemon

Trim the beets, leaving an inch of root and stem on each beet. (This keeps more of the nutrients inside the beets as they cook.) Set the greens aside. Scrub the beets and place in a steamer basket inside a pot of simmering water. Cover and cook, using a temperature setting that produces a steady release of steam. Add more water to the pot if necessary. Steam the beets until they are tender when pierced with a fork, approximately 40–60 minutes, depending on the size of the beets. Remove the cooked beets from the steamer basket and let cool.

While the beets are cooking, press or mince the garlic and set aside. Rinse the greens thoroughly, shake off excess water, and tear the leaves off the ribs in roughly 2-inch pieces. Discard the ribs. Dry the greens between layers of paper towels or in a salad spinner, then set aside.

Combine the olive oil and chopped onions in a medium-size skillet and sauté for 3–4 minutes over medium-high heat, stirring occasionally, until softened. Add the garlic and the beet greens. Toss the greens until they are coated with oil, cover, and cook over medium-low heat until the greens are wilted but still bright green, about 5 minutes. Set aside.

Bring the balsamic vinegar to a slow boil in a small saucepan over medium heat. Continue to boil, uncovered, until the vinegar has been reduced to about ¼ cup, approximately 4–5 minutes.

Trim the roots and stems off the cooled beets, then peel them. Slice them into uniform slices about ¼–⅓ inch thick, then distribute them evenly among four salad plates. Cover the beets with the sautéed beet greens and onions and drizzle with the balsamic reduction. Top with the crumbled cheese and grated zest. Serve warm or at room temperature. You can also refrigerate and serve chilled.

WHY SOME PEOPLE DO NOT LIKE BEETS

Despite their sweet flavor and silky texture, beets are not very popular in the United States. As a nation, we eat forty times more white potatoes than beets. One reason some people don't like beets is that they contain a chemical compound called geosmin, which has an earthy odor and flavor. (*Ge* is the Greek word for "earth." Geosmin means "earth smell.") After a rain shower, the air is permeated with the odor of geosmin. We humans are extremely sensitive to the aroma of geosmin and can detect it in concentrations as low as five parts per *trillion.* People who do not like the odor will have a hard time eating beets.

Geosmin has no effect on your health, positive or negative, but if you do not like earthy flavors, choose cultivars that are low in geosmin, such as Detroit Dark Red and Crosby Green Top. (You'll find them at farmers markets and in seed catalogs.) Avoid the easily recognized Chioggia beets, because they have twice as much geosmin as Detroit Dark Reds, and, as mentioned earlier, less betalain as well.

Whichever variety you buy, you can tone down the earthiness of the beets with the right condiments. Dark balsamic vinegar has a blend of sweet and acidic flavors that masks geosmin, as do condiments with sharp flavors, such as mustard and horseradish. One of the earliest known cookbooks, *De re coquinaria* (*The Art of Cooking*), written in the first century AD, recommends that boiled beets be served with a dressing of mustard, oil, and vinegar. Our taste sensibilities have changed very little.

Beets, as you may be aware, have an unusual side effect: eating them can turn your urine and stools red, a phenomenon known as beeturia. Not to worry. This harmless condition, experienced by between 10 and 15 percent of the population, is caused by the red pigments in the beet. You will experience beeturia if you lack the specific combination of genes that produces a compound that breaks down the red pigments.

SWEET POTATOES

Our common (Irish) potatoes and sweet potatoes are not closely related. Sweet potatoes (*Ipomoea batatas* L.) belong to the morning glory family, not the potato family (*Solanum tuberosum*). Sweet potatoes originated in Central America or northern South America, whereas our common potatoes originally came from Peru. When Christopher Columbus landed in the New World, sweet potatoes were a staple food in the West Indies. Botanists believe that the tubers had been cultivated for thousands of years by that time and were among the earliest of all domesticated plants. The sweet potatoes that Columbus brought back to Spain were not very sweet, and tasted more like carrots than like our modern sweet potatoes. The tubers were warmly received nonetheless. Spanish explorers who visited the West Indies in the 1500s discovered a sweeter variety, which the native people called batatas. Batatas soon replaced the earlier varieties throughout southern Europe.

Today, millions of people in Africa, Southeast Asia, the Pacific, and the Caribbean consume large amounts of sweet potatoes. The typical US adult eats only three to four pounds a year. Candied sweet potatoes make a guest appearance on Thanksgiving and Christmas menus, and southerners still make sweet potato pie, but the vegetable plays only a minor role in our diets.

We would do well to eat more of them. Despite their name and sweet taste, sweet potatoes have a much lower glycemic index than white potatoes—45 compared with 75–100. That's an important difference. People on low-glycemic diets can eat sweet potatoes without limitation. Sweet potatoes are also richer in antioxidants than common potatoes. A baked sweet potato has almost twice the antioxidant value of a baked russet potato. Yet another advantage is that they cook in half the time.

In most supermarkets, you will find two types of sweet potatoes, one with yellow flesh and another with darker, softer flesh, marketed as a yam. Despite the name difference, these so-called yams are just another variety of sweet potato. True yams are from a different species altogether, and are rarely sold in the United States outside of ethnic markets. (To avoid confusion, I will reserve the word *yams* for these less common vegetables.)

The deeper the color of the flesh, the greater the antioxidant content of the sweet potato. Those with intense, jewel-like colors are better for you than those with yellow or pale flesh. You can't see inside the sweet potatoes at the grocery store, of course. If the produce manager doesn't know the internal color, buy the variety with the darkest skin.

When you shop for sweet potatoes at a farmers market or buy seed potatoes for your garden, you can shop by specific variety. See the list of recommended cultivars on pages 134–35. Stokes Purple is high in anthocyanins. Carolina Ruby has red-to-purplish skin with moist, very sweet, dark orange flesh and a high antioxidant content.

STORING AND COOKING SWEET POTATOES

Sweet potatoes can be stored for a week at normal room temperature. They'll last longer if you store them in an unsealed bag in a dark and cool (fifty to sixty degrees) place with good air circulation. Refrigerating raw sweet potatoes can cause the flavor to go "off." Steaming, roasting, or baking them can double their antioxidant value, but boiling reduces it. Ounce per ounce, the skin is more nutritious than the flesh, so eat the whole root.

RECOMMENDED VARIETIES OF CARROTS

IN THE SUPERMARKET	
TYPE	COMMENTS
Orange carrots	Carrots with a deep orange color have the most beta-carotene. Carrots sold with their tops are fresher than carrots that have been trimmed. Baby carrots sold in bags have had their most nutritious parts whittled away.
Blue, purple, yellow, and red carrots	Some supermarkets now carry blue, purple, yellow, and red carrots, either separately or in a bag of mixed varieties. Most of them have more antioxidants than conventional orange carrots.

FARMERS MARKETS, SPECIALTY STORES, U-PICK FARMS, AND SEED CATALOGS		
VARIETY	DESCRIPTION	INFORMATION FOR GARDENERS
Atomic Red	Tapered roots (9 inches long) are light pink when raw but turn scarlet when cooked. Cooking improves the texture and flavor. High in lycopene.	Matures in 70–80 days. Good for fall planting. Imperator type.
Bolero	Sweet and crunchy, with a 7-inch tapered root. Rich in falcarinol.	Matures in 70–80 days. Excellent yield. Holds well in the ground. Nantes type.
Carlo	Orange carrot with uniform, smooth, blunt-tipped roots. Rich in falcarinol.	Matures in 90–120 days. Cold-tolerant. Excellent yield. Seeds can be hard to find. Nantes type.
Cosmic Purple	Long roots have dark purple skin and orange interior. Spicy and sweet. Good for slicing and juicing. High in anthocyanins and beta-carotene. Introduced in 2005.	Matures in 65–75 days. Will grow all winter in climate zones that do not dip below 25 degrees in winter. Imperator type.
Deep Purple	Purple throughout, except for a small, light-colored core. Roots are 12–14 inches long and tapered. Mild flavor, good for slicing, juicing, and eating raw. Rich in anthocyanins. Ten times more antioxidants than some other varieties.	Matures in 70–80 days. Imperator type.
Nutri-Red (also called Nutri Red)	Red inside and out, with 9-inch roots. Turns deep red when cooked. Strong, not sweet, flavor. Twice as much lycopene per ounce as tomatoes.	Matures in 70–80 days. Hardy. Grows best when day temperatures are between 45 and 75 degrees. Imperator type.
Purple Haze	Purple skin and orange centers; roots are 10–12 inches long and tapered. Sweet, with a tender crunch. Color fades with long cooking. Twice the antioxidants of Cosmic Purple.	Matures in 70–80 days. Imperator type.

RECOMMENDED VARIETIES OF BEETS

IN THE SUPERMARKET	
TYPE OR VARIETY	COMMENTS
Deep red or purple	When shopping in the supermarket, choose beets with deep red or purple roots. Golden, white, and multicolored beets, such as Chioggia, are less nutritious. Beets with their tops are fresher than beets that have been trimmed, and the greens themselves are very nutritious.

FARMERS MARKETS, SPECIALTY STORES, U-PICK FARMS, AND SEED CATALOGS		
VARIETY	DESCRIPTION	INFORMATION FOR GARDENERS
Bull's Blood	Roots have red rings alternating with dark pink rings. Deep red-purple leaves are sweet and flavorful; baby leaves provide pleasing flavor and color contrast in mixed salads.	Matures in 65 days. Tasty and tender when harvested early, as baby beets. Color intensifies as beets mature.
Cylindra	Dark red cylindrical beets. Sweet with a fine grain; good for eating fresh, canning, freezing, and pickling. Easy to peel and slice. Leaves are sweeter than those of other varieties of beets.	Matures in 60 days. Plant closer together than you would other beets because they grow longer rather than wider. Keeps well in the soil. Does not become tough or fibrous.
Detroit Dark Red	One of the most common varieties. Round, about 3 inches in diameter. Sweet and smooth, with fine-grained, deep red skin and flesh. Young beet tops taste good in salads and side dishes. Low in geosmin, so they do not have an earthy taste.	Matures in 58 days. Good for small gardens because the tops are relatively small, allowing the seeds to be planted close together.

VARIETY	DESCRIPTION	INFORMATION FOR GARDENERS
Red Ace	Sweet, tender, and smooth roots have up to 50 percent more red pigment than standard beets. Bright green, glossy tops make good salads and side dishes. Roots are good for slicing, dicing, and serving whole, especially when young.	Matures in 55 days. Hybrid vigor provides good germination, fast spring growth, uniform roots, and good disease resistance.

RECOMMENDED VARIETIES OF SWEET POTATOES

IN THE SUPERMARKET	
TYPE	COMMENTS
Dark-fleshed varieties	Sweet potatoes have a lower glycemic index and are higher in antioxidant value than conventional potatoes. The most nutritious varieties have orange, deep orange, or purple flesh, and are often marketed as yams.

FARMERS MARKETS, SPECIALTY STORES, U-PICK FARMS, AND SEED CATALOGS		
VARIETY	DESCRIPTION	INFORMATION FOR GARDENERS
Beauregard	Oblong tubers with dark red-orange skin and tender, moist, sweet, bright orange flesh. High in beta-carotene. One of the most popular varieties.	Matures in 90 days — early for a sweet potato. Good for cool climates.

VARIETY	DESCRIPTION	INFORMATION FOR GARDENERS
Carolina Ruby	Ruby skin and orange flesh. Higher in antioxidants than Beauregard.	Matures in 115–125 days. Drought-tolerant. Requires lots of space. Prefers warm or hot growing conditions.
Diane (also called Red Diane)	Red-orange skin and orange flesh.	Matures in 105 days.
Hawaiian (also Okinawan)	Native to the Japanese island of Okinawa. Drab gray skins and brilliant purple flesh. More anthocyanins than blueberries. Rare. Drier in texture and lighter in color than Stokes Purple.	Matures in 100 days.
Stokes Purple	Even higher in anthocyanins than the Hawaiian sweet potato. Deep purple, almost black flesh with brown skin. Rich, winey flavor. Rare. Available in some farmers markets.	Matures in 100 days. Patented variety licensed to only a few companies located primarily in Livingston, California.

ROOT CROPS: POINTS TO REMEMBER

1. ***Get the most out of orange carrots.***
   To get the most health benefits from orange carrots, choose whole fresh carrots rather than so-called baby carrots. Carrots with their tops still attached have a fresher flavor than other carrots. Cooked carrots are more nutritious than raw carrots. Include some fat or oil with the meal. If you steam or bake them whole and cut them after they're cooked, carrots are more flavorful and nutritious.

2. ***Purple carrots and purple-and-orange carrots are more nutritious than all-orange carrots.***
   Purple, red, and yellow carrots are found in some supermarkets and farmers markets. The purple varieties are your most healthful choice because they are rich in anthocyanins. In an animal study, the anthocyanins in purple carrots reversed many of the

health problems associated with a high-fat, high-carbohydrate, and high-fructose diet.

3. ***Eat more beets and beet greens.***
   Red beets are high in betalains, bionutrients that may reduce the risk of cancer and a number of other diseases. Red beet juice reduces the effort it takes to run and walk and can lead to better athletic performance. Beet leaves are even more nutritious than the roots. When you buy bunch beets, trim the leaves from the roots and store them separately in the refrigerator—the leaves in a bag pricked with about twenty tiny holes and the roots unwrapped in the crisper drawer. Roasting, steaming, or microwaving beets increases their antioxidant properties. To disguise the geosmin or earthy flavor of beets, serve them with mustard, horseradish, or vinegar.

4. ***Sweet potatoes are better for you than common potatoes.***
   Sweet potatoes are a different species from common potatoes. They are higher in antioxidants than ordinary potatoes and have a lower glycemic index. The most nutritious varieties have red, dark orange, purple, or deep yellow flesh. The so-called "yams" sold in United States supermarkets are not true yams but a different variety of sweet potato. If you store sweet potatoes in the refrigerator, they can develop an "off" flavor. Store them in a cool, dark location instead. Eating more sweet potatoes and fewer conventional potatoes is a healthful choice.

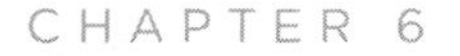

TOMATOES

BRINGING BACK THEIR FLAVOR AND NUTRIENTS

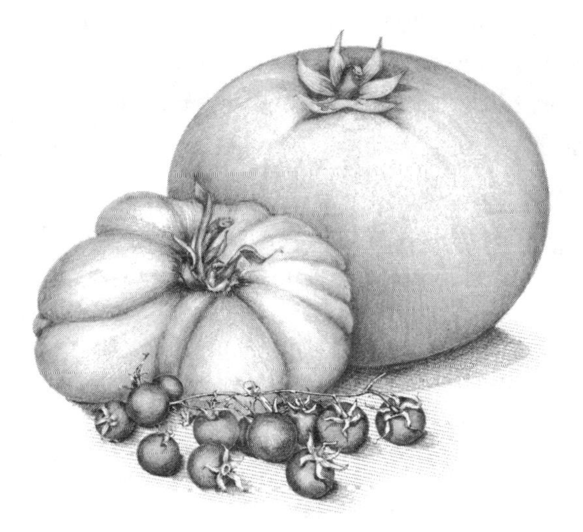

Modern, heirloom, and wild tomatoes

Tomatoes are wildly popular in this country. The typical American eats ninety-five pounds of them a year, half of this quantity in the form of ketchup, pizza sauce, pasta sauce, soup, tomato paste, and canned tomatoes. Although we eat more potatoes than tomatoes, tomatoes are dearer to our hearts. In the 1820s, an Italian painter named Michele Felice Cornè put it this way: "The potato grows in the dark with pale lank roots; it has no flavor, it lives underground. But the tomato grows in sunshine; it has a fine rosy color, an exquisite flavor; it is wholesome, and when put in the soup—you relish it."

Who today would write an ode to our supermarket tomatoes? Many of them look ripe and appealing, but they fail to satisfy. Compared with tomatoes fresh from the garden, they have little flavor or aroma. Although consumers continue to buy them, the thrill is gone. Food producers have also noted the loss of flavor. When designing a tomato-based product, they add a chemical concoction called "natural tomato flavor" to make up for what's missing. Tomato flavor is no longer *in* tomatoes; it's something we add *to* them.

While the loss of flavor is obvious, the loss of phytonutrients can be detected only by expensive, highly advanced technology. Lab tests show that most of the tomatoes in the supermarket fail to deliver the goods. Some heirloom varieties are equally low in nutrition. If you don't know which heirlooms to buy, you can end up bringing home some expensive tomatoes that give you very few health benefits. In this chapter, you will learn about modern and heirloom tomato varieties that are wildly nutritious *and* delicious. You will also discover new ways to increase their food value and flavor.

TWO THOUSAND YEARS OF REINVENTING TOMATOES

To understand what we've done to tomatoes, we need to go back to their origins. The wild ancestors of our tomatoes are native to the dry plateaus of South America that are bounded by the Pacific Ocean and the Andes mountain range. You could harvest some of these living treasures today—provided you had the time and resources. Here's what you would have to do. First, fly to Lima, Peru. When you arrive at the airport, hire a local guide who knows where to find wild tomatoes. Rent a four-wheel-drive vehicle and drive for many hours up steep, narrow, pockmarked, washed-out mountain roads that traverse five-thousand-foot passes. When you arrive at your destination, jostled and dusty, get out of the car and begin searching the rocky terrain for plants that have small, tomato-like leaves attached to long, sprawling vines.

When you spot the tomato vines, you will see at a glance that they are not the same as your backyard tomato plants. Most of our modern tomatoes are determinant, which means they grow to a certain height and then stop, a testimony to their civilized nature. Wild tomatoes are indeterminate—they keep growing all summer long and would mock your every attempt to stake them or confine them to cages. Stoop down and take a closer look at the vines and you will see sprays of tiny tomatoes. The tomatoes are so small that they look like red berries. Some of them are the size of blueberries and weigh less than half a gram. You would have to eat 450 of these bitty tomatoes to consume the equivalent of one modern beefsteak tomato.

The diminutive size of the wild tomatoes makes sense given the fact that all tomatoes are classified as a fruit, not a vegetable. (If a fruit or "vegetable" has seeds or a pit, it's a fruit.) Tomatoes are further relegated to the berry family. Those slabs of tomato that sit atop your BLT are, in reality, monstrous berries.

In recent years, several teams of researchers have made the trek to Peru to learn more about these tiny fruits. So far, they've identified eight different species. The most nutritious species is the deep red *Lycopersicon pimpinellifolium.* The nutritional differences between these wild tomatoes and our modern behemoths are stunning. Ounce for ounce, they have up to *forty times* more lycopene than the large slicing tomatoes we buy in stores. They are also miniature flavor bombs. Take a bite of one, and its delectable juice will ricochet around your mouth, giving you a refresher course in tomato flavor.

THE FIRST CULTIVATED TOMATOES

Two thousand years ago or more, South American farmers began to save the seeds of wild tomatoes and plant them in their terraced hillside gardens. Little is known about which varieties they planted, but we do have clues as to how they were eaten. The oldest existing recipe for tomatoes, blocked out in hieroglyphics, calls for tomatoes, chili peppers, and salt—the original salsa.

Over the next millennium, tomatoes spread into Central America, Mexico, and the Galápagos Islands, most likely from seeds that were transported by migrating birds, turtles, and farmers moving to new lands. Tomatoes remained confined to the New World until about five hundred years ago. Then, in 1519, Spanish conqueror Hernán Cortés sailed to the Yucatán peninsula and began warring with the Mayans. He took time out from his marauding to sample some of the local tomatoes. A Spanish priest named Bernardino de Sahagún happened to be living in the area at that time. At the request of the king of Spain, he wrote a detailed description of the "xitomatls" that were being sold in village markets. He wrote that the street merchants were offering "large tomatoes, small tomatoes, and leaf tomatoes" as well as "large serpent tomatoes" and "nipple-shaped tomatoes." He described their many nuances of color: "Quite yellow, red, very red, quite ruddy, ruddy, bright red, reddish, and rosy-dawn colored." He commented on their flavors as well. He reported that some were so bitter that "they scratch one's throat, or make one's saliva smack." Others "burned the throat." Clearly, not all the tomatoes had been made suitable for sensitive palates.

Cortés and his crew must have found a few varieties that they liked, because they brought tomato seeds back to Spain, along with their pirated treasure of emeralds and gold. The odds are that they selected seeds from the tomatoes that were the sweetest and most succulent, leaving the throat-burning and "saliva-smacking" (astringent) varieties behind. The tomatoes that would eventually spread throughout Europe would come from this select gene pool.

Just two decades after the seeds arrived in Spain, tomatoes were growing in gardens in Spain, Italy, and France. In the mid-1500s, Italian physician and naturalist Pietro Mattioli noted in his journal that his compatriots anointed tomato slices with olive oil, salt, and pepper. The first printed cookbook to mention tomatoes was published in Naples in 1692 and included a recipe for sauce alla spagnuola, or tomato sauce in the Spanish style. The French were so enamored with tomatoes that they called them pommes d'amour, or love apples.

The reception was much chillier in northern Europe. This wary population took one look at tomato plants and thought they resembled a number of toxic and potentially fatal plants from the nightshade family, including deadly nightshade (*Atropa belladonna*), mandrake (*Mandragora officinarum*), and jimsonweed (*Datura stramonium*). Tomatoes do indeed belong to this nefarious family, but they lack the toxicity of its other members. Tomatoes, though, were not given the benefit of the doubt. Many people were convinced that they were equally evil—guilt by association. It took several hundred years before tomatoes were embraced by the majority of northern Europeans.

TOMATOES ARRIVE IN THE UNITED STATES

Thomas Jefferson, a passionate foodie and gardener, was introduced to tomatoes in the 1780s while serving as the US minister to France. He loved the strange fruits and brought seeds back to plant in his extensive gardens at Monticello. According to Jefferson's gardening notes, he planted a "dwarf tomata" and a large, ribbed "Spanish tomata," which he described as "much larger than common kinds." Every year, he wrote down the date that the first tomatoes "came to table." Thanks to Jefferson and other epicurean travelers, dozens of European varieties soon arrived on our shores. Most of them, however, came from just one species—*Solanum lycopersicum*. The other seven species remained sequestered in South America, including the outrageously nutritious *Lycopersicon pimpinellifolium*.

Like the northern Europeans, many Americans were slow to

warm up to the new fruit. At first, people grew them as decorative plants, not as food. But Thomas Jefferson and others encouraged people to embrace the savory fruit, and it began to appear in more home gardens. Forty years later, however, some people still regarded tomatoes as oddities. Theodore Sedgwick Gold, secretary of the Connecticut Board of Agriculture, wrote that "we raised our first tomatoes about 1832, only as a curiosity, made no use of them though we had heard that the French actually ate them."

CREATING THE PERFECT TOMATO

Tomatoes, like most of our fruits and vegetables, were given a major makeover during the nineteenth and twentieth centuries. US tomato breeders had three main goals—making them more productive, uniform, and attractive. The fruit's appearance was given high priority. The varieties grown in our great-grandparents' day were nothing like our sleek, shiny orbs. Some had rough, sandpapery skins. Most were squat or ribbed. Some were hard-cored, some were hairy, and many had large open cavities, like a bell pepper. A few varieties were so gnarly that they were said to have "cat faces."

Alexander W. Livingston, a "seedsman" from Reynoldsburg, Ohio, took it upon himself to get rid of these flaws. His goal was to create superlative new cultivars that were flavorful but also more uniform and pleasing in appearance. He also wanted more controlled growth habits. No more sprawling vines! A perfectionist, Livingston spent two decades breeding hundreds of new varieties before he created one that met all his criteria. He named it the Paragon. Released in 1879, the Paragon was hailed as the world's first perfectly uniform and solid tomato. Livingston followed the Paragon with Acme, Royal Red, Favorite, and dozens of other cultivars.

Few of Livingston's varieties are grown today, but he and other tomato breeders set the standards for all tomatoes to come. By the early 1900s, US consumers expected store-bought tomatoes to be large, shiny, thin-skinned, juicy, solid throughout, and free of warbles and ridges. Just as important, tomatoes had to be a uniform color from top to bottom.

The nutritional consequences of creating uniformly red tomatoes were not known until a century later. The reason that the new varieties were a solid color, USDA researchers reported in the journal *Science* in 2012, is that they had a mutant gene that made them ripen uniformly. This gene had an unforeseen negative effect: it lowered the lycopene content of the tomatoes, making them less nutritious overall. Today, virtually all our modern varieties of tomatoes carry this mutant gene and are lower in lycopene as a result.

PREMATURE HARVEST—THE DEATH KNELL FOR FLAVOR

By the mid-1900s, tomato production had become highly industrialized. Most of the fruit was grown in megafarms in California and Florida or raised in hothouses in northern regions. For the first time, tomatoes were being shipped hundreds or even thousands of miles to reach their markets. Some fresh fruits and vegetables can be shipped long distances and arrive at their destinations undamaged—potatoes, onions, carrots, and iceberg lettuce among them. Fully ripened tomatoes, however, are impossible to ship. No matter how carefully one places them into a packing crate, the fruit is likely to split or become bruised during transport. Even if it arrives intact, it is likely to be overripe, festooned with fruit flies, or on the verge of rotting.

The tomato industry found a way to get around these problems: pick the fruit before its time. Through trial and error, producers discovered that if they harvested the tomatoes when the fruit showed the first hint of color—a point technically known as the breaker stage—it would turn red in about two weeks. Pick it a few days earlier, however, and it would never ripen. This left a narrow window of time in which to harvest the fruit. If all went well, the tomatoes would be firm enough to ship and would become red-ripe by the time they arrived at the stores.

Today, tomato production is a billion-dollar industry, and the ripening process has become an exact science. Tomatoes are still picked at the breaker stage, but now they are shipped to regional warehouses, where they are force-ripened with precise amounts of ethylene gas. When the warehoused tomatoes become red enough to satisfy consumers—but not fully ripe—they are distributed to nearby stores. Ideally, they will finish ripening in the stores or in the home kitchen.

Although force-ripened tomatoes can turn the requisite "tomato red," they are less sweet and more acidic than tomatoes that ripen under the sun. The aroma—an essential part of flavor—is all but gone. Even the most flavorful, garden-ripe, organic tomato will taste insipid if you eat it without inhaling.

In their search for the missing flavor, many consumers pay extra for high-priced "on-the-vine," or cluster, tomatoes. The logical assumption is that these premium tomatoes have ripened in the field. That's not the case. Cluster tomatoes are harvested only a week or two after conventional tomatoes, and they, too, finish ripening in storage. Those added days in the field do make them somewhat more flavorful. Nonetheless, they never attain the flavor or health benefits of tomatoes that are plucked at the peak of ripeness. If you buy on-the-vine tomatoes, taste them when you get home to make sure they justify the added cost. When you buy them, look for firm, dark red tomatoes on flexible, bright green vines.

TIME FOR A TWENTY-FIRST-CENTURY MAKEOVER

Clearly, it's time for another tomato makeover. This twenty-first-century revival needs to focus on flavor *and* nutrition, not just on productivity and ease of harvest and shipment. I am happy to report that this revival is already under way. A few pioneering researchers have begun using conventional breeding methods to create new varieties of tomatoes that restore much of the flavor and health benefits of the wild fruit.

Plant scientist Majid Foolad, from Pennsylvania State University, has gone one step further: he has mated modern tomatoes with wild tomatoes. When he discovered that our modern tomatoes lack the genes to produce high levels of lycopene, he went back to the source—South American wild tomatoes. He focused on the dark red *Lycopersicon pimpinellifolium*. Foolad planted and studied more than three hundred individual plants of the species. One particular plant, labeled LA722, stood out from all the others. It was very high in lycopene and resistant to several diseases. It had only two drawbacks: the vines refused to stop growing, and the fruit was the size of a marble. This wild child would have to be tamed and enlarged. Foolad spent years crossing LA722 with modern cultivars of tomatoes until he succeeded in creating a cherry variety and several larger varieties that have three times more lycopene than most supermarket tomatoes. These new cultivars will be available for home gardeners in the near future.

SHOPPING FOR TOMATOES IN THE SUPERMARKET

Fortunately, you don't have to wait for the release of new cultivars to enjoy flavorful and extra-nutritious tomatoes. If you know how to identify the most nutritious tomatoes currently in the supermarket, you can triple or quadruple your intake of lycopene the next time you shop for tomatoes. Many of these select varieties are also exquisitely flavorful. As of this writing, few supermarkets display the varietal names of their tomatoes. Instead, all the tomatoes are grouped together into four general categories: (1) large beefsteak tomatoes; (2) medium-size tomatoes, referred to as slicing, salad, or globe tomatoes; (3) Roma, or plum, tomatoes; and (4) assorted small tomatoes, including cherry, grape, and currant varieties. You can select the most nutritious in each category by following a few simple guidelines.

First, choose tomatoes by their color. In general, tomatoes with the darkest red color have the most lycopene. Look closely and you will see color differences among different varieties of tomatoes and also among individual tomatoes of the same variety. The darkest red fruits win the nutritional prize. Tomatoes that are yellow, gold, pink, green, or pale red have relatively little lycopene. Many people are especially fond of yellow cherry tomatoes because they are very sweet and low in acid. Of these, Sun Gold tomatoes are a perennial favorite. These bright gold tomatoes are a treat to eat and contrast beautifully with red tomatoes, but they have little antioxidant value. Enjoy them for their flavor and novel color.

Shopping by size is just as important as shopping by color. Small, dark red tomatoes have the most lycopene per ounce, and they are also sweeter and more flavorful. On average, beefsteak tomatoes contain between 3 and 5 percent sugar, medium-size tomatoes contain between 5 and 7 percent sugar, and cherry-size and smaller tomatoes contain between 9 and 18 percent sugar. Because tomatoes are a low-glycemic fruit, the higher amount of sugar in small tomatoes is not enough to raise your blood sugar—it just makes them more enjoyable to eat. Small tomatoes also have more vitamin C than their beefier relatives. When you downsize your tomatoes, you get more flavor *and* nutrients.

The smaller-is-better rule applies to varieties within a category as well. Some cherry tomatoes are half the size of other cherry tomatoes. As a general rule, the smallest ones are the most nutritious and flavorful. The smallest beefsteaks are also more nutritious than the largest ones, but they are still a long way from the tiny toms.

Grape tomatoes, relative newcomers to the market, are smaller than most cherry tomatoes and are more nutritious as well. They look like miniature plum tomatoes. One of their selling points is that you can pop them whole into your mouth, which makes them a natural for the hors d'oeuvre platter, salads, and after-school snacks. Typically, they are sold in plastic clamshells to keep them from drying out. (Their high ratio of skin to volume allows moisture to escape more easily.) Before you buy, examine them closely and reject tomatoes that are shriveled, dented, or have lost their gloss.

Currant tomatoes, the smallest of them all, are not just diminutive cherry tomatoes—they are a different species. In fact, they belong to the long-lost *Lycopersicon pimpinellifolium* species, the superstar of tomato nutrition. Currant tomatoes are now sold in most large supermarkets. They, too, are sold in plastic clamshells. Think of them as an oasis of wildness in our industrialized food desert. Eat these tiny fruits and enjoy their flavor, sweetness, and extra helping of lycopene.

Most people limit their consumption of cherry, grape, and currant tomatoes to salads, snacks, and hors d'oeuvres. I suggest that you invent other ways to use them. Slice or chop them and add them to sandwiches, burritos, tacos, salsas, guacamole, frittatas, omelets, and hamburgers. Cook them down and turn them into an intensely flavored, high-lycopene tomato sauce.

The following recipe for tomato salsa is easy to make, delicious, and beautiful. It has the high phytonutrient content and bright red color of tiny tomatoes plus the dark green color and nutritional benefits of scallions. Cilantro, a traditional ingredient, has more antioxidant properties than spinach or lettuce. If you don't like cilantro, substitute fresh basil. Make a double batch of this salsa and freeze half of it. If you add chopped avocados to the mixture, you will absorb more of the nutrients in the other ingredients.

TOMATO SALSA

TOTAL TIME: 15 MINUTES YIELD: 2 CUPS

1 pound cherry, grape, or currant tomatoes (about 2 cups)
½ cup chopped scallions (including white and green parts)
3 tablespoons freshly squeezed lime juice (from about 2 small limes)
½ cup finely chopped fresh cilantro leaves
1 small serrano pepper, seeded and finely diced, or ¼–½ teaspoon cayenne pepper, to taste
1 garlic clove, pushed through a garlic press
¼ teaspoon salt
⅓ cup chopped avocado (optional)

Rinse the tomatoes and remove any leaves or stems. Put them in the bowl of a food processor or blender and pulse a few times, until they reach the consistency of ¼-inch dice.

Transfer the tomatoes to a small, nonreactive bowl, add the remaining ingredients, and stir until combined. Serve at room temperature or chill and serve cold. Store in the refrigerator.

BEYOND THE SUPERMARKET

When you buy tomatoes at a farmers market, you can choose from the widest possible selection, including heirloom varieties that were bred for flavor, not for industry. All the tomatoes are grown by local farmers and picked when ripe. Buying tomatoes from local farmers is like growing your own tomatoes—without all the work.

At farmers markets, you will be able to shop by variety. Farmers know the varietal names of their produce, as do produce managers in specialty stores that sell local and heirloom tomatoes. The list of recommended varieties at the end of this chapter includes heirloom and hybrid varieties. Even though the hybrids did not grow in our grandparents' or great-grandparents' gardens, many of them taste great and are extra-nutritious. The new Juliet F1 hybrid variety, for example, is sweet and flavorful, and it has three times more lycopene than Stupice, a Czechoslovakian heirloom. My grandfather, for one, would have been eager to try Juliet.

Heirloom tomatoes vary greatly in their nutritional value. The intensely flavored Red Pear heirloom tomato has an astounding twenty-seven times more lycopene than the typical supermarket tomato. By contrast, the equally venerable Dona has fewer nutrients than most of the tomatoes sold in convenience stores. Shop with the list of varieties on pages 154–56 and you will bring home the most nutritious and delicious tomatoes.

HOMEGROWN TOMATOES

More than thirty-five million gardeners in the United States grow their own tomatoes. If you have room to grow a few plants, give it a try. Growing tomatoes has gotten much easier in recent decades. Years ago, most people had to grow tomatoes from seed. Today, you can buy tomato starts (young tomato plants, or seedlings) in nurseries, garden stores, discount stores—even supermarkets. Pick up a six-pack of tomato starts, take it home, plant the tomatoes in fertile soil in a sunny location, and water as needed. If you don't have room for a garden, plant them in large pots. From late July through September, you can be savoring your own homegrown tomatoes.

When you grow your own tomatoes, you can choose from more than one hundred varieties, both heirloom and hybrid. You'll get the most health benefits if you grow more red-colored grape, cherry, and currant tomatoes. Small tomatoes are well suited for cool climates because they ripen weeks earlier than full-size varieties; some years, they're the only ones that ripen in my Puget Sound garden. In warm climates, small tomatoes spread out the harvest. You can enjoy a rich harvest of cherry tomatoes before larger tomatoes begin to blush red.

ORGANIC TOMATOES

On nonorganic farms, tomatoes are sprayed with herbicides, insecticides, and plant growth regulators. The standard pesticides used in the industry include metam-potassium, metam-sodium, chloropicrin, 1,3-dichloropropene, chlorothalonil, and methyl bromide. All of them are classified as Bad Actors by the Pesticide Action Network (PAN). A Bad Actor, in their lexicon, is a chemical that is toxic, promotes cancer in lab tests or animal studies, interferes with reproduction, or contaminates the environment. Organic tomatoes are free of these undesirable compounds.

Does organic cultivation influence flavor and nutrition? One study determined that organic tomatoes have a more intense and balanced flavor than conventionally raised tomatoes. Some studies, but not all, show that organic tomatoes are also more nutritious. In all the research so far, however, the variety of the tomato has had far more influence on its nutritional content than the way it's been raised. The best of all worlds is to choose fully ripened, highly nutritious varieties that have been raised by organic farmers or that you have grown in your own garden.

STORING TOMATOES

Once you've brought home your excellent tomatoes from the market or harvested them from your garden, their fate is in your hands. What you do with them from that moment on can have a profound effect on their flavor and health benefits. In terms of flavor, the worst thing you can do is to store tomatoes in your refrigerator. When the internal temperature of a tomato dips below fifty degrees, it stops producing flavor and aromatic compounds. Worse, the flavor it has already acquired begins to fade. Within just two days of refrigeration, tomatoes are less sweet, more bitter, and almost devoid of aroma. The longer they are refrigerated, the greater the loss.

Eat tomatoes right away, or store them in an area of your apartment or house that is between fifty-five and seventy degrees. Remove any split or overripe fruit. Place the tomatoes stem side up to slow the softening and darkening of the fruit. (The stem end has a small depression.) Cover with cheesecloth or fruit netting to keep away fruit flies and other pests. Eat within two or three days.

If you buy semiripe tomatoes, store them in a closed paper bag (not a plastic bag) and leave them on the counter. Check them every day. The tomatoes are ready to eat when they are a deep red color but still somewhat firm.

PREPARING TOMATOES

When preparing tomatoes, think twice before removing the pulp, seeds, and juice, a procedure called for in many recipes. The juice is high in an amino acid called glutamate, which is part of the chemical flavor enhancer monosodium glutamate, or MSG. Like MSG, glutamate enhances the flavor of other foods. The skin and the seeds also provide about 50 percent of the tomato's vitamin C, lycopene, and overall antioxidant value.

Tomatoes, like a few other fruits, are better for you cooked than raw. In fact, *the longer you cook them, the more health benefits you get.* The heat increases their food value in two ways. First, it breaks down the fruit's cell walls, making their nutrients more bioavailable. Second, it twists the lycopene molecule into a new configuration that is easier to absorb. (The heat transforms a substance called trans-lycopene into cis-lycopene, which is more bioavailable.) Raw tomatoes are good for you, but cooked tomatoes are akin to medicine. Just thirty minutes of cooking can more than double their lycopene content, as shown by the graph below.

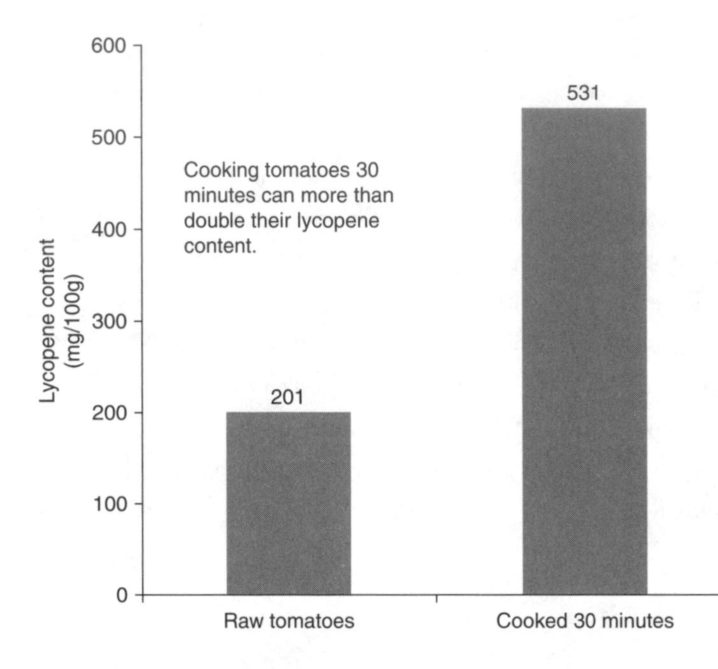

PROCESSED TOMATOES

I've saved one of the biggest surprises for last. The most nutritious tomatoes in the supermarket are not in the produce section—they're in the canned goods aisle. Processed tomatoes, whether canned or cooked into a paste or sauce, are the richest known sources of lycopene. The reason is that the heat of the canning process makes the lycopene more bioavailable. Interestingly, processed tomatoes are also more flavorful than the typical supermarket tomato. Tomatoes grown for the food industry are picked when red-ripe, and they are processed immediately, sometimes within a few hours. No flavor is lost along the way.

Tomato paste, the most concentrated form of processed tomato, has up to *ten* times more lycopene than raw tomatoes. Tomatoes produce lycopene to protect themselves from UV rays. Eating tomato paste has the same effect on us. In a German study, volunteers were divided into two groups. Half the participants made no changes in their eating habits. The other half added three tablespoons of tomato paste to their daily diets. When the volunteers were exposed to enough UV rays to produce a moderate sunburn, the people who had been consuming tomato paste were 40 percent less red overall.

Unlike most other canned tomato products, tomato paste has no added salt or sugar; it's the concentrated essence of ripe tomatoes. When you add the paste to prepared foods, such as canned soups, pasta sauces, salsas, and ketchup, the paste will add flavor, color, and nutrients and also dilute their high salt or sugar content.

Many chefs and knowledgeable cooks add small amounts of tomato paste to their non-tomato dishes as well. Tomatoes add a multidimensional flavor that enhances the taste of the other ingredients. Try adding a tablespoon or two to vegetable soups, stews, casseroles, and egg dishes. The tomato flavor will be barely detectable, but the flavor of the food will seem "rounder" and more balanced, thanks to the glutamate in the tomatoes.

Most tomatoes are packed in cans that have a plastic lining that contains a noxious chemical called BPA (bisphenol A). To lower your exposure to BPA, look for tomato products sold in glass jars or BPA-free cans. Another option is to buy them in aseptic containers—coated paper containers, such as Tetra Paks—which allow food to be stored for months without refrigeration.

RECOMMENDED TYPES AND VARIETIES OF TOMATOES

IN THE SUPERMARKET		
COLOR	TYPE	COMMENTS
Red	Cherry	Higher in lycopene than large red tomatoes. In general, the darker the color and the smaller the size, the more nutritious the tomato. Eat within a few days. Do not refrigerate.
Red	Grape or Currant	Smaller and even more nutritious than cherry tomatoes. Grape tomatoes look like miniature Roma tomatoes. Currant tomatoes are smaller and round. Both have thicker skins than cherry tomatoes, so they can be stored for a longer period of time. Typically, they are sold in plastic clamshells.

FARMERS MARKETS, SPECIALTY STORES, U-PICK FARMS, AND SEED CATALOGS			
VARIETY	TYPE	DESCRIPTION	INFORMATION FOR GARDENERS
Abraham Lincoln	Salad, or globe	Medium-size tomato that is bright red and slightly acidic. Good for juice, ketchup, and slicing. Very high in lycopene.	Matures in 80 days. Indeterminate.
Black Cherry	Cherry	Small round cherry tomato with dark purple skin and rich flavor. High in lycopene.	Matures in 65–75 days. Indeterminate.
Elfin	Grape	Tiny tomato with red fruit. Good for snacking and salads. High in carotenoids and lycopene.	Matures in 55–60 days. Determinate. Plants are only 9–18 inches tall. Can be grown in containers.

TOMATOES

VARIETY	TYPE	DESCRIPTION	INFORMATION FOR GARDENERS
Gardener's Delight (also called Sugar Lump)	Cherry	Small red tomato with strongly sweet flavor. Good for snacking and salads. Highest in lycopene of 40 varieties tested in a recent survey.	Matures in 65 days. Indeterminate. High yield.
Giant Belgium	Beefsteak	Large heirloom tomato. Higher in lycopene than most large varieties but lower in lycopene than smaller tomatoes. Dark pink meaty flesh and few seeds. Low in acid.	Matures in 85–90 days. Indeterminate.
Hawaiian Currant	Currant	Sweet; deep red color; marble-size heirloom. Very high in lycopene.	Matures in 75–85 days. Indeterminate. Vigorous, sprawling growth. Holds fruit on clusters until ripe. High yield.
Jet Star	Salad, or globe	Medium-size (6–8 ounces), globe-shaped, mild-flavored, firm, meaty fruit. Low acidity. Good for slicing and canning. High in antioxidants.	Matures in 72 days. Indeterminate. High yield.
Juliet (Also called Juliet F-1 Hybrid)	Grape	A small, deep red, shiny grape tomato with an intense, sweet flavor. Good for snacking and salads. Very high in lycopene.	Matures in 60 days. Indeterminate. Crack- and disease-resistant. Fruit holds on the vine when ripe. High yield.
Matt's Wild Cherry	Currant	Very small (1/2 inch), soft, round, deep red tomato with smooth texture and a sweet, robust flavor. Good for salsa, snacking, and salads. High in lycopene. A wild tomato discovered in Mexico in recent years.	Matures in 60–70 days. Indeterminate with a vengeance. In some climates, the vines will grow twenty feet long and keep producing tomatoes into the fall. Rare, but seeds are becoming more available.

VARIETY	TYPE	DESCRIPTION	INFORMATION FOR GARDENERS
Oxheart	Beefsteak	Large heart-shaped tomato. Meaty, solid, with a sweet flavor and few seeds. Fairly acidic. High in lycopene compared to other large varieties.	Matures in 85 days. Indeterminate. Continuously productive. Fernlike foliage. High yield.
Red Pear	Cherry	Small (up to 2 inches long), deep red, pear-shaped tomatoes. Heirloom. Sweet and juicy; good for snacking and salads. Among the highest in lycopene.	Matures in 90 days. Indeterminate. High yield.
San Marzano	Plum or Sauce	Medium-size plum tomato. Slim, red fruit with a pointy end. Heavy walls with little juice. Considered the best for sauce and paste by some chefs. High in lycopene.	Matures in 75–85 days. Crack-resistant. Compact plant size.
Sara's Galapagos	Currant	Wild variety discovered on the Galápagos Islands in the twenty-first century. Tiny (1/3 inch); red; intensely flavored; sweet. Very rare.	Matures in 75 days. Indeterminate. Keeps well on the vine.
Sun Cherry	Cherry	The red equivalent of the yellow cherry tomato, but much more nutritious because of high lycopene content.	Matures in 55–68 days. Indeterminate. Pick as soon as they ripen to avoid cracking. Grows in long clusters of 20 fruits.

TOMATOES: POINTS TO REMEMBER

1. ***Deep red tomatoes have more lycopene and overall antioxidant activity than yellow, gold, or green tomatoes.*** Choose yellow and green tomatoes for novelty, but choose red ones for their nutritional value.

2. ***As a rule, the smaller the tomato, the higher its sugar and lycopene content.***
   Red-colored cherry, grape, and currant tomatoes are the most flavorful and highest in lycopene. Use them in salsas, sauces, and soups as well as salads. Small beefsteak tomatoes are more nutritious than large beefsteaks.

3. ***On-the-vine tomatoes are not field-ripened tomatoes.***
   The so-called ripe-on-the-vine tomatoes are picked only a week or two after ordinary tomatoes. Taste to see if the increase in flavor justifies the cost.

4. ***Processed tomato products can be more flavorful and nutritious than fresh tomatoes.***
   Unlike fresh tomatoes, tomatoes grown for canning and for making tomato products ripen in the field and are processed shortly after harvest. The heat involved in canning increases the absorption of lycopene. Canned tomato paste has the highest concentration of lycopene of all the tomatoes and tomato products in the store.

5. ***Store fresh tomatoes at room temperature to preserve their flavor.***
   Chilling tomatoes below fifty degrees breaks down their flavor and aroma compounds.

6. ***Cooking tomatoes converts lycopene into a form that is easier to absorb.***
   Cooking concentrates the flavor of tomatoes and makes their nutrients more bioavailable.

7. ***Use the skin, juice, and seeds of tomatoes whenever possible.***
   The skin and seeds are the most nutritious parts of a tomato, and the juice is rich in glutamate, a part of the flavoring ingredient monosodium glutamate (MSG).

CHAPTER 7

THE INCREDIBLE CRUCIFERS

TAME THEIR BITTERNESS AND REAP THE REWARDS

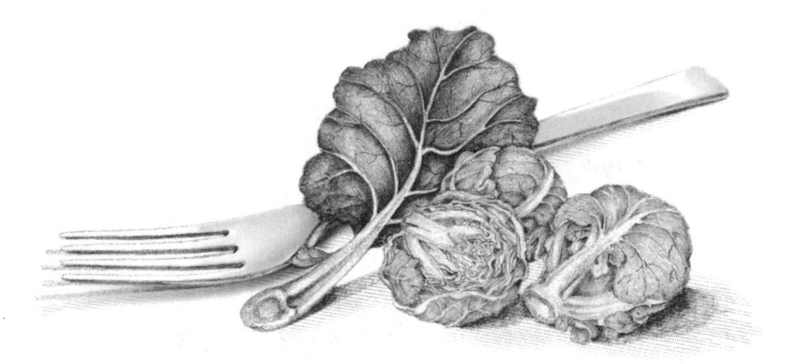

Brussels sprouts

The cabbage, cole, or cruciferous family is a big, bumptious clan of vegetables. There are more cruciferous vegetables than you might think. In a large supermarket you'll find arugula, broccoli, Brussels sprouts, cabbages, cauliflower, collard greens, kale, kohlrabi, mustard greens, radishes, and turnips.

Shop in specialty markets and you'll find rapeseed, a cool-climate crucifer, which is the source of canola oil. Mizuna is a frizzy Asian green. Wasabi, a root similar to ginger, adds green fire to sushi. Bok choy is a white-ribbed cabbage popular in the Far East that's gaining ground in the United States. What unites all these vegetables is the fact that their flowers have four petals arranged in the shape of a cross, which is why they became known as crucifers.

THE WILD ORIGIN OF CRUCIFERS

Most botanists agree that our modern crucifers developed from wild plants that grow in the eastern Mediterranean region. In nature, they are leafy greens without a crown or central head, much like our modern kale. According to Greek myth, the first crucifers sprang from beads of sweat on the brow of the god Zeus. Whether this is a positive or negative association is anyone's guess. Roman conquerors brought the vegetables to the British Isles around 500 AD. The Saxons were so taken with them that they named the second month of their calendar year Sprout Kale, in honor of the plants' annual sprouting. People living in the ancient Kingdom of Fife, a region of Scotland situated between the Firth of Tay and the Firth of Forth, were equally fond of crucifers. People in surrounding areas referred to the denizens of Fife as the "kale eaters."

Unlike most of our produce, crucifers have not been watered down or sweetened up. This is good news and bad news. The good news is that crucifers offer more health benefits than all but a few fruits and vegetables. The bad news is that many of them have a bitter or spicy taste that drives many consumers away, especially children and supertasters.

Compounds called glucosinolates are the main source of their health benefits and their off-putting flavor. The more glucosinolates in a vegetable, the better it is for you, but the more bitter it tastes. Kale and Brussels sprouts have the most glucosinolates, and they are also the least liked of all our fruits and vegetables. On average, adults in the United States manage to choke down only a half cup of Brussels sprouts per year. We eat 250 times more white potatoes.

Most crucifers are rich in antioxidants. The graph below shows the antioxidant value of some of our common fruits and vegetables relative to how much of them we eat per year. The gray bars show their antioxidant levels in terms of their ORAC value. (ORAC, which stands for oxygen radical absorbance capacity, is an effective and common way to measure the antioxidant content of food.) The black bars next to them show how much of them we consume. Study the chart and you will see that broccoli and kale are loaded with antioxidants, but we eat them in very small amounts. Iceberg lettuce, french fries, and bananas, on the left side of the graph, have the lowest antioxidant value, but we eat them in very large quantities. When the USDA says, "Eat more fruits and vegetables," most Americans are going to eat more french fries and bananas, not more broccoli and kale.

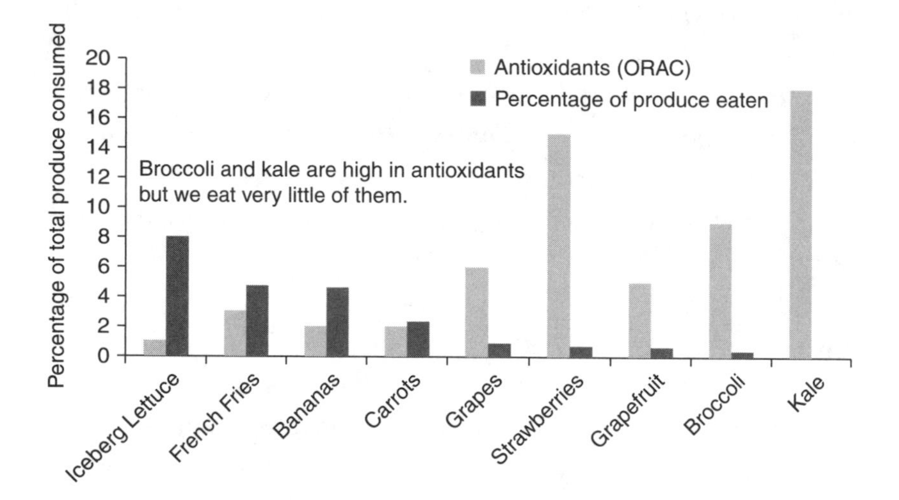

New research highlights another problem with crucifers. Even those people who crave them and eat them in large quantities may be getting only a fraction of what the vegetables have to offer. If the vegetables are freshly harvested, they are among the most healthful foods of all. But by the time they are shipped, warehoused, displayed in the supermarket, and stored in your home refrigerator, they can lose up to 80 percent of their beneficial nutrients. Their natural sweetness disappears as well, and their bitter flavors become more intense. Furthermore, if you cook the vegetables in the most common way, very few nutrients remain. In this chapter, you will learn new ways to select, store, prepare, and cook cruciferous vegetables that will give you all their health benefits, and—just as important—make them delightful to eat.

BROCCOLI

More than any other vegetable, broccoli has come to epitomize health itself. It graces the covers of health magazines, diet books, cookbooks, and health bulletins. At the moment of harvest, broccoli lives up to its reputation. It is rich in glucosinolates and antioxidants, which gives it a two-pronged attack against disease. Few people get to benefit from those nutrients, however, because these compounds are used up soon after harvest. Like other fruits and vegetables, broccoli continues to respire after it's been picked, but it does so at a very fast rate; it pants rather than breathes. Within a week's time, this heavy breathing can destroy its most beneficial nutrients.

This takes place even under ideal shipping and storage conditions, as a 2003 Spanish study revealed. Food scientists from Murcia, Spain, purchased freshly harvested broccoli and then exposed it to the same conditions that occur during normal storage and transport. For one week, the broccoli was stored in a climate-controlled warehouse that provided the ideal humidity and temperature conditions. Then, for the next three days, it was exposed to the warmer and drier conditions of a typical supermarket. At the end of those ten days, the broccoli had lost more than 80 percent of its glucosinolates, 75 percent of a class of phytonutrients called flavonoids, and 50 percent of its vitamin C. Although the broccoli still looked appetizing, it was much less nutritious than it had been when freshly harvested.

In order to preserve all the nutrients in broccoli, it must be chilled as soon as it is harvested, kept cool, and then eaten within two or three days. This is not possible given our current system of centralized production. Most of the broccoli consumed in this country is grown in California or Arizona and then shipped around the country.

It takes a week or more for it to arrive at its destination. Typically, it spends several more days on display in the supermarket. The broccoli that is imported from Mexico, which amounts to ninety million dollars' worth per year, spends yet more days in transport.

You can prevent some of the nutritional loss by choosing the freshest broccoli in the supermarket. Look for broccoli with dark green crowns and tightly closed buds. There should be no sign of yellowing. The stem should be firm and bright green. The cut end of the stem should be moist and smooth, not dry or pocked with holes. Whole heads of broccoli are more nutritious than pretrimmed florets. When broccoli is sectioned into florets, the vegetable responds to the injury by doubling its already rapid rate of respiration; it uses up so much of its sugar and antioxidants that little is left for you. When you buy a whole head of broccoli and trim it into florets before you cook it, you save money and get more health benefits in the bargain.

Once you get the broccoli home, chill it immediately and eat it that day or the next. If you're planning to keep it for more than one day, put it into a microperforated bag and store it in the crisper drawer of your refrigerator. If you follow these instructions, according to recent research, the broccoli will have *more than twice as much* antioxidant activity than if you had put it in the crisper drawer without any wrapping or if you had stored it in a tightly sealed bag. In some instances, storing vegetables in a microperforated bag can give you as many added health benefits as choosing a more nutritious variety.

BEYOND THE SUPERMARKET

Most of the broccoli sold in farmers markets is impeccably fresh and highly nutritious. There, you will also be able to shop by variety. Extra-nutritious varieties to look for include Packman, Brigadier, and Cavolo. Look for a vendor who has the broccoli on ice or in a cooler. Broccoli that has been held at warm temperatures for just one day has a 10 percent reduction in natural sugars, which makes it less enjoyable to eat. The vegetable also has fewer nutrients.

Purple Sprouting broccoli is another excellent choice. Instead of forming a head, the crucifer produces small purple florets on its side branches that can be harvested for several weeks. The purple color comes from anthocyanins. This now-rare variety was growing in Europe at least five hundred years ago and is believed to be one of the original forms of the vegetable. In fact, the word *broccoli* comes from the Latin word *brachium,* which means "arm" or "branch." Our present-day broccoli, with its large, green crown, is the result of intensive breeding efforts.

If you're a gardener, the freshest broccoli will come from your own garden. It's a good practice to plant several varieties that mature at different times so you can have a continuous supply throughout the summer and fall. Some of the hardiest varieties will last over the winter in mild climates.

Frozen broccoli is convenient, but it is less nutritious than fresh broccoli. Like all vegetables, broccoli contains natural enzymes that must be destroyed before it is frozen, or the flavor and overall quality will degrade. The standard way to deactivate the enzymes is to steam or boil the vegetable for a few minutes, a process called blanching. Recent tests have shown that blanching broccoli destroys a third of its glucosinolates before it even hits the freezer.

RAW AND COOKED BROCCOLI

Eating broccoli raw gives you up to twenty times more of a beneficial compound called sulforaphane than cooked broccoli. Sulforaphane provides much of the vegetable's anticancer properties. Eat raw broccoli as a snack, add it to salads, and feature it on the hors d'oeuvre tray along with a tasty dip.

How you cook broccoli also makes a major difference in how many benefits you get from it. If you cook broccoli in a pot of boiling water—the most common method—half the glucosinolates will leach out of the vegetable into the cooking liquid. If you deep-fry it in hot oil, you will lose even more. Cooking some vegetables in the microwave enhances their nutritional content. Nuking broccoli, however, can destroy half its nutrients in just two minutes.

One of the best ways to cook broccoli is to steam it for no more than four minutes. Steaming retains the most nutrients and also prevents the formation of unpleasant odors and flavors. To make perfect steamed broccoli, separate a head of broccoli into small florets, each about the size of an egg. Leave two-inch stems on each floret. Pour an inch of water into a saucepan and bring the water to a full boil. Meanwhile, arrange the florets in a single layer in a steamer basket, stems down. Place the basket in the saucepan and put on the lid. Reduce the heat to a temperature setting that produces a steady release of steam. Steam for four minutes. At the end of the cooking time, remove the broccoli from the steamer to keep it from overcooking. The broccoli stems will be slightly crunchy. If you cook it longer than four minutes, it will be less sweet and nutritious. Many of the best restaurants serve crisp broccoli.

Another recommended way to cook broccoli and other crucifers is to sauté them in extra virgin olive oil or a similar oil flavored with garlic. They don't lose any of their water-soluble nutrients that way, because they are in contact with oil, not water. Also, the vegetables absorb the phytonutrients in the oil and garlic, which can make them even more nutritious.

BRUSSELS SPROUTS

Brussels sprouts are a high-nutrient mutant. Researchers' best guess is that they came from a type of kale called Flanders kale, which underwent a spontaneous mutation and developed small cabbage-like structures along the stalk. Brussels sprouts were popular in England and France by the late eighteenth century. Thomas Jefferson, ever on the lookout for new adventures in food, brought the vegetable back to the United States in 1812.

If you don't like the taste of Brussels sprouts—and most people don't—you can blame it on sinigrin and progoitrin, two bitter chemicals. Brussels sprouts have more of them than any other crucifer in our supermarkets, which is why they are the least beloved. The sprouts offer so many health benefits, however, it's a good idea to eat more of them. For example, Brussels sprouts kill more human cancer cells than all other crucifers. In a 2009 test-tube study, extracts of the vegetable destroyed 100 percent of human cancer cells of the breast, pancreas, stomach, prostate, and lung.

The trick is to reduce the bitterness of the sprouts as much as possible. If you select them carefully and cook them properly, they can be surprisingly sweet, nutty, and mild-flavored. At the supermarket, look for bright green Brussels sprouts that have tightly wrapped leaves. If they look wilted, yellow, or have a strong cabbage odor, they were harvested long ago and will have used up most of their natural sugars and nutrients. Frozen Brussels sprouts are convenient and available year-round, but lab tests show they have only 20 percent of the cancer-fighting compounds of fresh sprouts.

Brussels sprouts respire rapidly, so treat them as you would broccoli. Refrigerate them as soon as you get them home and eat them that day or the next. Just before cooking, rinse and trim the stems. Cut a cross into the bottom of the larger stems so they will cook as quickly as the leaves. Steam on the stove top for six to eight minutes, depending on their size. Taste one to see if it's done. The sprouts should be tender but still lightly crunchy. If you steam them much longer than eight minutes, they will become limp, bitter, and lose their bright green color. To serve, toss with butter, olive oil, or a vinaigrette. Salt and pepper to taste. Serve with a cream sauce on special occasions—this will also make them palatable to people who don't like bitter flavors. In addition, you can roast Brussels sprouts in the oven or sauté them in olive oil and garlic. A chef I know recommends sautéing the vegetable in duck fat.

CABBAGE

Cabbage is the world's most popular vegetable. In the United States, however, it ranks after potatoes, tomatoes, iceberg lettuce, corn, peas, and green beans on the popularity scale. On average, we eat about eight and a half pounds of cabbage a year, one-fifth as much as people in eastern Europe and half as much as people in western Europe.

Most Americans prefer green cabbage, which is also called white cabbage because its inner leaves are so pale. Green cabbage has fewer antioxidants than all other types, but nonetheless it is one of our most nutritious vegetables. When you shop for cabbage, look for compact heads that are firm and heavy for their size. Rub two heads of cabbage together. If you hear a squeak, they are reasonably fresh.

Unlike broccoli and Brussels sprouts, cabbage does not respire very rapidly, so it can be stored in the crisper drawer of the refrigerator for weeks without losing many of its nutrients. (Also, you don't have to store it in a perforated bag.) Long storage does compromise its sweetness, however. In fact, in just a few days of refrigeration, *30 percent* of its sugar will be gone. If you eat cabbage soon after you buy it, it will be the most flavorful.

SWEETER, MORE NUTRITIOUS, AND LESS ODORIFEROUS CABBAGE

Onions become sweeter as they cook, but cabbage becomes more bitter. It also begins to produce hydrogen sulfide, a foul-smelling gas reminiscent of rotten eggs. There are dozens of folk methods for deodorizing cooked cabbage, most of which involve adding ingredients to the cooking water, such as unshelled walnuts, a rib of celery, slices of lemon, fresh strawberries, or vinegar. Some cooks just throw up their hands and get out the air freshener.

There's a better way. If you steam cabbage for five minutes or less, it produces only a small amount of hydrogen sulfide. Surprisingly, cooking cabbage just two minutes longer doubles the gas production. In order for cabbage to be done in five minutes, though, you need to cut it into half-inch slices or chop it roughly. As with all other vegetables, bring the water in the pot to a rapid boil before adding the vegetable-filled steamer basket. Remove the cooked vegetables from the heat as soon as they're finished cooking. For a memorable but easy side dish, toss steamed cabbage with a tablespoon of olive oil or butter and sprinkle with a tablespoon of lightly roasted cumin seeds. Salt and pepper to taste.

Red cabbage is the antioxidant king. It has six times more antioxidant activity than green cabbage and three times more than savoy cabbage. Most people use it as a decorative garnish in their green salads, but it deserves to play a starring role. Make borscht from red cabbage and red onions instead of green cabbage and white onions. Chop the cabbage and sauté it in olive oil flavored with garlic. Add it to stir-frys. Sauté red cabbage with red, orange, or purple carrots for a dazzling display of color. Make a red cabbage coleslaw.

CAULIFLOWER

Mark Twain once quipped: "Cauliflower is nothing but cabbage with a college education." In reality, cauliflower (*Brassica oleracea* var. *botrytis*) is cabbage with more antioxidants and greater cancer-fighting ability. White cauliflower is the most common variety. In fact, many Americans think it's the only color that exists. Although pale in color, it is rich in glucosinolates. Cauliflower is a good reminder that some wan-colored fruits and vegetables can be extraordinarily good for you. If you were to shop solely by color, you would leave cauliflower behind in the store.

The colorful varieties of cauliflower, however, are even higher in antioxidants. In some large supermarkets and produce stores you can find neon-green, orange, and purple cauliflower. Although new to us, these flashier varieties predate white cauliflower. In fact, botanists believe that white cauliflower is an albino mutant of these earlier forms. The intensely purple Graffiti cauliflower has two and a half times more antioxidants than the standard white variety. Keep your eyes open for the bright green Romanesca cauliflower, which some people refer to incorrectly as broccoli. It's a preposterous-looking vegetable made up of fractals that bring to mind the skyline of the Emerald City of Oz. Children will be awestruck. Romanesca cauliflower and other green cauliflowers have about four times more glucosinolates than white cauliflower.

When you're shopping for cauliflower, choose the freshest head you can find. It should have no spots, speckles, bruises, or traces of gray mold. The leaves should be bright green. Do not buy cauliflower that looks "shaved"—most likely it was scraped to remove mold. Cauliflower has a lower respiration rate than broccoli and can be stored for a week in the crisper drawer of your refrigerator without compromising its flavor or nutritional value.

Frozen cauliflower, like most frozen vegetables, has fewer nutrients than fresh cauliflower. The blanching process alone can destroy up to 40 percent of its cancer-fighting compounds. Steam or sauté cauliflower, don't boil it. Boiling, the most common cooking method, reduces its antioxidant value and its ability to fight cancer. To steam the vegetable, break the head into egg-size pieces and place them stem side down in a steamer basket. Bring a pot of water to a rapid boil, then place the basket with the cauliflower inside the pot. Cover and steam until the cauliflower is barely tender, no more than ten minutes.

KALE

Kale, the king of the crucifers, reigns over most other kinds of vegetables as well. Kale was first cultivated around 2000 BC and was grown extensively in ancient Greece and Italy. It has changed very little since that time, although we now have fewer varieties than we did just one hundred years ago. In 1895, researchers at Michigan

State University were growing nineteen cultivars of kale in their experimental gardens, including Red Flanders kale, Thousand-Headed kale, the white-ribbed Angers kale, and Red Jersey Cavalier kale, a variety that grew so tall it was as high as a man on horseback, thus the word *cavalier*.

Kale is one of the few vegetables that meets or exceeds the nutritional value of some wild greens. All varieties of kale grown today are good sources of cancer-fighting, heart-protective glucosinolates. In test-tube studies, extracts of kale have blocked the proliferation of six different kinds of human cancer cells. Kale is also high in antioxidant value, with red-leaved varieties being higher than green-leaved varieties. One serving of kale has more calcium than six ounces of milk and more fiber than three slices of whole-wheat bread.

These attributes have not made kale a popular vegetable, unfortunately. On average, each US adult eats six ounces of kale a year. Whether people like or dislike it is highly influenced by their sensitivity to bitter flavors. Supertasters rank kale as being four times more bitter than do people with a low sensitivity to bitterness. If you love kale, chances are you have a high tolerance for bitterness. Count your blessings.

Store kale in the crisper drawer of the refrigerator and use it within a few days. Raw kale is higher in vitamin C, antioxidants, and phytonutrients than cooked kale. Chop it and add it to salads. Steaming kale or sautéing it in olive oil just long enough to wilt the greens is the best way to cook it. Briefly cooked kale has a mild flavor and no sulfurous odor.

Making roasted kale chips is a growing trend among health-conscious consumers. The directions are simple. Children might want to help out. Make a large bowlful, because they go fast. Some recipes recommend a low oven temperature, but the longer it takes to bake the kale, the more nutrients are lost. A setting of 350 degrees results in more nutritious chips. If you use the convection bake setting, lower the temperature to 325.

BAKED KALE CHIPS

PREP TIME: 15 MINUTES
COOKING TIME: 8–10 MINUTES
TOTAL TIME: 23–25 MINUTES YIELD: 4 CUPS

8 ounces kale
2 tablespoons extra virgin olive oil, preferably unfiltered
Salt to taste

Preheat the oven to 350°F. Rinse the kale leaves thoroughly, shake off excess water, and tear the leaves off the ribs in roughly 2-inch pieces. Discard the ribs. Dry the leaves between layers of paper towels or in a salad spinner.

Transfer the leaves to a large mixing bowl and toss with the olive oil and salt, coating both sides. Place a single layer of leaves on one or more baking sheets and bake for 8–10 minutes, or until crisp but not too dry. Turn once. Cool and serve.

VARIATIONS: Use sesame oil instead of olive oil and sprinkle the kale with 2 tablespoons sesame seeds before baking. Or press 1 clove of garlic into the olive oil and let rest for ten minutes before mixing with the raw kale.

RECOMMENDED VARIETIES OF BROCCOLI

IN THE SUPERMARKET	
TYPE	COMMENTS
Green	All varieties of green broccoli in the supermarket are nutritious. For maximum nutrition, look for the freshest broccoli you can find. Intact heads of broccoli are fresher than pretrimmed florets.
Purple	Purple broccoli, which is available in some supermarkets, is higher in antioxidants than the more traditional green broccoli.

FARMERS MARKETS, SPECIALTY STORES, U-PICK FARMS, AND SEED CATALOGS		
VARIETY	DESCRIPTION	INFORMATION FOR GARDENERS
Atlantic	Well-rounded with solid, bluish heads. Flavorful. Introduced in 1960.	Matures 70 days after setting out transplants. Likes cool weather. Good for spring, midseason, or fall planting. Has abundant side shoots.
Brigadier	Medium-size broccoli. High in antioxidant value and in the cancer-fighting compound glucosinolate.	Matures in 70 days after setting out transplants. Midseason broccoli.
Cavolo (also called Cavolo Broccolo)	Medium-size yellow-green head. Tender, with abundant side shoots. Compact.	Matures 60–80 days after setting out transplants. Medium to late variety.
Majestic Crown	Large, firm head.	Matures 55–70 days after setting out transplants. Wait until after last frost to plant.

VARIETY	DESCRIPTION	INFORMATION FOR GARDENERS
Marathon	Large blue-green heads with a high, smooth dome.	Matures 75 days after setting out transplants. Needs lots of space. Highly tolerant to cold.
Packman	Dark green, tight buds with uniform heads up to 9 inches wide. Very common. Among the highest in antioxidant value.	An early maturing variety that is ready 55 days after setting out transplants. Ideal for spring planting. Heat-tolerant. Has abundant side shoots.
Purple Sprouting	Rich in anthocyanins. Believed to be the original form of broccoli. Very sweet purple side shoots that turn green when cooked.	Plant seeds in the fall and you can begin to harvest side shoots in March or April and for several months thereafter. Grows to 24–36 inches tall. Hardy to below 10 degrees.

RECOMMENDED VARIETIES OF CABBAGE

IN THE SUPERMARKET	
TYPE OR VARIETY	COMMENTS
Red cabbage, any variety	Red cabbage is rich in anthocyanins and antioxidants and is one of the most nutritious vegetables in the entire store. It has six times more antioxidants than green cabbage.
Savoy cabbage, any variety	Savoy cabbage has deeply netted, flexible leaves. It has three times more antioxidant value than standard green cabbage and makes a great sandwich wrap. Savoy cabbage is available in most large supermarkets.

FARMERS MARKETS, SPECIALTY STORES, U-PICK FARMS, AND SEED CATALOGS		
VARIETY	DESCRIPTION	INFORMATION FOR GARDENERS
Deadon	Red savoy cabbage with light green interior leaves. Delicious, sweet flavor.	Matures 105 days after setting out transplants.
Mammoth Red Rock	Uniform, red, round heads about 8 inches in diameter. Excellent for cooking, salads, and pickling. Heirloom introduced in 1889.	Matures 98 days after setting out transplants.
Red Express	Extra-early red cabbage. Good flavor.	Matures 65 days after setting out transplants. Compact plants. Recommended for northern areas.
Ruby Perfection	Bright magenta leaves. Medium-size heads.	Matures 85 days after setting out transplants. Mid- to late-season variety.

RECOMMENDED VARIETIES OF CAULIFLOWER

IN THE SUPERMARKET	
TYPE OR VARIETY	COMMENTS
White cauliflower, any variety	Traditional white cauliflower is a good source of cancer-fighting compounds.
Colorful varieties	Some large supermarkets carry orange, green, and purple cauliflower. All of them are higher in antioxidant value than white cauliflower.

FARMERS MARKETS, SPECIALTY STORES, U-PICK FARMS, AND SEED CATALOGS		
VARIETY	DESCRIPTION	INFORMATION FOR GARDENERS
Celio	Light green, pyramidal cauliflower highly recommended for taste and presentation.	Sow in April for a September or October harvest.
Emeraude	Bright green heads. High in antioxidants and glucosinolates.	Late-summer crop. F1 hybrid.
Graffiti	Bright purple heads. Very high in anthocyanins. Twice as many antioxidants as most other varieties. Retains color when cooked. Tender texture and mild flavor.	Matures 80–90 days after setting out transplants. F1 hybrid.

RECOMMENDED VARIETIES OF KALE

IN THE SUPERMARKET	
VARIETY	COMMENTS
All varieties	All varieties of kale in the supermarket are high in cancer-fighting compounds and antioxidants, providing extraordinary nutrition. Red-leaved varieties are especially high in antioxidant value.

FARMERS MARKETS, SPECIALTY STORES, U-PICK FARMS, AND SEED CATALOGS		
VARIETY	DESCRIPTION	INFORMATION FOR GARDENERS
Tuscan (also called Cavolo Nero, or Lacinato)	Long, narrow, deeply embossed, straplike leaves that are dark blue-green. Excellent source of sulforaphanes, the main anticancer ingredient in crucifers. Sweeter and milder than many other varieties. Excellent for making kale chips.	Matures in 60–80 days. Cold-tolerant. Can reach 3 feet tall, but is not as bushy as other varieties. Italian heirloom.

VARIETY	DESCRIPTION	INFORMATION FOR GARDENERS
Red Russian	Curly deep purple leaves with mauve-colored veins on large, upright plants with thick stems. Slightly more pungent and bitter than other kales.	Matures 50 days after setting out transplants (25 days if you want to harvest them as baby greens). Flavor sweetens after fall frosts. Very hardy. Consistently high yield.
Redbor	Rich, purple-red color. Finely curled. Twice the antioxidant value of Red Russian kale.	Matures 65 days after setting out transplants. Good for spring and fall crop.

CRUCIFERS: POINTS TO REMEMBER

1. ***Once harvested, broccoli loses its sugar and nutrients very rapidly.***
   Choose the freshest broccoli in the supermarket. Whole heads of broccoli have more nutrients than precut florets. Chill the vegetable as soon as you bring it home and eat it raw or cook it as soon as possible. If you keep the broccoli for more than a day, place it in a sealable plastic bag that you have pricked with about twenty tiny holes, then place it in the crisper drawer of the refrigerator. For even fresher broccoli, shop at a farmers market or grow your own. Steaming broccoli for less than five minutes preserves the most nutrients. Boiling it or cooking it in a microwave destroys a high percentage of its potential health benefits. Raw broccoli gives you the most sulforaphane, a potent cancer-fighting nutrient.

2. ***Shop for fresh Brussels sprouts in season.***
   Look for bright green, tight heads. Chill them immediately and eat them as soon as possible. Store in a microperforated bag if you plan to keep them for more than a day. To preserve the most nutrients, steam them for six to eight minutes. Brussels sprouts

become less sweet and more bitter the longer they cook. Serve in a cream sauce for special occasions.

3. ***Cut cabbage and steam it briefly to reduce odor and increase nutritional value.***
   Cabbages are the most popular members of the cruciferous family. Although they are lower in antioxidants than other crucifers, they are nutritious vegetables nonetheless. Cabbage can be stored weeks longer than broccoli or Brussels sprouts without losing its nutrients, although it is sweetest when eaten within a few days of purchase. Red cabbage is especially high in antioxidants.

4. ***White cauliflower has more cancer-fighting compounds than green and purple cauliflower, but the colorful varieties are higher in antioxidants.***
   In the supermarket, look for white cauliflower that has no spots or traces of mold. Cauliflower can be stored for up to a week in your refrigerator. Steam cauliflower rather than boil it to preserve the most nutrients. Sautéing cauliflower in extra virgin olive oil adds to its nutritive value. Fresh cauliflower is more nutritious than frozen cauliflower.

5. ***Kale is the most bitter and beneficial of all the crucifers.***
   Lab tests and animal studies show that kale is very effective not only for preventing cancer but also for slowing its growth. Store it in the crisper drawer of your refrigerator and use within a few days. It is most nutritious when eaten raw. Alternatively, steam kale briefly, sauté it in extra virgin olive oil until wilted, or make roasted kale chips.

CHAPTER 8

LEGUMES

BEANS, PEAS, AND LENTILS

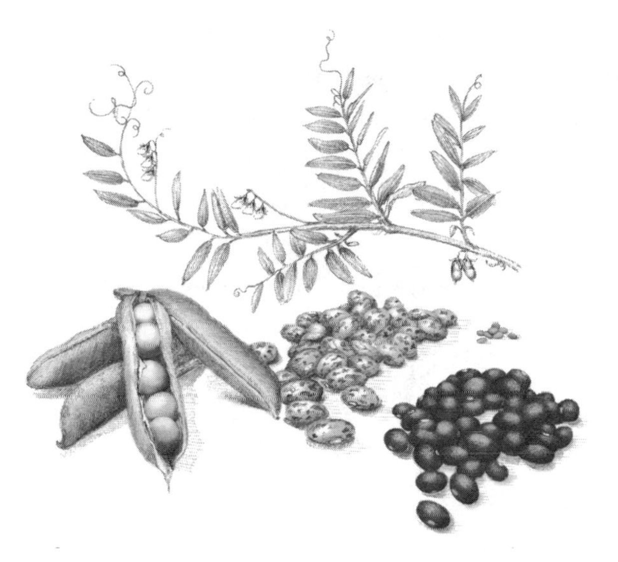

Peas, wild lentils, and beans

Hunter-gatherers were not wild about peas, beans, or lentils. If you tried to harvest them, you'd understand why. Wild lentils are a case in point. Domesticated lentils are the smallest legumes in the modern supermarket, but their wild ancestors were extremely small, each one weighing just a hundredth of a gram. It would take three hundred wild lentils to fill a soup spoon. To complicate matters, the seeds are ejected from their pods as soon as they are ripe. This is a great way for the plant to spread its seeds, but it's a bother for people trying to pick them up. The time it takes to harvest most other crops is measured in tons, bales, or bushels per hour. The wild lentil harvest is measured in *ounces* per hour. In 2008, a dedicated team of Israeli anthropologists challenged one another to see who could gather the most wild legumes in one hour. The winner harvested a mere four tablespoons. The job of gathering the beans burns up as many calories as can be gained by eating them. Want to lose weight? Try the "wild lentil diet."

Despite all the effort it took to harvest and prepare wild legumes, hunter-gatherers did consume them, albeit in small amounts. Remnants of wild legumes have been found in hunter-gatherer sites that were last inhabited twenty thousand years ago. The likely reason that our distant ancestors bothered to gather them is that they loved their flavor. Legumes have high amounts of an amino acid called glutamate, which, like sugar, triggers the "umami response," a flavor sensation that jangles the pleasure centers of our brains (see page 181). We humans are willing to work very hard if our bodies reward us with enough feel-good chemicals.

THE DOMESTICATION OF LEGUMES

Before lentils and other legumes could become staple crops, they had to undergo two major changes. First, the ripe seeds had to stay on the plants long enough for people to beat them into baskets or cut the plants down with sickles, which would make harvesting them much more efficient than picking the seeds up off the ground. Second, the seeds had to lose their dormancy. In nature, the seeds of a given species do not sprout at the same time. Some sprout early in the season, some late in the season, and some can remain dormant for years. This staggered germination insures that all the seedlings won't be destroyed by a single event, such as an early frost, a drought, or a plague of insects.

The plants' survival strategy was a problem for farmers, however. If they planted five hundred bean seeds in the spring and only one hundred of them germinated, they would have a meager harvest. To ensure a good yield, they would have to plant more seeds.

But it's hard to get ahead if you have to plant a high percentage of this year's harvest to ensure a reasonable crop next year. These two changes—the seeds clinging to the plants long enough to be harvested and the seeds germinating within a narrow window of time—came about as a result of spontaneous mutation and human selection.

Even when peas and beans became more productive and easier to harvest, there was still one problem to resolve. Many legumes contain a number of potentially toxic compounds, or antinutrients, such as trypsin inhibitors, phytic acid, tannins, and oligosaccharides. Early farmers learned by trial and error which varieties had the smallest amounts of these compounds. They also found ways to make legumes safer to eat. A common technique was to soak them in several changes of water and then cook them thoroughly before eating them.

BEANS, GRAIN, AND SQUASH IN TRADITIONAL FARMING COMMUNITIES

Legumes are very high in protein, but they are low in the amino acid methionine, which is necessary to form a high-quality protein. As luck would have it, most grains are rich in methionine but lack other essential amino acids that legumes have in spades. When grains and legumes are eaten in the same meal, a complete protein is formed that has the same high quality as the proteins in meat, eggs, and dairy products.

Early farmers were not aware of this chemistry, of course, but people in many traditional cultures grew both kinds of crops. The first farmers in the Middle East grew wheat and barley, which complemented their peas and beans. East Asian farmers combined rice with lentils, peas, beans, and chickpeas. African farmers consumed millet along with peanuts and cowpeas. In the New World, Native American farmers grew corn, squash, and colorful beans. In 1884, according to ethnologist and missionary Reverend James Owen Dorsey, the Omaha tribe was growing fifteen varieties of beans, including dark red, black, dark blue, white, and a mixture of these colors. The highly pigmented beans would have been a good source of phytonutrients.

A number of North American tribes planted corn, beans, and squash in a single mound, a technique we now refer to as companion planting. The Wyandot people, renamed Hurons by the French, were masters of this art. Each spring, the Wyandot women would walk to a cleared field and spread a mound of fish waste every three or four feet. They covered the fish with dirt and then planted a few corn seeds in the center of each mound. When the corn leaves reached hand height, they planted beans next to the corn, then sprinkled pumpkin seeds between the mounds. Thus they had planted the Three Sisters of Native American agriculture—corn, beans, and squash.

Throughout the summer, the three vegetables grew in sisterly symbiosis. The corn stalks grew tall and sturdy, providing support for the limply twining beans. The beans made their contribution by drawing nitrogen dioxide out of the air and converting it to a stable form of nitrogen that could be used by all three plants, but especially by the nitrogen-hungry corn. (The ability to perform this chemical feat, known as nitrogen fixation, is shared by all legumes.) The broad squash leaves fanned out beneath the corn and beans, preventing weeds from growing, cooling the soil, and slowing the evaporation of water. When the corn ripened enough to tempt the crows, young and old tribal members kept watch on platforms and scared them away. In some tribes, trained hawks aided the effort. Watering, staking, weeding, feeding, and pest control took minimal effort.

The nutritional benefits of the Three Sisters tradition went beyond creating a high-quality protein. The corn that the Wyandot planted was richly colored and high in antioxidants. The pumpkins provided carbohydrates, manganese, vitamin C, fiber, and a goodly amount of beta-carotene. The beans came in multiple colors, supplying yet more phytonutrients. The Three Sisters were a meal in a mound.

We All Love Umami

Eating an adequate amount of protein is essential for human health. For this reason, our tongues have sensors that detect an essential component of protein, an amino acid called L-glutamate, or glutamic acid. These sensors, like our sugar receptors, are hardwired to the pleasure centers of the brain. The flavor sensation that accompanies eating food rich in glutamate is called umami (pronounced *ooh-MAH-mee*). In 1985, umami was added to the list of four main taste sensations—sweet, sour, bitter, and salty. Some people refer to umami as the fifth taste.

Foods that trigger the umami response include legumes, red meat, chicken, seafood (especially crab), beans, tomatoes, mushrooms, and cheese (especially Parmesan cheese). A cheese and mushroom pizza with tomato sauce is a trifecta. Whenever we eat food that is naturally rich in umami, we want to eat more of it. People describe the flavor sensation as "brothlike," "meaty," "savory," and just plain delicious.

The chemical monosodium glutamate, or MSG, contains glutamate and is a potent trigger of the umami response. When food manufacturers and restaurants add MSG to their products, people eat more of them and are more likely to buy them again. Interestingly, one study shows that people consume MSG-seasoned food more quickly than the same food without MSG, even when the concentration of the chemical is below the limit of conscious detection.

Human breast milk is rich in umami. This is one of the reasons that infants are so highly motivated to suckle. The milk also contains fat and sugar, two other foods that trigger the release of feel-good brain chemicals. The look of bliss that you see on the face of nursing infants is, in part, a response to the chemical rewards they get from consuming these enticing flavors.

FRESH PEAS AND BEANS

While Native Americans were following their Three Sisters tradition, Europeans were enjoying their peas and beans. Fresh peas were rare in English gardens, however, until the late 1600s. Prior to that time, peas had been imported from Holland. According to an early edition of the *Journal of the Royal Horticultural Society,* peas were "dainties for ladies—they came so far and cost so dear." When peas began to be grown in England, they caused a mild sensation. King Louis XIV, for one, was passionate about the new peas, and his ardor swept through the French court. Madame de Maintenon, his mistress of eleven years and then, later, his wife, described the courtly obsession in a letter dated May 10, 1696: "The subject of Peas continues to absorb all others—the intense desire to eat peas, the pleasure of having eaten them, and the joyful expectation of eating yet more peas—these have been the three points of discussion for the last four days. . . . It is both a fashion and a madness."

By the eighteenth century, the French were savoring their haricots vert, white-bean cassoulets, and Sauce à la purée de lentilles à la reine—a red lentil puree fit for a queen. Germans were stolidly eating dried beans cooked with chunks of cured or smoked pork. The English were serving up pease porridge, some of which was—as the nursery rhyme says—more than nine days old. Traditionally, the soup was cooked in an iron kettle that hung close to the kitchen fire. When soup was ladled out of the kettle, dried peas and kitchen scraps were added to the kettle to top it off, creating an ageless, ever-changing soup.

All these food traditions and more were transported to the New World by the first European immigrants. Over time, they mingled with Native American traditions. During the eighteenth century, Americans were consuming a wide variety of fresh beans and peas. Thomas Jefferson grew nineteen cultivars at Monticello, including fava beans, a blue-hued pea called Blue Prussian, scarlet and crimson runner beans, and crowder peas—peas that are crowded so tightly together in their pods that their ends are squared off.

Today, two hundred years later, there are only a few varieties of fresh peas and beans in our supermarkets, and all of them are green. Indeed, their generic names are green peas and green beans. Eliminating the other colorful varieties has removed yet more nutrients from our diet. Green peas and beans are among the least nutritious of our common fruits and vegetables.

CHOOSING THE MOST NUTRITIOUS PEAS AND BEANS

One way to get more food value from green peas is to buy edible pod peas, also known as sugar snap peas and snow peas. The pods have more fiber and antioxidants than the peas themselves. Today, it is easier to find edible pod peas in the supermarket than it is to find the old-fashioned peas in a pod, because most people don't want to be bothered with the work of shelling them.

You will find more colorful and nutritious varieties when you shop in farmers markets or search the seed catalogs. Fresh black-eyed peas, for example, have almost five times more antioxidant activity than common green peas. The rare varieties of fresh beans that are purple, red, or blue in color are high in anthocyanins. Look for Royal Burgundy, Royalty Purple, and Black-Seeded Kentucky Wonder beans.

Many of the fresh, or snap, beans on the market today are more fibrous than beans were just a few decades ago. These tougher varieties are favored by producers because they are less likely to break during mechanical harvesting, packing, and shipping. When fresh peas and beans are canned, they lose much of their flavor and also become less nutritious. Freezing green beans and peas destroys about 25 percent of their antioxidants. Canning some vegetables maintains or enhances their antioxidant activity, but studies show that canning peas destroys 50 percent of it.

DRIED PEAS AND BEANS

The varieties of peas and beans that are raised for drying have far more phytonutrients than the ones sold fresh in the produce department. The extent of the difference was not known until 2004, when a USDA team surveyed the phytonutrient content of one hundred of our most common fruits and vegetables. To many people's surprise, three of the four top-ranked foods were dried legumes. The fourth was wild blueberries. The study determined that one serving of cooked pinto beans has more antioxidant activity than six cups of cooked cauliflower or twelve cups of cooked carrots. Dark red kidney beans, our most popular variety, have even more. Black beans, a staple in Hispanic, Asian, and African cuisines, have more antioxidants still. But nothing beats a bowl of lentil soup, as you can see by the following graph. Now that this information is beginning to percolate throughout the population, the plebian bean is gaining superstar status.

There is also a wide range of antioxidant value among dried peas. Make your pea soup from dried yellow peas instead of green peas, for example, and you will get six times more antioxidant protection. Chickpeas, also known as garbanzo beans, are relatively low in antioxidant activity.

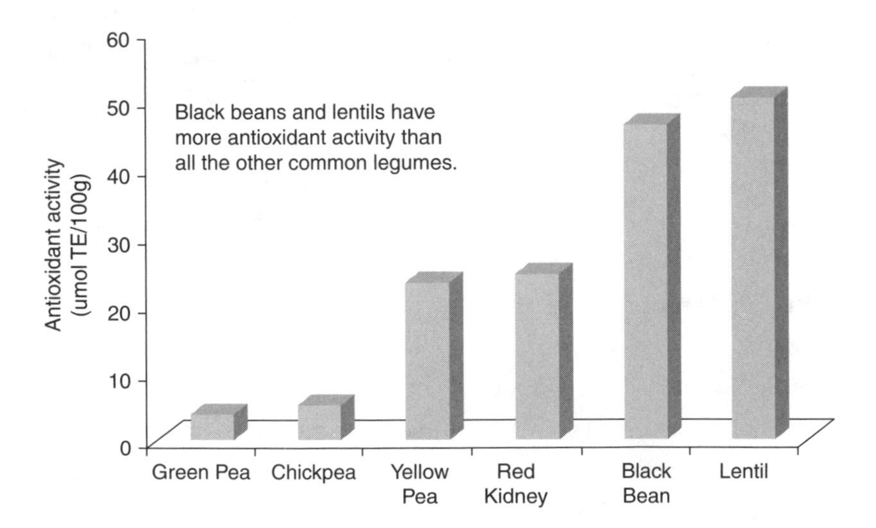

All dried peas and beans are high in soluble fiber. One cup of cooked navy beans has nineteen grams of fiber, making the beans the third best source of fiber listed in the USDA National Nutrient Database. Soluble fiber slows the emptying of your stomach and helps keep you feeling satisfied between meals. A big bowl of bean chili for lunch can keep the munchies away until dinner.

New research shows that legumes have the potential to lower your risk of several deadly diseases as well. Eat four or more servings of legumes a week and you could reduce your risk of heart disease by 22 percent, according to a 2006 European study. Legumes also have the potential to battle high blood pressure, cardiovascular disease, diabetes, obesity, cancer, and diseases of the digestive tract. In the Nurses' Health Study II, a 1989 survey of the health and eating habits of more than ninety thousand female nurses, those who consumed beans or lentils two or more times a week had a 24 percent lower risk of breast cancer.

A NEGATIVE SIDE EFFECT

Dried peas and beans are notorious for their malodorous byproducts—flatulence. The degree to which you are troubled by this socially awkward side effect depends on your genes and the kinds of beans you eat. Carbohydrates called oligosaccharides are the source of the problem. If you have inherited a deficiency in the enzymes that break them down, you will have difficulty digesting them. The carbohydrates will enter your lower intestines intact, where they will be digested by gas-producing bacteria. Unfortunately, the bacteria don't take the blame for the flatulence—you do.

Some beans are more likely to cause flatulence than others. Thanks to the rigors of twenty-first-century science, it is now possible to list them in "order of odor." Lentils produce relatively little gas, which makes them an even more desirable choice. In the following list, the worst offenders are at the top of the list.

1. Lima beans
2. Pigeon peas
3. Kidney beans
4. Green split peas
5. Black beans
6. Black-eyed peas
7. Pinto beans
8. Navy beans
9. Lentils
10. Great Northern beans

You can reduce gaseous emissions by discarding the soaking liquid before you cook dried peas or beans. You can also take over-the-counter remedies that contain the enzyme alpha-galactosidase, which breaks down the oligosaccharides and makes them more digestible. A clinical trial determined that the enzyme preparations are effective when taken as directed.

GETTING THE MOST FROM DRIED LEGUMES

How you cook dried beans has a major effect on how many health benefits you get from them. If you simmer them in water, the most common cooking method, up to 70 percent of the antioxidants will migrate into the cooking liquid. If you consume the liquid as a part of the dish, you will recoup the loss, but if you throw the cooking liquid away, the nutrients go down the drain. One way to retain their nutritional content is to simmer the dried beans until they are done *and then let them soak in the cooking liquid for an additional hour.* The beans reabsorb some of the nutrients from the cooking liquid and become plumper and more attractive as well.

Cooking beans in a pressure cooker—a great time-saver—is an even better option. In a study comparing different cooking methods, dried beans that were soaked and then cooked in a pressure cooker retained the most antioxidant activity. They also took the least time to cook and were tender and moist.

Ready for this? When dried beans are canned, they become far more nutritious—the opposite of fresh peas and beans. In a 2011 survey of the top one hundred antioxidant-rich foods in the United States, canned kidney beans and pinto beans were ranked first and second, respectively. They had a greater ORAC value than blueberries, black plums, red wine, red cabbage, spinach, and green tea. Canned beans have been around since 1813, when an Englishman named Peter Durand developed a method of sealing food into tin containers. Hundreds of millions of people have benefited from eating canned beans without any knowledge of their health benefits.

In the rest of this chapter, I focus on two legumes—lentils and edamame, or fresh soybeans. You'll learn how to prepare them so that all their nutrients are retained, and you'll discover new ways to serve them as well. Do try the recipe for Armenian lentil soup. It is one of the most nutritious and flavorful lentil soups you can make.

LENTILS

Strictly speaking, lentils (*Lens culinaris*) are not peas or beans but a close cousin of the two. All varieties of lentils are very high in phytonutrients, but some are superior to others. The tan-colored lentils that are available in supermarkets are an excellent choice, but others are better still. Black lentils—tiny lentils that are rarely found in supermarkets—are the most nutritious of all. They are also called beluga lentils because they look like beluga caviar, the most coveted and expensive variety. (James Bond prefers beluga caviar.) They are followed by Morton lentils, a brown variety developed by the USDA for winter hardiness. As of this writing, it is difficult to find Morton lentils, even on the Internet. The next most nutritious varieties are French (or green) lentils and red lentils, in that order. They are available in many large supermarkets. Look in the ethnic section.

Lentils are so small and absorbent that you don't have to soak them before you cook them. You can start with dried lentils at 5:30 p.m. and serve lentil soup an hour later. Each variety of lentil has a slightly different response to heat. The common tan-colored lentils cook within twenty to thirty minutes and hold their shape when cooked. French lentils take about fifteen minutes longer to cook; they, too, hold their shape. Red lentils cook in about thirty to forty minutes and become mushy when fully cooked. For this reason, red lentils are used to thicken soups and curries and to make the traditional East Indian dish called dal.

Hearty lentil soup is a favorite of vegetarians and omnivores alike. The following recipe for Armenian lentil soup was first popularized by the book *New Recipes from Moosewood Restaurant,* published in 1987. Since that time, it has won thousands of fans. Dried apricots, eggplant, and cinnamon—three unexpected ingredients—give the soup a complex and exotic flavor. Search the Internet and you will find dozens of variations of the recipe. The following version has been tweaked to give you the most nutritional benefits. The total preparation and cooking time is just one hour. Make a double batch and freeze some for later.

ARMENIAN LENTIL SOUP

PREP TIME: 30 MINUTES
TOTAL TIME: 1 HOUR YIELD: 6 CUPS (ABOUT 4 SERVINGS)

1–2 medium garlic cloves
1 cup dried lentils, preferably black, green (French), or red
4–5 cups low-sodium vegetable or meat broth
½ cup coarsely chopped dried apricots (see page 284)
3 tablespoons extra virgin olive oil, preferably unfiltered
½ cup chopped pungent red or yellow onion
1 red, green, yellow, or orange bell pepper, cut into ½-inch dice
3½ cups chopped fresh tomatoes, with their seeds, or 1 28-ounce can diced tomatoes, undrained
1 medium unpeeled eggplant, cut into ½-inch cubes
1 tablespoon dark brown sugar, firmly packed
1 tablespoon vinegar
½ teaspoon ground cinnamon
¼ teaspoon ground allspice or ground cloves
¼ teaspoon cayenne pepper, or more or less to taste
1 teaspoon salt, or more or less to taste
4 tablespoons chopped Italian (flat-leaf) parsley or chopped fresh mint for garnish

Push the garlic through a garlic press and set aside. Rinse the lentils and put them in a large pot. Add 4 cups broth and the apricots, bring to a boil, then cover and reduce the heat to low. Simmer while you prepare the remaining ingredients, about 20 minutes.

Heat the olive oil in a large saucepan over medium heat. Add the chopped onions and sauté 4–5 minutes, or until the onions are translucent. Add all remaining ingredients except the herbs. Bring to a simmer, cover, and cook for 10 minutes.

Add the vegetable mixture to the lentils and simmer for another 30 minutes, or until the lentils are tender. Adjust the seasonings. If the soup is too thick, add more broth. Ladle the soup into large bowls, garnish with the chopped herbs, and serve.

VARIATIONS: Top each serving with a dollop of sour cream or yogurt. Sprinkle the soup with a small amount of grated orange zest. Substitute chopped chives or cilantro for the parsley. For a meaty soup, add 1 pound of raw lean hamburger or chopped sirloin steak, preferably from grass-fed cows, and combine with the vegetables and the lentils. Heat until the meat is thoroughly cooked.

EDAMAME

Soybeans that are eaten while they are green and immature are called edamame (*eh-dah-MAH-may*). The first mention of them is in a Chinese medical text dated 200 BC. The cultivars used for edamame are larger, sweeter, and more digestible than the varieties used to make dried beans and animal feed. (They have fewer indigestible oligosaccharides and trypsin inhibitors.) Their flavor has been described as sweeter, more flowery, more buttery, and less "beany" than our common fresh beans. They contain all the essential amino acids, which makes them a good substitute for animal protein. Although most soybeans produced in this country are genetically modified, this is not true of edamame.

In Asian countries, the beans are sold on the vine. (The word *edamame* means "beans on branches" in Japanese.) The longer the beans stay attached to the vine, the more sugar and flavor they retain. Because the beans are faintly sweet and high in glutamate, they tickle both your sweet and your umami receptors.

Fresh soybeans are more nutritious than most other fresh beans and peas. One half cup gives you five grams of fiber, ten grams of protein, and significant amounts of vitamin K, folate, and manganese. A serving that size also contains zero cholesterol and only one hundred calories. Edamame are also high in isoflavones, compounds that have been linked with a reduced risk of prostate cancer and heart disease. The sale of edamame in the United States has more than tripled since 2003. You will find frozen edamame in many supermarkets, either shelled or unshelled. Most of the frozen edamame sold in their pods have been boiled and salted. Thaw the beans and they are ready to eat. But for the most nutrition and flavor, buy fresh edamame on the vine from Asian food markets.

The easiest way to prepare fresh, unshelled edamame is to boil them in salted water for five minutes. (The pods prevent the nutrients in the beans from leaching into the water.) To eat them in the traditional manner, squeeze the beans out of the pods directly into your mouth. The beans go well with beer and rice crackers. Although this combo is not going to replace potato chips and beer any time soon, it is being served in a growing number of households and restaurants.

You can create a savory dish by sautéing shelled fresh edamame in olive oil or peanut oil along with a clove of garlic. (Press or slice the garlic, and then let it rest ten minutes before adding it to the oil). Finish with a splash of low-sodium soy sauce. If you want more heat, stir in a dab of wasabi. You can also turn this simple dish into a dip. Once the ingredients are cooked, puree them in a blender or food processor, along with two teaspoons of lemon juice, until smooth. Then top with chopped garlic chives, parsley, or fresh cilantro. Serve with rice crackers, rice cakes, or fresh vegetables. Rice crackers made from black rice, a type of rice that is loaded with anthocyanins, are now available in some supermarkets.

RECOMMENDED VARIETIES OF FRESH PEAS AND BEANS

IN THE SUPERMARKET

TYPE	COMMENTS
Pod peas	Because you eat the pod as well as the peas, you get more antioxidants and fiber than you would eating peas without the pod. Fresh peas are more nutritious than frozen peas.
Dried peas	Yellow peas are more nutritious than green peas.
Fresh or frozen edamame	Edamame, or fresh soybeans, are higher in antioxidants and protein than other fresh beans. They also have compounds called isoflavones that are linked with a lowered risk of cancer. Look for frozen edamame in the freezer case.
Lentils	All varieties are very nutritious. Look for black, French (green), or red lentils for the greatest antioxidant value.
Common dried beans	The most nutritious varieties are black beans, red beans, kidney beans, and pinto beans, in that order. Canned beans are especially high in antioxidants and are convenient to use. Stock your shelves with canned beans of the above varieties.

FARMERS MARKETS, SPECIALTY STORES, U-PICK FARMS, AND SEED CATALOGS

VARIETY	DESCRIPTION	INFORMATION FOR GARDENERS
Royal Burgundy	Violet-purple skin and green interior. Beans grow to 5 inches long. Excellent flavor. The burgundy color fades the longer the beans are cooked. Add raw beans to salads for maximum color and maximum anthocyanin value.	Matures in 55 days. Upright, 2-foot-tall bushes keep the beans off the ground. A good bean for cool climates.
Royalty Purple	Pods of these snap beans are 5–6 inches long. Beautiful purple color.	Matures in 50–60 days. Short runners and purple flowers. Sow after the last frost. Needs wide row spacing or a fence for climbing.

LEGUMES: POINTS TO REMEMBER

1. ***Choose pod peas over traditional shelled garden peas.***
   When you eat the pods along with the peas, you get more nutrients and fiber.

2. ***Frozen peas and beans are not as nutritious as fresh ones.***
   Blanching the vegetables, freezing them, and thawing them reduces their antioxidant properties.

3. ***When shopping in farmers markets or choosing seeds for your garden, look for the most colorful varieties of peas and beans.***
   Although rare, fresh peas and beans that are red, blue, or purple have more phytonutrients than traditional green varieties.

4. ***Dried peas and beans are very high in phytonutrients.***
   Dried peas and beans have more antioxidants than all but a few fruits and vegetables. Varieties with the highest antioxidant activity include lentils, black beans, small dark red beans, dark red kidney beans, and pinto beans.

5. ***Steam or pressure-cook dried beans to retain their antioxidant value.***
   If you simmer beans and do not plan to use the cooking water, let them soak in the cooking liquid for an hour after they are done so they will reabsorb some of the nutrients. Steaming beans lessens their exposure to water, which also preserves more nutrients. Cooking them in a pressure cooker is better still.

6. ***Canned beans are even higher in antioxidants than home-cooked beans.***
   The heat of the canning process enhances the nutritional content of dried beans, making canned beans among the most nutritious foods in the supermarket.

7. ***There are ways to increase the digestibility of dried beans.***
   Some people have difficulty digesting a type of carbohydrate in beans called oligosaccharides. One solution is to choose varieties that are low in this compound, such as lentils and pinto beans. Another remedy is to discard the soaking liquid before cooking them.

CHAPTER 9

ARTICHOKES, ASPARAGUS, AND AVOCADOS

INDULGE!

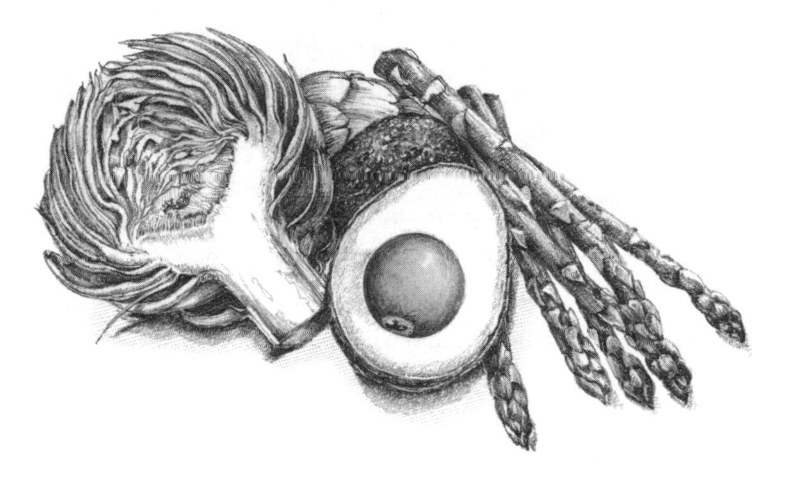

Artichoke, avocado, and asparagus

Artichokes, asparagus, and avocados belong to three different families of vegetables. What unites them—other than the fact they all begin with the letter *a*—is that they are wonderfully nutritious and deserve to play a larger role in the American diet. All three are rich in bionutrients and fiber, which are in short supply in our modern diet. They are also low in sugar, making them a good addition to a low-glycemic diet.

ARTICHOKES

Our modern artichokes are related to wild plants called cardoons (*Cynara cardunculus* L. var. *sylvestris*), which are native to North

Africa. Cardoons have spines that look like dogs' teeth, and their heads are the size of tangerines. People in most traditional cultures eat the leaves of the plant. Today, we eat a different part of our domesticated varieties—the leaflike bracts of the unopened flower.

Cardoons were domesticated during the Middle Ages. They became very popular in Mediterranean countries, where they were valued as food and medicine. One of the most common uses was for "liver complaints." Modern science is catching up with the folklore. Two compounds in cardoons and artichokes—silymarin and cynarin—may indeed promote liver health. An animal study conducted by the US Army revealed that silymarin protects the liver from toxic compounds that can cause severe damage.

In 2007, food researchers learned something else about cardoons: they have six times more phytonutrients than our cultivated artichokes. Nonetheless, our modern cultivars are extraordinarily nutritious. Artichokes have a higher ORAC value than all the other fruits and vegetables in the supermarket. You would have to eat eighteen servings of corn or thirty servings of carrots to get the same benefits. The fact that artichokes are a drab olive color makes their nutritional content all the more surprising.

Artichokes have another virtue. They are high in inulin, a probiotic (beneficial microorganism) that nourishes the growth of "good" gut bacteria that can compete with deadly strains of E. coli and other disease-causing bacteria. Finally, artichokes are an unheralded source of fiber. One medium-size choke gives you between eight and ten grams of fiber, which is as much as two bowls of bran cereal with raisins. People in this country consume half the amount of the fiber recommended by the USDA and one-seventh as much as hunter-gatherers did. Eating more artichokes can help bridge the gap.

Currently, we eat minuscule amounts of this prickly thistle. On average, each US adult consumes less than one ounce a year. One reason for the vegetable's almost nonexistent sales is that artichokes are relatively expensive, largely due to the fact they are handpicked, which results in high labor costs. They also don't store very well, which limits their market season. Another impediment is that the most popular cooking method takes a full hour. Then, once they're cooked, they have little flavor other than a hint of nuttiness and a faint bitter note. To make them taste more appealing, most people use the leaves as handy scoops to transport mayonnaise, aioli, or melted butter into their mouths, turning a low-fat vegetable into a high-fat dish. Later in this chapter you will learn how to speed up the cooking of artichokes and also create a low-fat dip.

Most of the artichokes sold in the United States are grown in Castroville, California, the self-proclaimed "artichoke center of the world." Marilyn Monroe was crowned Castroville's first Artichoke Queen in 1948—a fitting choice given the fact that artichokes have been used as an aphrodisiac since early times. According to Dr. Bartolomeo Boldo, writing in 1576, the artichoke "has the virtue of provoking Venus for both men and women; for women making them more desirable, and helping the men who are in these matters rather tardy." Norma Jean Baker must have eaten a lot of artichokes to become Marilyn Monroe.

SHOPPING FOR ARTICHOKES IN THE SUPERMARKET

The most common type of artichoke, the globe artichoke, or French artichoke, is also one of the most healthful. You'll find it in most supermarkets. The choicest artichokes are the ones that grow at the very top of the plants, because they have densely packed bracts, the leaflike petals that surround the heart. The bracts curl inward and form a tight head. These top-growing artichokes have larger hearts and broader bracts than the slim, pointed chokes that grow on the sides of the plants. Some of our modern cultivars have a small thorn at the ends of the leaves, a throwback to their wild ways. Newer cultivars are thornless—a small gap in the leaf marks the place where the thorn would have been. Thornless varieties have softer flesh than artichokes with thorns, but lack the nutty flavor of traditional varieties.

Artichokes, like broccoli, have a very high respiration rate; their flavor and health benefits decline with each passing day. For this reason, it's important to buy the freshest artichokes you can find. A fresh artichoke feels firm when you squeeze it. Rub two artichokes together, and they should squeak. The brown streaks on artichokes come from exposure to cold temperatures during the growing season and do not detract from their flavor or nutritional content. Store the artichokes in the crisper drawer of your refrigerator as soon as you get them home and eat them within two or three days. The vegetables may look armor-plated, but they spoil very rapidly. If you shop for artichokes in a farmers market or grow your own, look for violet-colored varieties, such as Violetto or Violet de Provence. Their anthocyanin content makes them even more nutritious.

COOKING ARTICHOKES

There is one "tired" and true way to cook artichokes: simmer them in water seasoned with salt and a pinch of thyme, with perhaps a few slices of lemon or onions for added flavor, then serve them with melted butter or mayonnaise. There's nothing wrong with this approach. In fact, boiling artichokes *increases* their antioxidant levels, an exception to the general rule that boiled vegetables are less nutritious. But steaming the vegetables boosts the antioxidants even more. Steamed artichokes give you almost three times more antioxidant protection than boiled artichokes.

It can take up to an hour to steam artichokes on the stove top. But steaming them in the microwave takes between fifteen and twenty minutes. Whichever way you steam them, the preparation steps are the same. First, rinse the vegetables well. Remove the outermost layer of bracts to make the vegetables more compact and to shorten their cooking time. Trim the stems to one half inch. Don't worry—

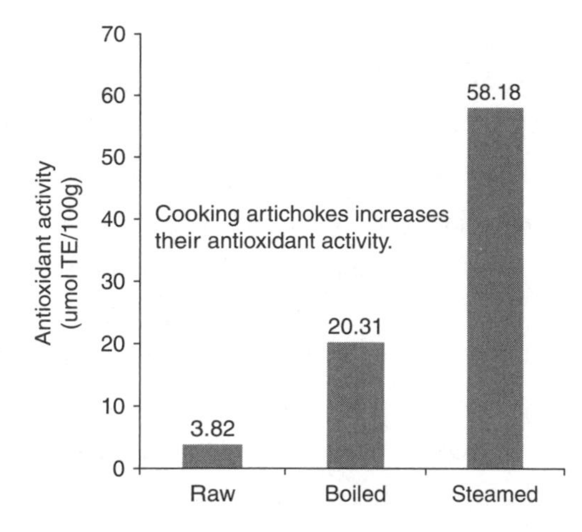

you won't be throwing away many nutrients. In contrast to those of most other fruits and vegetables, the outside leaves of artichokes have only one-tenth as many bionutrients as the tender inner leaves. If the bracts have thorns, use cooking shears or a sharp knife to trim off the top half inch of each bract. (Even though the thorns are small, they can cause painful pricks if you don't handle them carefully.)

To steam artichokes on the stove top, pour an inch of water into the bottom of a large pot and bring the water to a rapid boil. Take the pot off the heat, fit a steamer basket inside it, and arrange the artichokes in the basket stem side down. Put the pot back on the stove and cover with a lid. Bring the water back to a boil and then reduce the heat to the temperature setting that maintains a steady release of steam. Check every fifteen minutes or so and add more water if necessary. After fifty minutes of total cooking time, test a middle bract for doneness. If it is not tender, steam for an additional ten minutes, or until the vegetables are done.

To steam artichokes in the microwave, prepare them as directed above. Then pour an inch of water into a deep microwave-safe dish. Heat the water for two minutes on the highest setting. Add the artichokes, *stem side up,* and cover with a microwave-safe lid or ceramic plate. (If you cook them stem side down, the tips of the leaves will dry out.) If the dish is not deep enough, lay the chokes on their sides. The number of artichokes in the steamer and the power of your microwave will determine how long they cook. After fifteen minutes, test a middle leaf for doneness. If the leaf is not tender, cook a few minutes more and test again. Add more water if needed.

Most people serve artichokes whole or in halves. Alternatively, you can remove the leaves and serve them separately from the hearts. To do this, prepare and cook the artichokes as described above. Let them cool, and then strip off the bracts. Retain the heart, but discard the papery inner leaves and the fibrous portions that surround it. Put a small ceramic or glass bowl in the center of a large platter and arrange the leaves in concentric circles around it, placing the largest leaves on the outside and the smaller ones on the inside. The arrangement will look like a flower. Chop the artichoke hearts and combine them with the dip of your choice. Transfer the mixture to the bowl in the middle of the platter and serve. For a quick dip, mix two parts salsa, homemade or prepared, with one part mayonnaise.

ARTICHOKE HEARTS

I used to consider artichoke hearts a guilty pleasure. I'd order them on pizzas or add them to the occasional salad or dip, but I did not know they had any significant health benefits. How *could* they, with their pale, yellowish-gray color? Another reason I was hesitant to eat more of them is that the hearts are never sold fresh. They are usually canned or jarred, and they can linger on the grocery shelves or in my own pantry for months.

As it turns out, none of that matters. A 2006 analysis of the antioxidant content of common US foods revealed that canned artichoke hearts are loaded with antioxidants. It's not often that the tender heart of a plant is as nutritious as the leaves. Artichoke hearts are also very low in calories. Four ounces of water-packed hearts (half a cup) have four grams of fiber and only sixty calories. They are free of fat and cholesterol as well. Add them to pizza toppings, salads, sauces, soups, sandwiches, dips, and egg dishes. They are somewhat expensive, however. To save money, buy them on sale.

Artichoke hearts packed in glass jars—with water, oil, or a seasoned marinade—are free from the unwanted chemicals that can leach from the lining of conventional cans. Oil-packed artichokes have added calories, of course. Also, their food value is influenced by the type of oil that is used. Artichoke hearts packed in extra virgin olive oil are a healthful choice. Marinated artichoke hearts are also nutritious, but their overall food value will depend on the specific ingredients in the marinade.

ASPARAGUS

People have been gathering wild asparagus since ancient times. The Greeks were among the first to cultivate it. Cato the Elder (234–149 BC), a Roman statesman, wrote detailed instructions on how to grow asparagus in his book *De Agri Cultura* (*On Agriculture*), one of the first comprehensive books on farming. He even specified which kind of manure to use—sheep manure rather than horse or cow manure, because sheep dung has the fewest weed seeds.

In 2011, an Italian research team discovered that wild asparagus has almost twice as many phytonutrients and five times as much vitamin C as our domesticated varieties. But is it truly worth stalking? Europeans think so. I talked with Adolfo Rosati, a lead investigator of the study. "Wild asparagus tastes stronger than cultivated asparagus," he told me. "It is also less sweet and more bitter, but pleasantly so to most Europeans. It is a very popular wild vegetable here in Italy, even among our children. But you North Americans do not like bitter foods like chicory or wild vegetables because you have gotten used to such bland and sugary food."

Our modern varieties of asparagus may not measure up to their wild ancestors, but they are among the most nutritious vegetables in the grocery store nonetheless. In a nutritional analysis of eighteen vegetables, asparagus was found to have more antioxidants than all but three of those tested—broccoli, green peppers, and burdock, a wild root vegetable. (Artichokes were not tested.)

BUYING ASPARAGUS IN THE SUPERMARKET

Buying freshly harvested asparagus is of paramount importance. Asparagus has a very high respiration rate, just as broccoli and artichokes do. It can lose much of its flavor and nutritional value within just a few days. Remarkably, fresh-picked asparagus has *four times* more natural sugar than asparagus that has been stored for just one day, which gives it a very appealing flavor without boosting your blood sugar. After three days of storage, the vegetable becomes twice as acidic. Asparagus stored for longer periods develops tougher and more elongated stalks. (Asparagus can lengthen an inch or two during storage.) Because just-picked asparagus is sweet, tender, and low in acid, it is an exquisite treat.

Fresh asparagus has a number of distinctive qualities that are easy to recognize. First, the spears are dark green and shiny. Rub them together and they will squeak. In addition, the spears are straight, not bent. (When asparagus is stored in a dark warehouse or closed crate for a week or more, the spears lengthen and bend upward in search of light, giving them a contorted appearance.) Also, the tips are tightly closed and either green or purplish in color. If the tips are starting to separate ("fern out") or have a yellowish cast, the asparagus has been stored far too long. Finally, the cut end of the stalk should be smooth and moist. I have seen asparagus spears that were so old that the cut ends were dry and pockmarked with gaping holes; I left them behind in the store.

Many people think that thick asparagus spears are older and tougher than slimmer spears. That's not the case. In fact, the description of the highest USDA grade for asparagus states that the butt end should be at least a half inch in diameter. The very thin asparagus that is sold at a premium in early spring is harvested from newly established plants. It is very tender, but so are freshly harvested plants with thicker butts.

White asparagus is ordinary green asparagus that has been heaped with soil before it emerges from the ground. Because the spears never see the light of day, they do not manufacture chlorophyll; they're a ghostly version of the real thing. They are tougher as well. The clincher is that white asparagus is not as good for you. According to the USDA's calculations, green asparagus has seven times more antioxidants than sun-deprived asparagus.

AT THE FARMERS MARKET

You'll find the freshest asparagus when you shop in farmers markets and other markets that specialize in fresh produce. You'll also have more choices. Some of the most common varieties of green asparagus, including Jersey Knight, Apollo, and Rhapsody, are among the most nutritious. Purple asparagus, however, is superior to all of them. A variety called Purple Passion has up to three times more antioxidants than the standard green varieties. Look for the names of more varieties on page 210.

When you buy asparagus at an outdoor market, look for growers who keep the spears on ice or in a refrigerated cooler. Surprisingly, if the chilling is delayed by just four hours, the stalks can toughen by as much as 40 percent. Commercial growers superchill asparagus as soon as it is harvested by plunging it into ice water. They keep the vegetable chilled during transport and storage. Home gardeners and people who sell their fruits and vegetables at farmers markets would do well to follow these practices.

EAT ASPARAGUS—DON'T STORE IT

Asparagus loses its flavor and phytonutrients so rapidly that it is best to eat it the day you get it. If you plan to keep the vegetable for more than a day, place the spears in a microperforated bag and store them in the crisper drawer of your refrigerator. Some people put asparagus in a container of water, cut end down, and then store on a refrigerator shelf. The asparagus will stay moist, but it will be exposed to the high-oxygen environment inside the refrigerator and will respire very rapidly. In short order, it will burn its way through its stored sugar and phytonutrients.

GROWING ASPARAGUS

Asparagus is one of those vegetables that is best grown in a home garden. When you harvest it just moments before you cook it, you get peak levels of nutrients and fabulous, fresh-picked flavor. When you cook your homegrown asparagus, treat it as you would old-fashioned sweet corn: put the water on to boil before you harvest the spears!

When you grow asparagus, you can take advantage of another flavor-enhancing technique. Asparagus that is harvested when only six or seven inches of stalk have emerged from the soil is much sweeter than asparagus that is harvested when it is ten inches above ground. Amazingly, the tips of the shorter spears are ten times as sweet! Picking asparagus at the right time makes it more delicious for everyone, especially children and adults who dislike bitter flavors. (The sweetness is not a health problem; asparagus's overall sugar content is very low.)

COOKING ASPARAGUS

Research shows that cooked asparagus is better for you than raw asparagus. If you steam asparagus, the recommended method, you increase its antioxidant value by about 30 percent. To steam asparagus, fill a pot with about one inch of water and bring it to a rapid boil. Rinse the asparagus and arrange it in a steamer basket. Take the pot off the heat, fit the basket into the pot, put on a lid, and bring the water back to a boil. The asparagus is done when the spears bend slightly when you hold them in the middle. It will take about four or five minutes. The spears may be firmer than you are used to, but this method ensures that the spears will have the sweetest taste and highest nutritional content.

One simple and tasty way to serve steamed asparagus is to top it with a dressing made from one tablespoon orange juice, one tablespoon balsamic or red or white wine vinegar, one tablespoon extra virgin olive oil, and a dash of salt. Top with festive curls of orange zest or grated orange peel. You could also follow the new trend of shaving asparagus spears and adding them to salads. To make the shavings, rinse raw asparagus, cut off the tips, and use a vegetable peeler to make four-inch-long peels. Toss the tips with the salad greens and arrange the shavings on top.

AVOCADOS

Avocados are subtropical fruits—not vegetables. Like tomatoes, they are characterized as berries. Wild avocados, native to Central America, are about half the size of a hen's egg. These little fruits grow on evergreen trees that reach eighty feet in height. Like our modern varieties, they are between 15 and 30 percent oil—an anomaly in the fruit world. A major difference between wild avocados and the avocados in our supermarkets is that the wild ones have such large seeds that they leave little room for the flesh.

Avocados were cultivated as early as 6000 BC. By the first century BC, they were being grown in great quantity in a number of Mesoamerican cultures. In some regions, corn, beans, and avocados were the three staple crops. Together, these three foods provided a generous supply of starch, protein, and fat.

Generation by generation, farmers began to improve the palatability and amount of pulp in the fruit. As late as the seventeenth century, however, the fruit was still more seed than flesh. In 1653, a Jesuit friar named Bernabé Cobo described the avocados he had observed in his travels in the New World. "They have the largest seed that I have ever seen in any fruit, either in the Indies or

Europe," he said. "Between the seed and the rind is the meat, slightly thicker than one's finger except at the neck where it is very thick. It is of whitish green color, tender, buttery, and very soft."

PRESENT-DAY AVOCADOS

Our modern varieties still have very large seeds for their size, but the seeds are now enveloped in a reasonable amount of succulent flesh. California supplies most of the avocados in this country. The trees are pruned to keep the fruit at a convenient height for picking—no eighty-foot behemoths. Even though our modern varieties are more palatable than their wild ancestors, they have retained most of their nutrients. One serving gives you more antioxidants than a serving of broccoli raab, grapes, red bell peppers, or red cabbage. Avocados are also a good source of vitamin E, folate, potassium, and magnesium.

I was surprised to learn that avocados are an excellent source of fiber as well. How can something so smooth and creamy have *any* fiber at all? The explanation is that avocados, like most fruits, contain *soluble* fiber, a type of fiber that has a gel-like consistency. Half a medium-size avocado gives you six grams of soluble fiber—more than is in a bowl of oatmeal.

What about all that fat? The fat in avocados is in the form of monounsaturated oils, the same "good" fat that abounds in olive oil. In one study, women with diabetes who consumed one large avocado every day lowered their triglyceride levels but had no increase in weight. The fat in avocados also aids in the absorption of fat-soluble nutrients. Adding sliced avocados to a salad can increase the amount of beta-carotene and lutein you absorb from the greens by as much as 1,500 percent.

Half a medium-size avocado has 160 calories. You can make a fabulous 250-calorie salad by cutting an avocado in half, removing the seed, and heaping the cavity with fresh crab or shrimp topped off with tomato salsa and a drizzle of lemon or lime juice.

CHOOSING AVOCADOS IN THE SUPERMARKET

Some varieties of avocados have more phytonutrients than others. The Hass avocado, the large, black, bumpy-skinned variety sold in most supermarkets, has from two to four times more antioxidant value than most of the other varieties in the store. All Hass avocado trees that grow around the world are carbon copies of an avocado tree developed by Rudolph Hass, a mail carrier who lived in La Habra Heights, California. Hass patented the variety in 1935.

An avocado is ready to eat when it is soft at the top but yields only a small amount in the middle. The fruit will feel heavy and the pit will be anchored firmly in the flesh. If the middle of the avocado feels as soft as the top, or if the avocado rattles like a gourd, it is over the hill. Avocados that have dents in the upper half of the fruit are likely to be black and mushy inside. The skin of a Hass avocado is nearly black when ripe; the skin of green-colored varieties stays green.

If you buy unripe avocadoes, put them inside a paper bag, close it, and store at room temperature until the stem end begins to soften, about two or three days. You can speed-ripen them by adding a banana to the bag. The ethylene gas produced by the banana shortens the ripening time by a day or more.

Whole ripe avocados can be stored in the refrigerator for up to two days without losing their eating quality. Cut avocados do not store as well because the surfaces oxidize, or brown, very rapidly. There are two ways to keep them from browning. First, if you plan to use only half an avocado, slice the fruit open and keep the stone in the half that you are storing. (The stone helps slow the browning.) Next, squirt the cut surface with lemon or lime juice. Place the avocado in a plastic bag and press out most of the air before sealing it. Store it on a shelf in your refrigerator.

An even more effective way to prevent browning is to store cut avocados with sliced onions. Roughly chop or slice one-quarter of a large onion or one very small onion and place the pieces in the bottom of a small container. Place the avocado half (with the pit) skin side down on the onions. Top with a lid and store in the refrigerator. Even though the cut surface of the fruit is not in contact with the onions, the volatile oils of the onion have enough antioxidant activity to prevent browning. Try it and see. The avocado will have only a slight trace of onion flavor, because only the skin touches the fruit. Eat within two days.

RECOMMENDED VARIETIES OF ARTICHOKES

IN THE SUPERMARKET	
VARIETY OR TYPE	COMMENTS
Green Globe (also called French)	The most popular variety of globe artichoke, found in virtually all supermarkets, is also one of the most nutritious.
Purple artichokes	Some large stores carry purple artichokes as well as the Green Globe. Purple is the more nutritious choice, because it contains a significant amount of anthocyanins.

FARMERS MARKETS, SPECIALTY STORES, U-PICK FARMS, AND SEED CATALOGS		
VARIETY	DESCRIPTION	INFORMATION FOR GARDENERS
Green Globe (also called French)	Four-inch round globes. Heartier flavor than Imperial Star.	Start with crowns, not seeds. Does not do well in cool climates. Buds are edible 75–100 days after setting out the crowns.

VARIETY	DESCRIPTION	INFORMATION FOR GARDENERS
Imperial Star	Sweet, round, mild-flavored, and free of thorns.	Annual artichoke is started from seeds indoors. Transplant when soil temperature is 50 degrees or higher. Good yield the first year.
Violet de Provence	A medium-size globe artichoke with violet-tinged bracts. Three times higher in phytonutrients than most other varieties. French heirloom.	A hardy perennial that grows in USDA zones 7 and above. Start seeds indoors in late winter and transplant when soil temperature is above 55 degrees. Or begin with crowns and plant after all danger of frost has passed. Harvest the first crop in the fall, approximately 100 days after transplanting.
Violetto	Called the artichoke of aristocrats. Small, oval, slightly elongated heads up to 5 inches long. Tender and flavorful. Northern Italian heirloom.	Matures in 85 days. Not recommended for zones 5 and below. Produces an abundant crop for at least 4 years.

RECOMMENDED VARIETIES OF ASPARAGUS

IN THE SUPERMARKET	
TYPE	COMMENTS
All green varieties	Freshness is more important than the specific variety.
All purple varieties	Some large supermarkets and natural-food stores carry purple asparagus, which is more nutritious than green asparagus. Freshness is paramount.

FARMERS MARKETS, SPECIALTY STORES, U-PICK FARMS, AND SEED CATALOGS		
VARIETY	DESCRIPTION	INFORMATION FOR GARDENERS
Apollo	Highest in the family of phytonutrients called flavonoids.	Early and productive. The first spears appear early in the spring and spears continue to emerge for several weeks.
Guelph Millennium	A newly released green variety known for its uniform spears with tight tips.	Plant the crowns in the fall. Tolerates cold winters but also does well in warm climates. Highly productive for up to 6 years.
Jersey Knight	Tender and succulent bright green spears are 3/8 inch in diameter or more. The tips have a purple cast.	Matures from early April through mid-May. Produces high yields in small spaces. Good in warm climates.
Jersey Supreme	Average-size spears are sweet and tender.	One of the earliest varieties. Good yield. Resistant to rust and fusarium.
Purple Passion	Burgundy spears with creamy green interiors are larger and more tender than most green asparagus. Sweet, mild, and nutty flavor when cooked. Makes a distinctive salad garnish. One of the highest in phytonutrients.	Early-season variety. Hybrid and heirloom varieties are available. Smaller yield than other varieties. Fronds reach 4–5 feet.

ARTICHOKES, ASPARAGUS, AND AVOCADOS: POINTS TO REMEMBER

1. ***Artichokes are high in antioxidants and fiber.***
   The French, or globe, artichoke is the most common variety and one of the most nutritious. Artichokes lose their food value rapidly, so buy the freshest ones you can find, chill them as soon as possible, and eat within one or two days. Steaming artichokes retains more nutrients than any other cooking method. Canned or jarred artichoke hearts are nutritious as well. Add them to salads, dips, pizzas, and egg dishes.

2. ***Asparagus does not keep well.***
   Buy the freshest asparagus you can find, keep it chilled, and eat it within a day or two. Look for short, straight spears with tightly closed tips and moist ends. Steam until the spears bend slightly when you hold them in the middle. Do not overcook. Add shaved raw asparagus to a salad or use it to garnish other dishes.

3. ***Avocados contain soluble fiber and "good" fats.***
   Avocados are surprisingly nutritious and high in fiber. Although they are also high in fat, the oil is monounsaturated. The Hass variety is the most common and also one of the most nutritious. Ripen firm avocados in a closed paper bag. Add a banana to speed up the process. Avocados are ready to eat when they are soft at the stem end but have only a slight "give" in the middle. Store whole ripe avocados in your refrigerator for up to two days. Cut sections will stay fresh for two days if you drizzle them with lemon or lime juice, wrap them tightly in plastic, and store in the refrigerator. You can also store a cut avocado on a bed of onions.

PART II

FRUITS

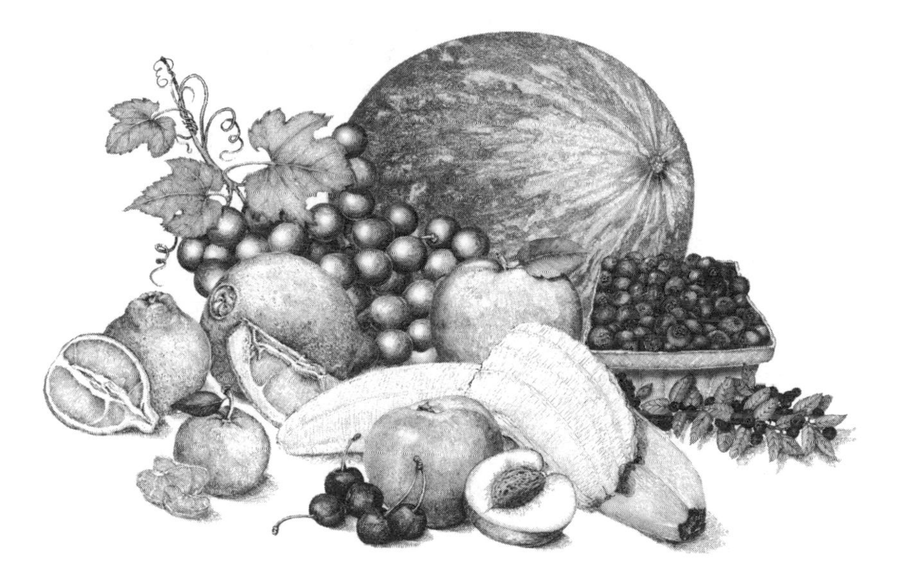

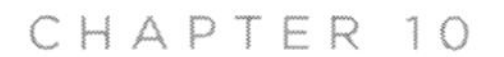

CHAPTER 10

APPLES

FROM POTENT MEDICINE TO MILD-MANNERED CLONES

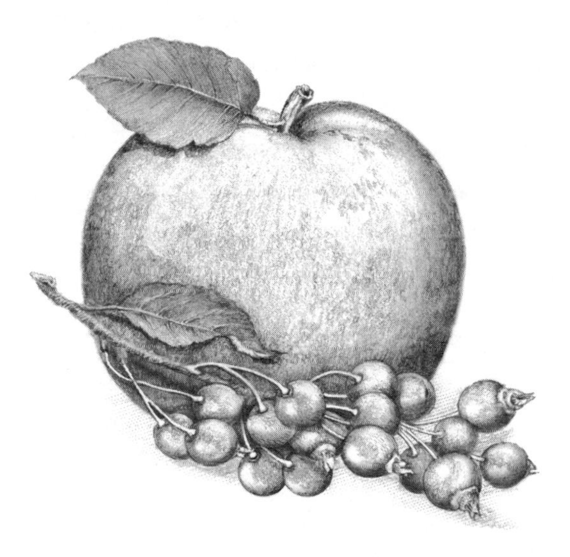

Honeycrisp and wild apples

People have been touting the health benefits of apples for at least five thousand years. Our well-known rhyme "An apple a day keeps the doctor away" is a remake of a nineteenth-century Welsh saying: "Et an apple before gwain to bed maketh the doctor beg his bread." During the Middle Ages, northern Europeans recounted a legend about a box of golden apples that granted eternal life: when the gods feel old age approaching, goes the story, one bite of the apples makes them young again. In 900 AD, Scandinavians were burying baskets of apples with their dead to nurture them in the afterlife. Egyptians had the same idea three thousand years earlier, as witnessed by the mummified apples found inside the tombs of the pharaohs. Apples have symbolized health and longevity throughout recorded history.

Wild apples—apples the way that nature made them—may indeed help us live longer and healthier lives. In a 2003 survey, USDA fruit researchers measured the phytonutrient content of apples from 321 wild and domesticated apple trees. The lab tests showed that the wild apples were vastly more nutritious than our cultivated varieties. One wild species had fifteen times more phytonutrients than the Golden Delicious variety. Another species had sixty-five times more. The show stealer was the Sikkim apple (*Malus sikkimensis*), native to Nepal. Ounce for ounce, the fruit had *one hundred times* more phytonutrients than our favorite apples. People living in remote villages in Nepal still gather these fruits today. One day's harvest gives them as much apple nutrition as most of us get in a lifetime.

Even though the Nepalese apples are extraordinarily nutritious, don't expect to see them in your grocery store any time soon. First of all, they are too bitter for our modern tastes. If the fruit is left on the tree until autumn, it becomes soft and somewhat sweet, but even then it tastes like tart applesauce—with skin and seeds. Second, each apple weighs only half a gram, the weight of half a raisin. You would have to eat five hundred of them to get the same amount of fruit as in one medium-size Honeycrisp. To match the Honeycrisp's *phytonutrient content,* however, you would need to eat only five of them—an amount that would nestle into a teaspoon. What the wild apples lack in size, they make up for in potency.

To get a broader sense of the stark contrast between the phytonutrient content of wild apples and the varieties we've created over the millennia, look at the following graph. The vertical bars on the left represent the phytonutrient content of six species of wild apples. The much shorter bars on the right represent the phytonutrient content of six modern varieties. For the most dramatic comparison, look at the difference between the Sikkim apple on the far left of the graph and the Ginger Gold, on the far right. The wild apples have *475* times more phytonutrients! In fact, Ginger Gold, a relatively new variety, has so few phytonutrients that it fails to register on the scale. Throughout our long history of cultivating apples, we have squandered a wealth of nutrients.

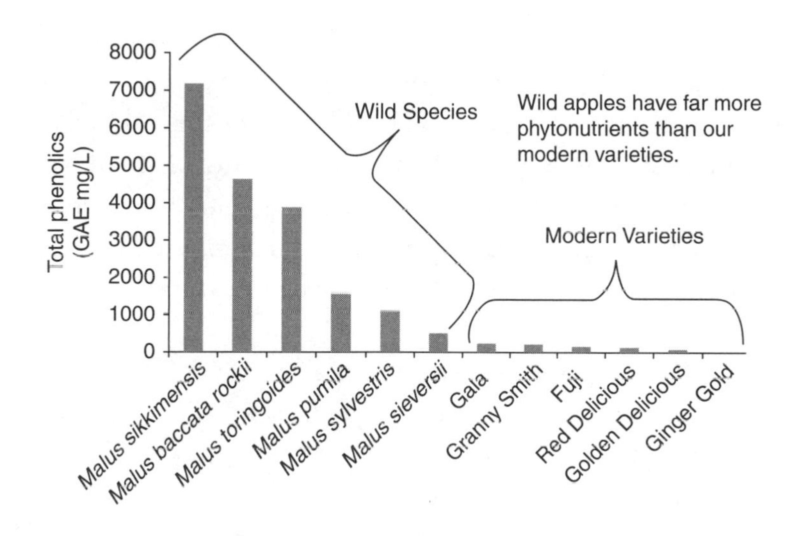

One of the consequences of this dramatic decline in bionutrients is that we may be more vulnerable to cancer. In a 1994 study, Japanese researchers compared Fuji apples, one of our most popular varieties, with apples from two other species. On average, the apples from the other species had five times more antioxidant activity than the Fuji, including four times more vitamin E. More compelling, they were much more effective at fighting leukemia cells. One species had eighty times more cancer-fighting compounds than the Fuji. The researchers concluded that the Fuji had "almost no anticancer activity." Our supermarkets have large, luscious, and sweet apples, but some of the varieties may offer relatively little protection against cancer and other diseases.

THE SALISH LOVE AFFAIR WITH APPLES

Hunter-gatherers the world over savored wild apples despite their tart flavor and minuscule size. This was true for the Coast Salish Nation, a family of tribes that once stretched along the West Coast from Northern California to British Columbia. The Salish gathered Pacific crabapples (*Malus fusca*), which are about the size and shape of small olives. (Any apple that is less than two inches in diameter is called a crabapple. If you can wrap your fingers around an apple, it's a crabapple.) The apples taste bitter until after the first frost, when they become somewhat sweet. Because most of the wild plants in the Salish diet were very low in sugar, even this small amount of sweetness was welcome. Today we are awash in sugar and high-fructose corn syrup, so crabapples no longer tempt us. In fact, the US apple industry classifies all our native apples as "spitters"—one bite and you spit them out.

The Salish prepared their apples in a multitude of ways. They dried them, grilled them, and smoked them. They stewed the fruit by putting it into watertight woven baskets filled with water and then bringing the water to a boil by adding red-hot rocks. They consumed the stewed apples as is or spread them on flat wooden trays to dry, creating a high-phytonutrient fruit leather. They mixed dried apples with dried fish or meat to make pemmican, an aboriginal trail mix. To provide food for long journeys, the women stitched deer hides into long, narrow tubes and filled them with pemmican, creating three-foot-long energy bars with reusable wrappers.

The Salish also found a clever way to store the crabapples over the winter. They crafted watertight cedar boxes and filled them to the top with apples and fresh water. They smeared the rims of the boxes with bear fat and then sealed them with tight-fitting lids. The water kept the apples from spoiling and drying out, and the sealed container kept the water in and the insects out. As an added bonus, the apples became sweeter the longer they stayed in the water bath. Children waited eagerly for the boxes to be opened the following spring; the stored apples were their equivalent of candied apples. On special occasions, stewed apples were served with a whipped topping. Although the topping looked like whipped cream, it was made from fish oil, not cream. Whatever we might think of their ceremonial dessert, it gave them a phenomenal dose of phytonutrients along with a generous dollop of omega-3 fatty acids.

THE MOTHER SPECIES

The tiny Pacific crabapple is not the wild ancestor of our present-day apple. Nor did the mother species come from anywhere in North America, South America, or Europe. The vast majority of apples produced in the United States and around the world can be traced back to a single wild species called *Malus sieversii,* which is native to central Asia. This one species produces the largest and sweetest apples of all the thirty-five known species around the world.

Some of the most extensive forests of these wild trees are in Kazakhstan, just north of the Tian Shan mountain range (the words *tian shan* mean "heavenly mountains"). The forests are so densely packed with trees that their branches interlock. Broken limbs show where bears have clambered up the apple trees to harvest the fruit. Bears, like humans, favor large, sweet apples, and they find them in abundance in the Kazakhstan forests. Visitors to the area say that some of the wild apples are so large and delicious that they would rival our supermarket apples. When mother nature created *Malus sieversii,* she jump-started the domestication process for us, giving us one glorious species that had the potential to satisfy our every desire.

Malus sieversii may be the fairest apple of them all, but it is also one of the least nutritious. In the 2003 USDA survey mentioned earlier, lab tests revealed that the central Asian species has fewer phytonutrients than all but a handful of others. The European species, *Malus sylvestris,* has twice as many phytonutrients as *Malus sieversii. Malus floribunda,* native to Japan, has ten times more. The superstar from Nepal, *Malus sikkimensis,* has fifteen times more. Unintentionally, when our distant ancestors chose the sweet apples from the Heavenly Mountains, they were reducing their protection against cancer and cardiovascular disease.

HERE COME THE CLONES

Despite the fact that wild *Malus sieversii* apples were the sweetest and largest of all, our ancestors were not satisfied with them for long. As early as three thousand years ago, farmers in Persia and other central Asian regions had begun to create new varieties of the fruit that were even more to their liking. This proved to be a more difficult task than domesticating other plants. Unlike most fruits, apples do not "breed true to type." This means that if you were to find a great-tasting apple and plant five of its seeds, each seed would grow into a tree that produced its own size, flavor, color, and shape of fruit. The odds are high that none of the trees would bear fruit as tasty as the one you started with. Botanists call this phenomenon extreme heterozygosity. In other words, each seed has its own idea of an apple. Our ancestors could not produce consistently high-quality fruit until they had removed this element of chance.

Fruit growers accomplished this feat more than two thousand years ago by creating a technique called grafting. Through grafting, they could choose an apple tree with superior fruit and multiply it into a limitless number of clones. To do this, they selected a tree that was producing superlative apples and cut off one of its buds or young branches. Next they selected a second apple tree that had less desirable fruit and cut it back to a one- or two-foot stump. They carved a notch into the top of the stump and inserted the bud or branch from the superior tree. If the tissues were aligned just right—cambium layer to cambium layer—the grafted tissue would be filled with rising sap and sprout new branches. In a few years' time, the tree would have hundreds of branches that produced carbon copies of the apples on the chosen tree.

ALEX APPLESEED

For all its glory, *Malus sieversii* and its man-made variations would have remained cloistered in Asia for a very long time but for an accident of geography. Several of the ancient silk and spice trade routes that connected China, India, and Europe skirted north around the Heavenly Mountains into southern Kazakhstan. The horse and camel caravans snaked their way through large forests of native trees. The travelers must have been enthralled by the apples, because *Malus sieversii* trees began to appear east, west, and south along the trade routes. Wherever people had a chance to compare the large sweet apples with their own smaller and more bitter fruit, they, too, chose the central Asian species.

In 328 BC, the apples got a speedy ride all the way from Kazakhstan to Greece, thanks to the military commander Alexander the Great. During his campaign against the Persians, his army passed through southern Kazakhstan near the town of Almaty, where he first encountered the apples. He was so taken with them that he sent seeds and cuttings back to northern Greece to be planted in his own gardens and to be studied by his mentor Aristotle, the renowned philosopher. Warmongering Alexander was the original Johnny Appleseed.

Once *Malus sieversii* trees were established in Greece, the Greeks began to try their hand at producing more favorable fruit. Not surprisingly, they chose to clone the trees that had the sweetest fruit. This preference was noted by Theophrastus, another one of Aristotle's students, who is now known as the "father of botany." In his book *Enquiry into Plants,* Theophrastus wrote: "Apples grown from seeds produce an inferior kind which is acid instead of sweet . . . and this is why men graft."

Once the central Asian species had spread to Rome, it was soon growing throughout the Roman Empire. By 400 AD, the sweetest varieties of the sweetest species were growing in orchards from Egypt to England. The species did not take root in North America, however, until twelve hundred years later, when the first colonists brought along seeds and cuttings of their favorite English varieties. The first apple orchard in North America was established in 1625 by Bostonian Reverend William Blaxton. By the 1700s, large orchards of the species from the Heavenly Mountains were growing up and down the East Coast.

The new apples won the hearts of Native Americans as well. Tribes from the Iroquois Nation sampled the large sweet fruit growing in the colonists' orchards and were quick to embrace it. By the time of the Revolutionary War, the tribes were managing dozens of their own orchards of *Malus sieversii,* including one large orchard with more than fifteen hundred trees. The central Asian fruit, once a rare and isolated species, had become the dominant species worldwide. All the other species would be left for the birds, bears, insects, and cider makers.

THE LOSS OF APPLE DIVERSITY IN THE UNITED STATES

At first, American farmers were content to grow the varieties of apples they had imported from the Old World. Then they began creating the first made-in-America clones. To do this, they surveyed the wide variety of apple trees that had grown from the seeds of the Old World fruit and selected the best ones to clone. One of the earliest creations was the Roxbury Russet, a medium-size apple with rough, or russeted, skin; our modern obsession with large, smooth, shiny apples had yet to take hold. The variety was so popular in the 1700s that it was given the affectionate nickname the Roz. The Newtown Pippin, another beloved apple, was grown as a cash crop by Thomas Jefferson. In 1837, the American minister to England presented Queen Victoria with several barrels of Newtown Pippins. She was so enamored with the fruit that she persuaded the British Parliament to lower the import tax on all American apples.

By 1910, more than fifteen thousand named varieties of apples were growing in US orchards. That number began to dwindle in the next few decades, as large orchards began to supply more of the nation's apples. The growers found it was much more efficient to grow a small number of varieties and to favor those that produced sweet, glossy fruit that was uniform in color, size, and shape. Small apples like the Roz, with its rough green-and-yellow skin, did not make the cut. The Newtown Pippin was rejected for similar reasons. The apple that captivated Queen Victoria is now growing in only a few dozen US orchards that specialize in heirloom varieties.

Today, the number of varieties growing in the United States has been winnowed down to five hundred—3 percent of the original fifteen thousand. At first glance, five hundred varieties may seem like ample diversity, but there's a catch—fewer than *fifty* of these varieties are being produced in any quantity. It gets worse. Nine out of every ten apples we eat come from a mere dozen varieties. We've gone from fifteen thousand varieties to twelve in just three generations. You see the same assortment of apples in store after store: Red Delicious, Golden Delicious, Fuji, Gala, Braeburn, Granny Smith, Jonagold, Idared, Gravenstein, McIntosh, Cortland, and the newly popular Honeycrisp. These varieties—the twelve most common in America—are making inroads around the world as well, squeezing out more nutritious heirloom apples. The low-nutrient Golden Delicious is not only the most popular apple in the United States, it is now the top-selling apple in the world.

At long last, the loss of nutrition and variety in our modern apples is coming to the attention of food activists, pioneering apple breeders, and USDA fruit researchers. A team of fruit specialists from the Agricultural Research Service of the USDA has mounted an aggressive campaign to collect buds and cuttings from all the known species of wild apples. Their primary goal is to create new varieties that are more resistant to disease. For the first time, however, they are also gathering information about their nutritional content. As a part of this work, they've gone back to Kazakhstan and tested the composition of apples from a large number of *Malus sieversii* trees. They discovered that some of the wild apples have six times more phytonutrients than our present-day variations of the same species. By going back to the source, it will be possible to begin the domestication process all over again, only this time, apple breeders will have the information they need to create twenty-first-century varieties that retain more of the health benefits of the original fruit.

Another encouraging sign is that heritage orchards are making a comeback, to the delight of people who choose to eat locally as well as those who are searching for apples with more complex and varied flavors than those found in the supermarket. Slow Food USA, a nonprofit organization based in Brooklyn, New York, is doing its part by fighting to preserve select varieties that have a rich history and great flavor. The Newtown Pippin is a new addition to their apple protection program. Queen Victoria would have approved.

More good news comes from New Zealand. In April of 2000, Mark Christensen, an accountant and longtime advocate of heirloom fruits and vegetables, discovered one of the most nutritious apple varieties in the world. Christensen was driving on North Island when he spotted an old apple tree growing by the side of the road. He stopped to take a closer look at the fruit. The apples were unlike any variety he had ever seen. Intrigued, he ate one of the apples and was pleased with its juiciness and flavor. He gathered some up to take home.

In addition to being a connoisseur of apples, Christensen has a keen interest in nutrition. He operates on the belief that "for every disease affecting human health, there will be a plant with the necessary compounds to treat the disease." To test the disease-fighting potential of his apples, he sent some to the New Zealand Institute for Plant and Food Research for nutritional analysis. The institute tested the apples and compared them with 250 other varieties. The apples from the roadside tree had exceptionally high levels of phytonutrients. In fact, the skin of the apples had more flavonoids than any other known variety of apple and the second highest amount of beneficial compounds called proanthocyanidins. In 2006, Christensen sent the apples to the French National Institute for Health and Medical Research to see if the fruit had any potential to fight cancer. Lab tests showed that extracts of the apples reduced the growth of many different types of cancer cells, and it was more effective at destroying colon cancer cells than any other apple tested.

Christensen named the new variety Monty's Surprise. New Zealanders call it the Full Monty because this apple has it all—great flavor, beauty, size, a bounty of phytonutrients, and the promise of being a potent weapon against cancer. Instead of patenting his find, as most plant breeders do today, Christensen and others formed the nonprofit Central Tree Crops Research Trust to spread the news about the new variety and to give away young trees. To date, the foundation has donated more than eight thousand trees to New Zealanders. Plans are under way to export Monty's Surprise to other countries, including the United States. When the apples arrive here, you will read about it in the news.

START YOUR OWN APPLE REVIVAL

What can you do right now to get more nutrients from apples? The first and easiest step is to choose the most nutritious varieties in the supermarket. The good news is that all supermarkets display the names of the apples, so it is easy to shop by variety. The varieties that are the most nutritious include Braeburn, Cortland, Discovery, Gala, Granny Smith, Honeycrisp, Idared, McIntosh, Melrose, Ozark Gold, and Red Delicious. Each variety has a different flavor and texture, so you are sure to find one that pleases you. If you like sweet and mild-tasting apples, choose a Honeycrisp or Red Delicious. If you like apples with more sass, the Granny Smith is a good choice. Braeburns are a blend of sweet and tart. Bring home one apple of each of the recommended varieties and discover which ones you like best. Varieties that are among the least nutritious include Elstar, Empire, Ginger Gold, Golden Delicious, and Pink Lady.

You can get even more phytonutrients if you choose the most colorful fruit of a given variety. If you are shopping for Braeburns, for example, survey all the Braeburns on display. The skin of the fruit will range in color from uniformly red to a blend of red and green. The reddest fruits are your best choice. These are the apples that grew at the top of the tree or on the outer limbs, where they were exposed to direct sunlight. To ward off ultraviolet rays, they had to produce an extra supply of red-pigmented phytonutrients. The apples retain this extra supply of phytonutrients even when they are stored for months in the dark. When you eat the apples, you absorb those compounds, strengthening your own protection against chronic inflammation, high cholesterol, cancer, and cardiovascular disease.

Apples that grow on the lower limbs or in the interior of the tree are more sheltered from the sun, so they do not produce as many bionutrients. According to Egyptian botanist Mohamed Awad, "Apples at the top of the tree contain twice as many antioxidants as apples that are hidden among the leaves and as much as three times more quercetin, the most powerful flavonoid." Happily, other researchers have found that sun-drenched apples are also sweeter and less acidic than apples that grow in the shade. When it comes to choosing apples and many other fruits, you want to *avoid* the low-hanging fruit.

Interestingly, a marked difference in nutrients can also be found on different sides of the same apple. If one side of a red apple is shaded by leaves and the other is in direct sunlight, the fruit becomes bicolored—green or yellow on the shaded side and bright red on the other. A bite from the sunny side can give you twice as many nutrients as a bite from the pale side. (Note that I'm not suggesting you eat only half the apple!) The most nutritious apples are the ones that are highly pigmented on *all* sides.

Uniformly red apples have become more common in recent years because of a change in the way many apple growers prune their trees. Instead of letting the trees grow into the customary apple tree shape, they prune them into tall, narrow spindles and plant them three feet apart in long rows. Each acre of spindle-shaped trees is two thousand dollars more profitable than each acre of traditionally pruned trees. Pruning the trees into a spindle shape also makes the canopy of leaves smaller, which exposes more of the apples to direct sunlight. Few growers realize that this produces not only more apples but, coincidentally, more nutritious ones as well.

What about Granny Smiths and other green- or yellow-skinned apples? They, too, become more nutritious with greater sun exposure, but they don't turn red. This makes it more difficult to judge where they grew on the tree and their degree of ripeness. Granny Smith apples, however, have more phytonutrients than many of the reddest apples, so they are always a good choice.

STORING APPLES

Apples last up to ten times longer when you store them in your refrigerator as opposed to on the kitchen counter. They do best in the crisper drawer. If you can regulate the humidity of the drawer, set it to high. The harvest date of an apple is a reasonable indicator of how long it will maintain its optimum crispness and flavor. As a general rule, early apples that ripen in July and August stay fresh and crisp for only two or three weeks; apples that ripen late in the season can be stored for several months.

Given the limited amount of space in the typical refrigerator, it might not be the ideal place to store more than a dozen apples. Instead, I recommend that you buy them as needed. Commercial storage facilities provide the ideal humidity, temperature, and concentration of gases for keeping apples fresh. They do a much better job than you could do at home. No matter how apples are stored, however, their nutritional content declines with each passing month. A team of Italian researchers estimated that you would have to eat two long-stored apples to get the same anticancer benefits as one freshly harvested apple. This is another excellent reason for eating locally produced fruit in season.

EAT THE SKINS

The skin is only a small portion of the whole fruit, but it is densely packed with nutrients. An unpeeled apple can give you 50 percent more phytonutrients than a peeled apple. It might also lower your risk of cancer. In an animal experiment, extracts from peeled apples inhibited the growth of human cancer cells by 14 percent, but extracts from *unpeeled* apples blocked the growth by *45* percent.

One concern about eating the skins is that apples have more pesticide residues than any other fruit or vegetable, according to the Environmental Working Group, and the concentration is greatest in the skins. The reason apple growers spray their trees so heavily is that they want to produce the large, blemish-free fruit that consumers have come to expect. The sight of one blemish is enough to put many people off. Trees grown in areas where a common fungal disease called apple scab is prevalent are treated with fungicides up to fifteen times a year. If you plan to eat the skins, scrub the apples thoroughly or buy organic apples. When you buy organic fruit, you reduce your intake of pesticides, and you also reduce the number of orchard workers who are exposed to the toxic chemicals.

When you combine all the suggestions listed above — choose a deeply pigmented apple of an extra-nutritious variety and then eat the whole fruit, including the skin — you will be getting the maximum amount of phytonutrients, vitamins, minerals, and fiber. For little cost or effort, you will be taking a giant step toward eating on the wild side.

The following recipe for apple crisp is a delicious way to begin. Most cooks peel apples before using them in a dessert because the skins have a sharp and chewy texture. In this recipe, you will be blending the peels with the sugar in a food processor until the peels are finely chopped and then adding them back to the filling. The peels add a bonus supply of phytonutrients, but do not distract from the overall texture of the apple crisp. If you taste carefully, you may notice that the peels add a pleasing tang to the dessert. You can use this "stealth" technique when you make applesauce, apple pies, cakes, cobblers, and pastries.

Traditionally, apple desserts have been made from varieties that are a mix of tart and sweet. If the apples are tart, more sugar is added. If they are sweet, a tablespoon or two of lemon juice perks up the flavor. Dry apples benefit from the addition of a few tablespoons of cream. The phytonutrient content of the apples has not been a consideration until now. For maximum nutrition, pick one of the varieties recommended on pages 234–37. You might start with the Granny Smith, which is high in phytonutrients and universally available.

APPLE CRISP WITH APPLE SKINS

PREP TIME: 30 MINUTES
BAKING TIME: 50–60 MINUTES
TOTAL TIME: 80–90 MINUTES YIELD: 6–8 SERVINGS

Apples

2½ pounds apples, preferably Granny Smith or another nutritious variety
½ cup honey
1 tablespoon unbleached all-purpose flour, whole-wheat flour, or rice flour
1 teaspoon ground cinnamon
½ teaspoon ground nutmeg

Topping

¾ cup unbleached all-purpose flour, whole-wheat flour, or rice flour
¾ cup rolled oats (not instant)
½ cup chopped walnuts
½ cup dark brown sugar, firmly packed, or ½ cup honey
½ cup (1 stick) unsalted or salted butter, melted

Preheat the oven to 350°F. Peel and core the apples, but do not discard the peels. Slice the peeled apples into ¼-inch slices and place into a large mixing bowl.

Combine 1 cup of the sliced apples, the apple skins, the honey, 1 tablespoon flour, cinnamon, and nutmeg in the bowl of a food processor. Process on high speed until the skins are finely chopped, about 3 minutes. (This will seem like a long time.) Stop and scrape the sides of the bowl as needed. Stir the chopped mixture into the bowl of sliced apples, then spoon into a greased 8-inch square baking pan. Set aside.

To make the topping, combine all the topping ingredients in a medium mixing bowl. Stir until blended, then spoon over the apples. Place the pan on the middle rack of the oven and bake 50–60 minutes, or until the top is golden brown and the apple slices are tender. Cool 10–15 minutes. Serve warm or at room temperature.

VARIATIONS: Add a teaspoon of grated lemon peel to the apples. Add ¼ teaspoon ground allspice or ground cloves. Use pecans instead of walnuts.

CHOOSE CLOUDY APPLE JUICE

You've heard this before. If you eat whole fruits rather than fruits that have been processed into juice, sauces, or other prepared products, you get more nutritional benefits. This is especially true for apples. Clear apple juice can contain as little as 6 percent of the phytonutrients of the original apple. The other 94 percent is left behind at the processing plant.

You will get more nutrients if you drink unfiltered, or "cloudy," apple juice. Cloudy apple juice has up to *four times* more phytonutrients than crystal-clear juice, according to research from the University of Warsaw, Poland. The scientists who conducted the study made the following comment: "Cloudy juices also taste better and have amazing body. . . .But the fact that cloudy juices have more health benefits is extra-exciting."

If you drink apple juice, go for the murk. Unfortunately, some juice makers are now labeling their products as "unfiltered" even though a significant amount of the phytonutrients and pectin has been removed. You can spot these impostors by holding a bottle of apple juice up to the light. You should not be able to see through it.

There should also be a layer of sediment at the bottom of the bottle.

At the present time in this country, there is no legal distinction between apple juice and apple cider. In most European countries, by contrast, cider must be made from traditional cider varieties, which are a blend of sweet and tart and, as a rule, have more phytonutrients than dessert apples and cooking apples. The juice is never filtered. But some of the "cider" sold in our supermarkets is made from sweet dessert apples, and the juice is refined. In fact, some commercial juice makers use the words *apple juice* on their labels in the spring and summer and then slap cider labels on the very same juice in the fall and winter. True cider is unfiltered and cloudy, so it's easy to "see through" this ruse.

Happily, a resurgence of artisanal apple cider is now under way. Hundreds of orchard owners are producing their own private-label cider. Some of the cider is fermented and turned into hard cider. In the early fall, look for this authentic cider at farmers markets, wine and liquor stores, and on the Internet. Stock up. The juice freezes well.

BEYOND THE SUPERMARKET

If you live in apple-growing country, spend some time getting to know your local varieties. The harvest season lasts from July through November, with most varieties ripening between August and late October. During peak harvest season, there might be as many as two dozen varieties in your local farmers market. You will be able to sample the apples as you go from booth to booth. As you will see, some of the heirloom varieties have overtones of pear or hints of banana, melon, or pineapple. Some taste like wine, including the aptly named Winesap. A few have what is known as melting flesh—a texture so delicate that it seems to melt in your mouth. Many are a balanced blend of sweet and tart. Attending an apple tasting is another way to expand your horizons. Many natural-food stores host these events in the early fall. When I've gone to apple tastings, I've heard comments like "*This* is how an apple should taste!" and "I'd forgotten that apples could be this crisp and juicy!" and "Where can I get a box of these?"

Some of the best-tasting and most nutritious varieties of apples were created more than one hundred years ago, including the Spartan, Gravenstein, and McIntosh, but many are modern hybrids. The Ozark Gold apple, for example, was released in 1970, making it a relatively new variety. Ozark Gold resembles the heirloom Golden Delicious in many ways—it is sweet, low in acid, and has a honeyed flavor. The winning difference is that Ozark Gold has four times more phytonutrients. Ozark Gold is most widely available in Missouri, where the variety was developed. It deserves more widespread distribution.

When you harvest apples from a U-pick apple orchard, you get to choose the variety you want and harvest the fruit at peak ripeness. Call ahead to make sure the orchard has the varieties you are looking for and that the fruit is ready to pick. If you have difficulty finding a specific variety, search online. The Orange Pippin website (http://www.orangepippin.com/apples) is an invaluable resource for apple lovers. The site lists more than a hundred different varieties, describing their flavor, texture, history, and appearance. It also lists the names of orchards around the country that produce each variety. (There's a British version and a US version. Make sure you log on to the right site.)

PLANT OR GRAFT AN APPLE TREE

If you grow your own apple trees, you can select from hundreds of varieties, both heirloom and modern. You can buy trees that are between two and five years old in pots from local nurseries, or you can have younger trees shipped to you from across the country. The trees are packed carefully so they arrive with moist roots and no broken limbs. If the trees are damaged during transport, the nursery will replace them.

Grafting a tree requires a greater level of skill and care than simply growing a tree. There are dozens of videos on the Internet that illustrate the technique of grafting. You can also get good information from the library, gardening magazines, and local gardening groups. When you learn how to graft, you can retrofit an existing apple tree with worthier fruit. The grafting material, called scion wood, is available from local tree nurseries and on the Internet. Scion wood is available for hundreds of varieties, both common and rare. Some suppliers will custom-graft a tree for you. Tell them which variety of apple you would like and whether you want the tree to be a dwarf, semidwarf, or standard size. It's nutrition, size, and flavor made to order.

RECOMMENDED VARIETIES OF APPLES

IN THE SUPERMARKET	
VARIETY	COMMENTS
Braeburn	Bicolored apple discovered in New Zealand in 1952. Excellent eating quality. Crisp and juicy with a balanced blend of sweet and tart. Keeps well. Lower in phytonutrients than most of the following varieties.
Cortland	Juicy, tender, snow-white flesh and thin skin. Good dessert and salad apple. Does not brown readily. Commonly available in New York State and surrounding areas. Very high in phytonutrients.
Discovery	Sweet and crisp. Discovered in England in the 1940s. Pink-tinged flesh. Does not store well. One of the most nutritious varieties. Rare.
Fuji	Sweet, crisp, and a good keeper. Widely available. Developed in Japan. A cross between the Red Delicious and another nutritious heirloom variety, Ralls Janet. One of the most nutritious of the 12 most common varieties.
Gala	Another New Zealand creation. Sweeter than the Braeburn and slightly higher in phytonutrients. Good dessert apple with mild flavor.
Granny Smith	Large, green, tart apple that is the most nutritious of the 12 most common varieties. It has 13 times more phytonutrients than Ginger Gold.

VARIETY	COMMENTS
Honeycrisp	Now one of the most popular varieties in the United States. Crisp, sweet, subacid flavor. It is one of the more nutritious varieties in the supermarket, provided you eat the peel. (The peel is especially high in phytonutrients.)
Liberty	Liberty is a medium-size red apple that was once rare but is now becoming more common. Higher in phytonutrients than Granny Smith. Crisp, hard apple with a balanced blend of tart and sweet. Good for eating and cooking.
Melrose	One of the best keepers. Its flavor improves during storage. Good for pies and baking. Lower in phytonutrients than most of the apples on this list.
Red Delicious	Once the most popular apple in the United States, Red Delicious now takes a backseat to Fuji and Honeycrisp, crisper varieties that are equally sweet. This American heirloom is relatively high in phytonutrients — provided you eat the dark red skin. Modern variants have even darker skin.

FARMERS MARKETS, SPECIALTY STORES, U-PICK FARMS, AND NURSERIES

VARIETY	DESCRIPTION	INFORMATION FOR GARDENERS
Belle de Boskoop	Large, greenish-yellow fruit with rough skin. Firm; fragrant; tangy. Very nutritious. Hard-to-find Dutch heirloom developed in 1856. Stores well.	Best for zones 6–9. Late-season apple. Needs two different apple varieties for adequate pollination.
Bramley's Seedling	One of the world's best cooking apples, but hard to find in the United States. Very high in phytonutrients (3 times higher than the Fuji). The apples do not keep their shape when cooked.	Best for zones 5–7. Matures in midseason or late season. Needs two pollinators. Vigorous tree produces a heavy crop. The apples store for 3 months or more.
Golden Russet	Small heirloom variety with rough, yellow-gold skin. Intense, sweet-and-tart flavor. Considered the best-tasting of its type. Ideal for making cider. Rare.	Best for zones 4–10. Late-season apple. Scab-resistant. Vigorous; winter-hardy.

VARIETY	DESCRIPTION	INFORMATION FOR GARDENERS
Haralson	Bright red, medium-size fruit. Crisp; firm; juicy. Mildly tart. Good baking, eating, and cider apple. Holds its shape when cooked. Extra-high in phytonutrients. Heirloom variety introduced in the United States in 1922.	Best for zones 3–7. Does well in cold climates. Stores for 6 months. Biennial bearer. Resists apple scab and cedar-apple rust.
Liberty	Medium-size red apple that is becoming more common. Crisp with a good balance of tart and sweet. Good for eating and cooking. Very high in phytonutrients.	Best for zones 4–10. Midseason apple. Resistant to scab, rust, mildew, and fire blight, so ideal for organic production.
McIntosh	Round, red, sweet, mildly tart fruit with white flesh. Good for eating and cooking. Discovered in Ontario, Canada, in 1798.	Best for zones 3–7. Midseason apple. Cold-hardy. Partially self-fertile but does best with a pollinator.
Northern Spy	Red-green apple good for eating fresh, cooking, and making juice. Stores very well. Very high in phytonutrients. Heirloom variety developed in the United States in the 1840s.	Best for zones 3–7. Late-season apple. Biennial tendency. Slow to start bearing.
Ozark Gold	Sweet, honeyed flavor. Juicy and low in acid. Very high in phytonutrients. Introduced in 1970. Comparable to an extremely nutritious Golden Delicious.	Best for zones 4–9. Early-to-midseason apple. Highly disease-resistant.
Redfield	Dark red skin with dark red flesh and juice. High in acid. Used for cider and baking, not for eating fresh. Very high in antioxidants. Rare. Short storage life.	Best for zones 3–4.
Red Jonagold	Large red-skinned apple rich in phytonutrients; good for eating and baking. A good blend of sweet and tart. Aromatic.	Best for zones 5–8. Late-season apple. Vigorous tree that is early to bear fruit. Requires a pollinator.
Rhode Island Greening	One of the best American cooking apples. Highest in major phytonutrients of six apples tested. Heirloom introduced in the United States in 1650s; perhaps the oldest variety of all. Rare.	Best for zones 4–10. Late-season variety. Takes long to go into bearing. Deserves a place in more home orchards.

VARIETY	DESCRIPTION	INFORMATION FOR GARDENERS
Spartan	Red-skinned medium-size apple. Crunchy, sweet, with a delicate winelike flavor. Rich in antioxidants, especially in the skin. Heirloom introduced in the United States in 1936.	Best for zones 4–8. Early fall apple and a heavy bearer. Benefits from having a pollinator that also blooms in midseason.
WineCrisp	Medium-sized, dark red, nonglossy fruit similar to Winesap. Firm and crisp with a good mix of sweet and tart. Stores well. Debuted in 2009.	Best for zones 4–8. Midseason apple. Scab-resistant. Just now becoming available in tree nurseries.

APPLES: POINTS TO REMEMBER

1. ***Choose the most nutritious varieties in the supermarket.***
   Our most popular apples vary widely in their nutritional value. The names of the varieties are displayed in the store, so it is easy to select the ones that are highest in nutrients. See the list of recommended varieties on pages 234–35.

2. ***Choose the most colorful fruit on display.***
   When you are shopping for red-skinned apples, choose those that are red on all sides. The red color comes from direct exposure to sunlight, which gives the fruit an added allotment of phytonutrients. As a general rule, apples with dark red skin are more nutritious than those with light red or bicolored skin. Granny Smith apples and a number of other varieties are high in antioxidants even though they have green or yellow skin.

3. ***Eat the skin.***
   The skin has a greater concentration of phytonutrients than the flesh. Eating the whole apple doubles your health benefits.

4. ***Lower your exposure to pesticides.***
   Conventionally grown apples have more pesticide residues than any other crop. The residues are most highly concentrated in

the skin of the apple, which is also the most nutritious part. Rinse the apples thoroughly or buy organic apples.

5. ***For the widest selection, shop off the grid.***
   During peak apple season in your area, you can expand your choices by shopping at farmers markets, farm stands, or natural-food stores. You can also harvest apples at U-pick orchards. Take along the recommended list of varieties on pages 235–37 to help guide your choices.

6. ***Store apples in a cool, humid environment.***
   Apples keep best if you store them in the crisper drawer of your refrigerator. Apples that are harvested in the summer can be stored for one or two weeks. Fall apples can be stored for a month or more. Commercial warehouses do a better job of preserving the eating quality of apples than your home refrigerator, so consider buying them as you need them. No matter how apples are stored, however, they will be less nutritious than freshly harvested ones.

7. ***Choose cider or cloudy apple juice.***
   Cloudy apple juice has up to four times more phytonutrients than clarified juice. It also has more body and a more authentic apple flavor. Traditionally, apple cider is not refined. Hold the bottle up to the light. If you can see through it, the juice has been filtered.

8. ***Grow or graft your own apple trees.***
   Plant an apple tree this year and you will be harvesting ripe fruit in three to four years. If you already have an apple tree, you can graft a new variety onto the tree to give it a nutritional makeover.

CHAPTER 11

BLUEBERRIES AND BLACKBERRIES

EXTRAORDINARILY NUTRITIOUS

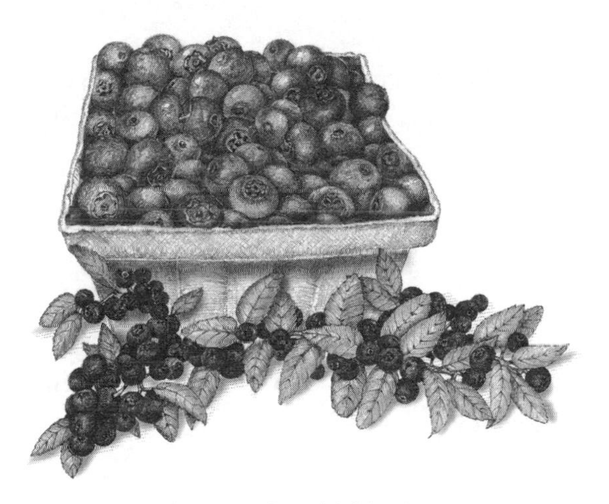

Modern and wild blueberries

Hunter-gatherers valued wild berries above all other fruits because they were abundant, naturally sweet, and easy to dry for later use. Some North American tribes gathered a dozen or more varieties. The Iroquois filled their woven baskets with wild blackberries, strawberries, elderberries, huckleberries, black raspberries, red raspberries, blueberries, thimbleberries, cranberries, nannyberries, mulberries, gooseberries, Juneberries, sumac berries, currants, dewberries, and wintergreen berries. If a berry didn't make them sick, they ate it.

Berries, like apples, were eaten fresh, stewed, and dried. They were also used to sweeten other foods, including pemmican. Most pemmican recipes combined three basic ingredients—dried meat or fish, dried fruit, and some type of oil or fat. Berries were the most commonly used fruit. The Ojibwa Nation, a family of tribes from the Great Lakes region, made pemmican from dried cranberries, bison, and bone marrow. Northwestern Coast Salish tribes used wild salal berries, smoked salmon, and fish oil. The Blackfeet made their pemmican from dried chokeberries, bison meat, and animal fat.

In most tribes, berry picking was woman's work. As each variety of berry came into season, the women would collect their baskets and walk to their traditional picking areas. Some baskets held as much as six gallons of fruit. The older children were outfitted with gallon-size backpacks. Today's pint-size plastic baskets are a joke in comparison. According to Arthur C. Parker, a noted early-twentieth-century observer of Native American culture, women of the Seneca tribe would carry two large baskets at a time, one slung in front and the other in back. When a woman had filled the front basket, she would swap it for the empty one on her back. "Everyone laughed or sang," Parker noted, "and they picked as fast as their two hands could touch the berries."

Native Americans living on the East Coast of North America gathered large amounts of chokeberries (*Aronia melanocarpa*). They are now called aronia berries, a more appetizing name. The pea-size fruit comes in a red variety and a black variety. The black variety has five times more antioxidants than our most nutritious blueberries. Wild Saskatoon berries, also known as serviceberries or Juneberries, were another popular fruit. Saskatoons have five times more antioxidants than the typical domesticated strawberry. Because hunter-gatherers consumed large amounts of extraordinarily nutritious berries, they benefited from an armor of antioxidant protection that we lack today.

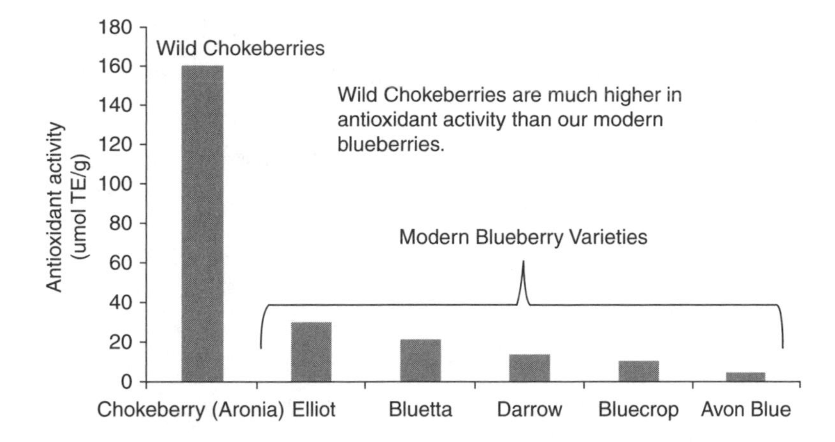

Although few of our cultivated varieties measure up to native berries, most of the berries in our stores are nutritional superstars nonetheless. As a rough estimate, berries have four times more antioxidant activity than the majority of other fruits, ten times more than most vegetables, and forty times more than some cereals. We need to eat more of them. The typical US adult consumes the equivalent of one medium-size white potato each day, but a paltry one tablespoon of berries per *week*. The health benefits of berries have been making news since 2005, so it's surprising our consumption remains so low. Yes, berries are more expensive than most other fruits, but if you think of them as medicine—not just food—the added cost is more than justified.

BLUEBERRIES

Until 150 years ago, people in this country were eating wild blueberries, not domesticated varieties. The wild berries were so delicious and abundant that no one bothered to cultivate them. People who lived in the country or in small towns could walk to a nearby berry patch and come home with buckets of fruit. This began to change in the early 1900s as millions of people moved into larger towns and cities, leaving their berry patches behind. The only source of berries for city dwellers was the wild fruit harvested by professional pickers that sold for a premium in metropolitan markets. The time was right for the commercialization of berries.

The taming of wild blueberries began in earnest in 1910. Most of our fruits and vegetables were domesticated over a period of hundreds or thousands of years; blueberries were tamed in just eight years. This blitzkrieg campaign was spearheaded by Frederick Coville, a USDA fruit researcher who had developed an effective way to propagate blueberries, and Elizabeth White, a self-taught scientist and the daughter of the owner of a large cranberry company. The Whites' cranberry farm was located in the Pine Barrens, a forested region that stretches across southern New Jersey. The area is called a barrens because the soil is acidic, sandy, and low in nutrients, making it unsuitable for most crops. Acid-loving cranberries and blueberries are two noteworthy exceptions.

The domestication of any fruit or vegetable begins with the selection of a promising species of wild plant. White suggested that a good candidate was the "wild swamp huckleberry" (*Vaccinium corymbosum*), technically a blueberry, which is native to the Pine Barrens. As a child, she would scout the woods for the largest and best-flavored berries and imagine fields full of this extraordinary fruit.

The main flaw of the wild fruit, White and Coville agreed, was its size. On average, each berry was about the size of a pea. Because it takes as long to pick a small berry as it does to pick a berry five times its size, growing large blueberries reduces labor costs. White devised a simple and cost-effective plan to create a bigger berry: she offered three dollars to any professional berry picker who found berries that were more than five-eighths of an inch in diameter. (Three dollars would be equivalent to seventy-five dollars today.) By 1916, one hundred superior wild bushes had been located. The bushes were cloned and planted in an experimental garden on White's property. When the transplants bore fruit, a round of elimination took place. First, White and Coville rejected bushes with the darkest berries. Light-colored berries, in their opinion, looked fresher and more appealing than dark blue or black ones. The next cut got rid of bushes that were susceptible to disease or produced mediocre-tasting fruit. When this rigorous selection process was over, only six plants remained. Coville and White devoted the next few decades to hybridizing these exceptional plants to create even better varieties of blueberries. As time went on, other breeders began to create their own hybrids of these superb specimens. Today, more than seventy-five hybrids are growing on commercial berry farms that are direct descendants of one of the original six plants.

It was not known until early in the twenty-first century that choosing the largest and palest blueberries had left the most nutritious ones behind in the Pine Barrens. Most dark blue berries have more anthocyanins than light-colored berries, and anthocyanins are the most beneficial phytonutrients in the fruit. Choosing the largest berries also diminished their nutritive value. In this particular species, the smaller the berry, the more anthocyanins it contains per ounce. Yet again, our desire to make wild plants more productive, attractive, appetizing, and easier to harvest diminished their healing properties.

There was one holdout in this century-long grand redesign of the swamp berry—the Rubel blueberry. This variety is a clone of one of the original six bushes selected by White and Coville. The fruit was so pleasing that it was released to growers without being crossed with other varieties or modified in any way. In a recent nutritional analysis of eighty-seven different varieties of blueberries, the Rubel had the highest antioxidant value and the second highest anthocyanin content. The Rubel is still available today. You won't find it in supermarkets, but you might find it in farmers markets and U-pick berry farms. You can also order Rubel berry bushes from some plant nurseries or over the Internet. I grow them in my own garden and marvel at their intense blueberry flavor. Some wild plants are so exquisite that the best thing we can do to them is nothing at all.

THE BENEFITS OF EATING MORE BLUEBERRIES

Blueberries, more than most other fruits and vegetables, show great promise in fighting our so-called diseases of civilization. In animal studies, the fruit has prevented tumor formation, slowed the growth of existing tumors, lowered blood pressure, reduced arterial plaque buildup, and soothed inflammation. It has also prevented obesity and diabetes in rats that were fed a high-fat, high-calorie, and high-sugar lab chow—in other words, a replica of the typical American diet.

The potential of blueberries to slow age-related dementia may be the most exciting news of all. Alzheimer's disease is the sixth leading cause of death in this country. The annual cost of caring for Alzheimer's patients is an estimated two hundred billion dollars a year. To date, the most advanced antidementia medications have done little more than slow the rate of mental decline. What's more, many of those drugs have serious side effects. For example, a class of antidementia drugs known as cholinesterase inhibitors is linked with a greater risk of heart rate disturbances, fainting, and hip fractures.

It is possible that eating more blueberries might be a better solution. Researchers at the USDA's Human Nutrition Research Center on Aging at Tufts University pioneered this line of research in the late 1990s. In an early study, they tested the antiaging effect of blueberries on middle-aged rodents. At the beginning of the eight-month research project, they placed the rats on one of four different diets. One group stayed on the standard lab diet and the other three groups were given daily supplements of either spinach, strawberries, or blueberries. At the end of the study, the now much older rodents were subjected to a series of tests. The blueberry-fed rodents triumphed. Compared with the other groups, they had better physical strength, balance, and coordination. Most remarkable, their brain chemistry was more youthful than it had been when the study began. This means that eating the fruit had done more than slow the aging of their brains: it had *reversed* it. In the summary of the study, the researchers commented: "This illustrates a surprisingly prompt and powerful effect of an antioxidant dietary intervention." When researchers write a scientific paper and use words like *surprising* and *powerful* in the same sentence, it means that the findings blew their minds.

THIS IS YOUR BRAIN ON BLUEBERRIES

The evidence is mounting that eating more berries might help us humans reverse some aspects of age-related mental decline as well. In a 2010 study, the same Tufts University researchers worked with a small group of men and women whose average age was seventy-six. The participants were showing early signs of memory loss and impaired cognitive ability. For three months, some of the volunteers drank two glasses of wild blueberry juice every day and the others drank the same amount of a nonberry drink. At study's end, the wild blueberry juice drinkers scored 30 percent higher on tests of memory and cognition than those who had been given the other juice. Intriguingly, they also had significantly better moods—a happy side effect that was not seen in the nonberry group.

Understandably, researchers are cautious about making antiaging claims for berries or any other natural substance, even when they get such promising early results. James Joseph, MD, was one of the lead researchers on the blueberry studies. In his 2003 book *The Color Code,* Joseph talked about the health potential of blueberries: "Does [our research] guarantee that blueberries will have the same effect in humans? Of course not. But I'm not waiting for the evidence to come in. I'm eating blueberries now. They taste good. And compared to some widely touted 'anti-aging remedies' like growth hormone injections, they are considerably safer."

BERRIES FOR YOUR HEART

Eating more blueberries might reduce the risk of cardiovascular disease as well. The more berries people consume, according to several dietary surveys, the less likely they are to die from a heart attack or stroke. The results from a two-month clinical trial in 2008 suggest why this is so. In this study, seventy-two overweight men and women at high risk for cardiovascular disease were divided into two groups. Each day, one group consumed a half cup of high-nutrient blueberries plus a small glass of berry juice. The other group stayed on their regular diets. At the end of the brief study, the berry eaters had lower blood pressure, a reduced risk of blood clotting, and higher levels of protective HDL cholesterol than the nonberry eaters. The investigators noted: "Compliance with the study protocol appeared to be excellent." If I were in a study in which I "had" to eat berries every day, I'd cooperate, too!

EAT MORE BERRIES

In all the berry studies conducted to date, the volunteers have eaten more berries than they normally would, or they were given concentrated berry extracts or extra-nutritious varieties. Eating a small amount of blueberries once a week is not going to give you the same results. Still, eating *more* blueberries—no matter the variety—will improve your odds of enjoying optimum health. Set a reasonable goal, such as eating a half cup of blueberries a day. You might begin your day with a bowl of yogurt topped with blueberries. Add berries to muffins, pancakes, waffles, quick breads, and scones. Don't skimp. Use twice the amount the recipe calls for. Serve fresh blueberries for dessert. Blueberries and other berries can be made into savory sauces for meat and poultry dishes.

Blueberry juice is not as refined as some other fruit juices, making it a good source of anthocyanins. Just make sure the juice you are buying is 100 percent blueberry juice. A drink labeled "blueberry juice" can contain 40 percent apple juice, 30 percent white grape juice, and only 30 percent blueberry juice. White grape juice is a common addition to many fruit juices because it is sweet and inexpensive. It is also relatively low in antioxidants, so it dilutes the nutritional content of the drink.

CHOOSING THE FRESHEST BLUEBERRIES IN THE SUPERMARKET

Some supermarkets sell fresh blueberries three or four months out of the year. Typically, only one variety is available at any given time, and the name of the variety is not given. You have to go farther afield to shop by variety. But in the supermarket, what you can do is choose the freshest of all the berries. Examine the boxes and reject those that contain soft, moldy, leaking, or shriveled fruit. Blueberries, like all berries, do not store well. They are picked when fully ripe and begin to spoil within a week. If you buy blueberries and don't eat them right away, store them in the crisper drawer of your refrigerator, where they will stay cool and moist. Don't rinse off the bloom (the natural waxy coating) until you eat the fruit, because it preserves its juiciness and fights surface bacteria. Eat the berries as soon as possible.

During the height of your local berry season, look for supermarkets and specialty stores that sell locally grown fruit. The berries are picked when fully ripe and delivered to the stores within a day or two of harvest. Save money by buying the berries by the flat. Get several flats and freeze the fruit in half-pint or pint-size freezer bags. In the months to come, you can reach into your freezer and pull out a meal-size portion.

FROZEN BLUEBERRIES

Frozen blueberries are available in supermarkets year-round. Research shows that they are almost as nutritious as fresh berries. The highest-quality frozen berries are those that are "flash-frozen." The industry term is individually quick frozen, or IQF. The speedy freezing slows down enzymes called polyphenol oxidases, which can destroy the berries' phytonutrients and vitamin C. If you buy berries in two- or five-pound bags, you pay less per pound. Some stores carry frozen *wild* blueberries, which are an even better choice.

One new and important finding is that berries and many other foods should be *"flash-thawed"* as well as flash-frozen. Thawing the fruit in the microwave is the best way to do this. Intuitively, one would think that microwaving frozen berries would destroy their nutrients, but the opposite is true. In fact, berries thawed in the microwave retain twice as many antioxidants as berries that thaw at room temperature or in the refrigerator. The thawing happens so rapidly that the nutrient-destroying enzymes have little time to work.

If you're freezing your own blueberries or other berries, you will preserve more of their nutrients if you dust them with granulated or powdered sugar, vitamin C powder, pectin powder, or any combination of the three. All of them slow the rate of oxidation. You can also buy commercial "stay-fresh" preparations in your supermarket.

The best way to freeze blueberries and other berries is to spread them out in a single layer on a cookie sheet and freeze them for a few hours. Once the berries are frozen, transfer them to individual freezer bags and put them back in the freezer. The berries freeze quickly when spread out on a tray, which preserves more of their phytonutrients. They also freeze individually, not in a clump. When you open the bags weeks or months later, the berries will tumble out.

COOKED BLUEBERRIES ARE BETTER FOR YOU THAN RAW BERRIES

Cooked blueberries, believe it or not, have greater antioxidant levels than fresh berries. Even canned blueberries are better for you than fresh-picked fruit, provided you consume the canning liquid along with the berries. The reason that cooking and canning increases their nutritional content is that the heat rearranges the structure of the phytonutrients and also makes them more bioavailable. Many other berries respond in a similar fashion. This is as good an excuse as any to make berry tarts, cobblers, scones, pancakes, sauces, syrups, and pies. It's also a good reminder that new scientific discoveries can overturn many of our most enduring beliefs about food and nutrition.

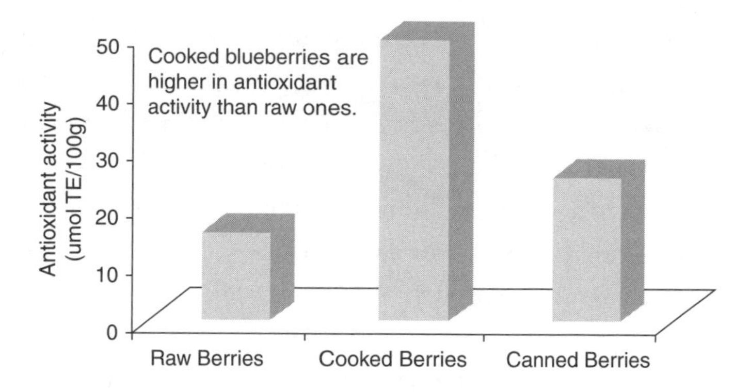

DRIED BERRIES ARE LESS NUTRITIOUS THAN FRESH BERRIES

Dried berries make convenient snacks, but from 50 to 80 percent of the antioxidant value of the berries is lost during the drying process. As the berries are drying, polyphenol oxidases are breaking down their phytonutrients. The longer it takes for the berries to dry, the more thorough the destruction. The ancient practice of drying berries in the sun is the slowest and most damaging method of all. Fruits that are dried more rapidly in a hot air tunnel retain more of their original health benefits. Look for the words *hot-air dried* or *tunnel-dried* on the package. A newer technology for drying fruit preserves the most phytonutrients of all. Called radiant energy vacuum drying, or REV drying, it uses a microwave oven to dry the fruit while a vacuum pump evacuates the moisture.

You may have noticed that most dried fruits in the supermarket are softer and sweeter than they have been in the past. Sales have increased as a result. Whenever food is made sweeter and easier to chew, there is a ready market for it. But this greater palatability comes at a cost—literally. To soften and sweeten the berries, producers have been infusing them with fruit juice, cane syrup, or high-fructose corn syrup before they are dried. Some of the sugar solution remains in the berries after drying, which is why they are extra-soft and moist. The problem is that you are paying for the inexpensive sweeteners at the same price per pound as the expensive berries. The following candid comment appeared in a food science journal: “The syrup loads the costly fruit with inexpensive sugar and increases product weight.” In other words, pump in the high-fructose corn syrup and you will pump up your profits. But if you shop around, you will find dried berries that have had nothing added to them — no sugar, syrup, oil, or concentrated white grape juice.

If you have a food dehydrator, you can make more nutritious dried berries than you can buy in the store. One reason they will be more nutritious is that you won’t be adding any sugar or syrup. In addition, you can decrease the drying time and preserve even more nutrients. The standard temperature setting for home-dried fruit is 120–130 degrees Fahrenheit. If you increase the temperature to 190 degrees, you will shorten the drying time and preserve twice as many nutrients. Monitor the fruit closely so it does not become too dry.

BEYOND THE SUPERMARKET

When you shop at farmers markets, harvest at a U-pick farm, or grow your own, you can select extra-nutritious berry varieties. It could make a significant difference in your health. For example, a half cup of the Aliceblue variety has the same antioxidant value as one cup of Beckyblue berries, yet the two varieties cost the same and are equally tasty. To learn about other stellar varieties, consult the chart on pages 254–57. If you can’t find a particular variety in your local market or U-pick farm, consider starting your own berry patch. Adding edible food to traditional plantings in the urban landscape is a rapidly growing trend. Blueberry bushes can be scattered throughout the landscape or grouped together to form a hedge. The leaves of some varieties turn a brilliant red in the fall, making the plants a feast for your eyes as well as for your table.

Most blueberry varieties do best in the cool climates of the northern states and Canada, but some do well in hotter climates. If you live in the South and are in USDA plant hardiness zones 8 through 10, plant the following varieties: Sharpblue, Floridablue, Avonblue, Blue Ridge, Cape Fear, Gulf Coast, O'Neal, or Georgia Gem. You can find your plant hardiness zone by going to the USDA site http://planthardiness.ars.usda.gov/PHZMWeb/ and entering your zip code.

BLACKBERRIES

In all the excitement over blueberries, blackberries have been given short shrift. It's time they shared some of the limelight. Many varieties of blackberries have more anthocyanins than blueberries and a lower glycemic load. They have from eight to ten grams of fiber per cup, making them one of our top ten sources of fiber.

Blackberries, like blueberries, were not domesticated until between one hundred and two hundred years ago. Since that time, blackberry breeders have focused their efforts on removing the fruit's punishing thorns, reducing the size and number of seeds, and increasing their overall size and shelf life. So far, no one has seen fit to create a lighter-colored blackberry, so most domesticated varieties have retained the rich black color and high anthocyanin content of their wild ancestors.

A new blackberry variety called Wild Treasure (*Rubus* subg. *Rubus* spp. Watson) is a sign of the times to come. Developed at the USDA's Horticultural Crops Research Unit at Oregon State University, it is a cross between a small but delicious wild blackberry (*Rubus ursinus*) and a domesticated thornless blackberry named Waldo. The new hybrid has larger berries than the wild fruit and is free of thorns, but it has retained the excellent flavor and nutritional content of the native species. Crossing a domesticated variety with a wild plant is proving to be an excellent way to bring back some of the nutrients we've lost over the millennia.

All blackberries are soft, perishable, and easily damaged during shipment. They are impossible to store for more than a few days, which makes them more costly and less available than firmer berries. To get your fill of them, you may need to harvest them at a U-pick berry farm, buy frozen berries (which are almost as nutritious as fresh berries), or grow your own. For a wild food adventure, gather a group of friends or family members and head to the woods to harvest your native blueberries or blackberries. (For more information on harvesting wild berries, go to http://www.eatwild.com.)

LOGANBERRIES, BOYSENBERRIES, AND MARIONBERRIES

Loganberries, boysenberries, and marionberries are man-made varieties of blackberries. They're the result of complex breeding experiments that mixed and matched different species of berries, not just different varieties. Surprisingly, all three of these human inventions are more nutritious than most blackberries. In terms of their antioxidant value, marionberries rank highest, followed by boysenberries and then loganberries.

Loganberries **(Rubus × loganobaccus)**

The loganberry is the result of an accidental cross between a blackberry bush and a red raspberry bush that happened to be growing next to each other in the garden of James Harvey Logan (1841–1928), a lawyer and horticulturalist. Logan planted the seeds of the naturally cross-pollinated plants and began growing a new fruit that had never existed before. The loganberry is large, somewhat tart, and dark red in color. It has smaller seeds than either of its parents.

Boysenberries **(Rubus ursinus × idaeus)**

Boysenberries are a man-made cross between a European raspberry, a blackberry, and the loganberry—which itself is a mix of species. Boysenberries look like large maroon raspberries. They are rich in anthocyanins and a compound called ellagic acid, giving them an ORAC value twice that of the typical blueberry. They are also sweeter than most blackberries. They were created by Rudolph Boysen in the late 1800s. He could not make a profit from the fruit, however, so he stopped producing it. By the 1930s, only a few struggling vines remained on his abandoned farm. Those vines were discovered by a Californian named Walter Knott, who transplanted them, nurtured them, and found them worthy enough to grow in quantity. Later, his farm would be known as Knott's Berry Farm. It is now an amusement park that features an enormous restaurant that can serve chicken dinners to nine hundred guests at a time. Fresh boysenberries are no longer on the menu.

***Marionberries* (Rubus *L. subg.* Rubus)**

Marionberries (or marion berries) have the most complex pedigree of all. Created by the USDA's Agricultural Research Service, they're a melting pot of red and black berries. Their lineage includes four different kinds of blackberries plus raspberries, dewberries, and loganberries. Released in 1956, marionberries are known for their glossy black color and intense, complex flavor, undoubtedly a reflection of their complex genetics. They have been called the Cabernet of blackberries. Marionberries make terrific pies.

STORING AND FREEZING BLACKBERRIES

Most blackberries can be stored in the refrigerator for only a few days before they begin to spoil, so eat them soon after you buy or harvest them. If you have a surplus of berries, freeze them. As is true for blueberries, you will preserve more of their nutrients if you sprinkle them with sugar, pectin, and/or vitamin C and then freeze them in a single layer on a cookie sheet. When they're frozen, transfer them to freezer bags. Thaw the berries in your microwave using the defrost setting.

RECOMMENDED VARIETIES OF BLUEBERRIES

IN THE SUPERMARKET	
TYPE OR VARIETY	COMMENTS
Blueberries, fresh or frozen, all varieties	Few supermarkets display the names of their blueberry varieties, but all blueberries are good sources of anthocyanins. Frozen blueberries are almost as nutritious as fresh ones. Some stores sell frozen *wild* blueberries, a bit more expensive but more nutritious. Buy flats of blueberries in peak season and freeze them at home.

FARMERS MARKETS, SPECIALTY STORES, U-PICK FARMS, AND NURSERIES		
TYPE OR VARIETY	DESCRIPTION	INFORMATION FOR GARDENERS
Aronia berries, dark blue	Pea-size, astringent, dry-tasting dark blue berries with dark blue flesh. Also known as chokeberries. Among the most nutritious of all fruits. Fresh aronia berries are rare.	Best for zones 3–7. Each bush can grow to 6 feet high, 6 feet wide, and bear 40 pounds of fruit. Takes 4 years to produce high yields.
Bluechip	Large, firm berry. One of the most nutritious in a study of 15 varieties.	Best for zones 3–7. Early-to-midseason variety. Vigorous, upright bush with medium-large clusters. Ornamental.
Bluegem	Medium-size light blue berry with a mild flavor. Among the highest in antioxidant value in a 2011 study of 42 varieties.	Best for zones 6–9. Rabbiteye type. Grown primarily in Florida. Vigorous plants.

TYPE OR VARIETY	DESCRIPTION	INFORMATION FOR GARDENERS
Bluegold	Firm, light blue berries, flavorful and uniform in size. Very high in antioxidants.	Best for zones 4–7. Northern highbush type. Late-season variety. Cold-hardy, compact, round bush grows to 4–6 feet tall. Productive.
Brightwell	Medium-size, juicy, almost seedless dark blue berries with good flavor. Considered one of the top varieties in the world. Can be frozen or dried. High in antioxidants.	Best for zones 6B–9. Rabbiteye type. Midseason variety. Bush grows to 6–8 feet tall. Good for hedges or borders. Plant several varieties for better pollination.
Brunswick	Wild blueberry originally from Nova Scotia. Small fruits with a wild flavor. Rare.	Best for zones 3–6. Lowbush type. Spreads through underground stems. Red-orange leaves make a great addition to the fall landscape.
Burgundy Maine	A wild blueberry from Maine known for its great flavor. The small berries have the high phytonutrient content found only in wild varieties. Rare.	Best for zones 3–6. Lowbush type. Available in plant nurseries that specialize in native plants. Spreads through underground stems. Burgundy leaves brighten the landscape in the fall. Plants are about 1 foot tall.
Burlington	Medium-to-light blue berries known for their firmness and good flavor. High in antioxidants.	Best for zones 4–7. Northern highbush type. Late-season variety. Extremely hardy. Very vigorous, upright, moderately productive. Easy to grow.
Centurion	Medium-to-large dark blue berry. Among the highest in antioxidants in a 2011 study of 42 varieties.	Best for zones 6–9. Rabbiteye type. Late-season variety. Upright growth. Easy to manage.
Chandler	Very large, light blue berry with a fine, sweet flavor. Despite its size, it is high in antioxidants.	Best for zones 4–8. Late-season variety. Strong growth and vigor; reaches 5–6 feet high. Produces fewer but larger berries.
Climax	Large berries that ripen uniformly and have a sweet flavor. Rich in antioxidants.	Best for zones 6B–9. Extra-early variety. Abundant crop. Good ornamental.

TYPE OR VARIETY	DESCRIPTION	INFORMATION FOR GARDENERS
Coville	Sweet, large berries, usually eaten fresh or used in cooking, preserves, and cakes. One of the most nutritious in a study of 15 varieties.	Best for zones 5–7. Northern highbush type. Ripens in late July or early August. Grows to 3–4 feet high and 4–5 feet wide. Needs two pollinators.
Darrow	Sweet but robust flavor. One of the largest of all blueberries. Also one of the most nutritious in a study of 15 varieties.	Best for zones 5–7. Northern highbush type. Ripens in August. Mature size is 5 feet by 5 feet.
Earlyblue (also called Early Blue)	One of the first to ripen. Sweet and light in color. Good for fresh eating or cooking. Ranks slightly below Coville in antioxidant value.	Best for zones 4–7. Northern highbush type. Early-season variety. Moderate yield. Grows to 4–5 feet tall.
Early May	Medium-size berries. Rare. Among the highest in antioxidant value in a 2011 study of 42 varieties.	Best for zones 6–9. Rabbiteye type. Needs two pollinators.
Elliot	Small-to-medium, firm, light blue fruit. Among the highest in antioxidants in a 2011 study of 42 varieties.	Best for zones 4–8. Northern highbush type. Late-season variety. Upright growth. High yield. Good ornamental.
Northcountry	Small-to-medium berries with a waxy, sky-blue bloom. Sweet and mild, with a wild blueberry flavor. High in antioxidants.	Best for zones 3–7. Northern highbush type. Early-to-midseason variety. Hardy, compact bush grows to 4 feet tall. High yield. Good ornamental.
Northsky	Small, sky-blue berries with a wild, sweet flavor. Slightly higher in antioxidants than Northcountry.	Best for zones 3–7. Northern highbush type. Midseason variety. Very hardy. Reaches 2 feet tall and can be grown in a container.
Rancocas	Small berries with a high sugar content and a hint of lemon. High in antioxidants.	Best for zones 4–8. Northern highbush type. Cold-hardy. Midseason variety. Leaves turn red in fall. Ripens over 7 weeks. Good yield.
Rubel	Small, dark blue berries with a sweet and intense wild flavor. Twice the antioxidants of many varieties. A wild plant that has been cloned but not altered.	Best for zones 4–8. Northern highbush type. Late-to-midseason variety. Strong, upright bush that reaches 6–7 feet tall. Consistent producer. Good fall color.

TYPE OR VARIETY	DESCRIPTION	INFORMATION FOR GARDENERS
Sharpblue (also called Sharp Blue)	Medium-sized, sweet, dark blue berries. Rich in antioxidants.	Best for zones 7–10. Southern highbush type. Good for warm climates. Needs a pollinator.

RECOMMENDED VARIETIES OF BLACKBERRIES AND BLACKBERRY HYBRIDS

IN THE SUPERMARKET	
TYPE	COMMENTS
Blackberries, boysenberries, loganberries, and marionberries, fresh or frozen	Few supermarkets display the varietal names of their blackberries, but all blackberries are good sources of anthocyanins and overall antioxidant value. Boysenberries, loganberries, and marionberries are also excellent choices. Frozen berries are almost as nutritious as fresh ones. Buy flats of berries in peak season and freeze them at home.

FARMERS MARKETS, SPECIALTY STORES, U-PICK FARMS, AND NURSERIES		
TYPE OR VARIETY	DESCRIPTION	INFORMATION FOR GARDENERS
Boysenberries	Very large, soft, deep maroon berries with a good sweet-tart flavor. Cross between a European raspberry, a blackberry, and a loganberry. Higher in antioxidants than many blackberries.	Best for zones 6–10. Midseason berries that tolerate heat. Canes have thorns and require trellis.

TYPE OR VARIETY	DESCRIPTION	INFORMATION FOR GARDENERS
Chester Thornless blackberries	Juicy, full-flavored, firm blackberries. Great for eating fresh and baking.	Best for zones 5–8. Ripens in July. Semierect thornless berry. Exceptionally cold-tolerant. Self-pollinating. Very productive (20 pounds per plant).
Hull Thornless blackberries	Large-to-very-large firm blackberry with a mild flavor. Sweeter than most other thornless varieties and higher in antioxidants. Introduced in 1981.	Best for zones 5–8. Midseason variety. Ripens from mid-June through July. Good yield. Semierect canes require trellis. Moderately hardy and disease-resistant.
Jumbo Thornless blackberries	Highest in anthocyanins and overall phytonutrients of 4 varieties tested.	Best for zones 3–9. Requires trellis.
Loganberries	Medium-size, long, dark red, soft berries with an excellent unique flavor. More nutritious than many varieties of blackberries.	Best for zones 5–9. Canes have thorns, but thornless types are available. Frost- and disease-resistant. Fruits from midsummer to midautumn, earlier than other blackberries.
Marionberries	One of the most widely cultivated hybrid blackberries in the world. Higher in antioxidants than loganberries and boysenberries. Intensely aromatic.	Best for zones 7B–9B. Fruits in mid- to late summer.
Waldo blackberries	Good-size berries are sweet and aromatic. High ORAC value, equivalent to the marionberry.	Best for zones 6–10. Midseason variety. Vigorous, thornless, trailing blackberry. Good yield.
Wild Treasure blackberries	A new thornless variety with small-to-medium-size berries, small seeds, and an excellent flavor reminiscent of its wild parent, the Western dewberry. Released in 1998. High ORAC value. Just now becoming available.	Best for zones 5–8. Cold-tolerant. A trailing blackberry as vigorous as the marionberry. Fragile canes require careful handling.

BLUEBERRIES AND BLACKBERRIES: POINTS TO REMEMBER

1. ***Eat more blueberries and blackberries.***
   Blueberries and blackberries are among the most nutritious foods you can eat. They are rich in vitamin C and anthocyanins, have a low glycemic load, and are rich in fiber. Eat them several times a week, or even more often, for the most health benefits. Studies show they have the potential to slow brain aging, fight cancer, and reduce the risk of cardiovascular disease.
2. ***Frozen berries are available year-round and are almost as nutritious as fresh berries.***
   If berries are flash-frozen, they are as nutritious as fresh berries. Thawing them, however, destroys many of their nutrients unless it's done very quickly. Thawing berries in the microwave is the fastest and most effective method.
3. ***For the greatest variety, shop in farmers markets, specialty stores, or harvest berries at a U-pick farm.***
   You can find extra-nutritious varieties when you shop in farmers markets, harvest them at U-pick farms, or grow your own bushes. Some of our present-day varieties are on a par, nutritionally, with wild berries. Round up friends or family members and harvest the berries that are native to your region.
4. ***Eat berries right away or freeze them.***
   Blueberries and blackberries spoil very rapidly. Eat them right away or store them in your refrigerator for up to three days. If you have a large quantity of berries, freeze them. To preserve their phytonutrients, spread them in a single layer on a cookie sheet, freeze, and then transfer them to freezer bags.
5. ***Cooking and canning blueberries can increase their phytonutrient content.***
   Cooked or canned blueberries can have greater antioxidant levels than fresh blueberries. The effects of cooking on blackberries are less well known.

CHAPTER 12

STRAWBERRIES, CRANBERRIES, AND RASPBERRIES

THREE OF OUR MOST NUTRITIOUS FRUITS

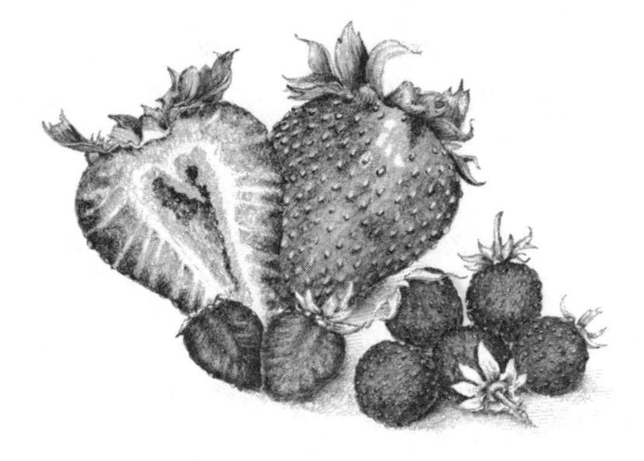

Modern and wild strawberries

Wild strawberries covered large areas of the eastern seaboard when the English colonists arrived in the early 1600s. Inhabitants of the Jamestown Colony were amazed by the abundance of berries and raved about them in their letters and journals. One man wrote that "it was impossible to direct the foot without dyeing it in the blood of this fruit." He noted that his horse would have berry-stained legs as well. Roger Williams, a religious leader and prominent member of the Plymouth colony, was so impressed by the flavor of the berries that he penned this accolade: "Doubtless God could have made a better berry, but doubtless God never did."

He, too, was overwhelmed by the abundance of fruit. He reported that he saw as many wild strawberries within the distance of a few leagues "as would fill a good ship." Strawberry fields forever.

As you might expect, Native American tribes consumed large quantities of wild strawberries. They were the first berries to ripen, so their arrival was celebrated as a rite of spring. To the Iroquois, they were a symbol of the Creator's annual promise of goodwill. The Iroquois marked each spring's harvest with an annual "strawberry thanksgiving," a ceremony of great importance. A common way for the Iroquois to prepare the berries was to bruise them in a mortar, mix them with cornmeal, and use the paste to make strawberry flat bread. Native Americans valued strawberries for their medicinal properties as well. The Huron consumed dried strawberries every January to ward off sickness. We now know that strawberries are high in vitamin C and anthocyanins, which have antiviral properties.

Some tribes did more than harvest the wild berries—they also fostered their growth. Every few years they would burn the berry fields to rid them of the tall bushes and young trees that were shading the berries. In just a few months' time, the strawberries from outside the burned area would lay claim to the now open field by casting out a profusion of bright red runners, each runner creating a new strawberry plant.

DOMESTICATED STRAWBERRIES

The ancestor of our modern strawberries was an accidental cross between two wild species, the small but delicious wild strawberry of the eastern United States, *Fragaria virginiana,* and a larger, hardier, but less flavorful strawberry native to the West Coast, *Fragaria chiloensis.* As luck would have it, the unplanned nuptials took place in the mid-1700s in a botanical garden in the Netherlands, where the two species happened to be growing side by side. One spring, the pollen of one of the species drifted onto the flowers of the other, and a natural hybrid was born. The new crossbreed had fruit as large and hardy as the West Coast fruit but with some of the flavor and bright red color of the East Coast species. People liked this natural hybrid so much that it became the ancestor of most of the domesticated strawberries grown worldwide.

The nutritional fallout of the botanical merger was not discovered until 2007. The wild Virginia berry, USDA researchers discovered, is higher in phytonutrients than the West Coast fruit and is also a more potent cancer fighter. When we opted for the chance hybrid, we got a bigger, hardier berry, but we lost the incomparable flavor and superior health benefits of the Virginia fruit.

BREEDING AN EVEN LARGER, MORE DURABLE BERRY

For the next 225 or so years, plant breeders around the world were hard at work creating new and improved varieties of the new hybrid. Until recent times, the strawberries were delicate and relatively flavorful. This is true where I live, Vashon Island in Washington State. Before the 1940s, the island boasted several hundred acres of strawberry fields. The most popular variety was the Marshall strawberry, which James Beard declared the most delicious strawberry ever grown. The community held an annual strawberry festival to celebrate the harvest. We still have the festival, but most of the strawberry fields have gone back to forestland or have been subdivided into smaller parcels and "planted" with houses. The Marshall strawberry is no longer grown in this region—or anywhere else in the country, for that matter. In fact, it is so close to extinction that Slow Food USA has included it in their list of the ten most endangered varieties of fruits and vegetables.

The reason that the Marshall and other old-fashioned varieties are so rare is that they don't meet the needs of large-scale berry producers. Eighty percent of our strawberries now come from the coastal regions of California. Most of the commercial varieties grown in this area are twice as large as the Marshall, a characteristic that was bred into them in order to reduce the amount of time it takes to harvest them. Although many varieties have a pleasing flavor when fully ripe and freshly harvested, few consumers get to taste them that way. To keep the berries from spoiling or becoming damaged in transport, producers now harvest them when they are only three-quarters ripe. Unlike peaches, avocados, and bananas, strawberries do not get any riper or sweeter once they've been harvested; they only soften and spoil. Semiripe strawberries are also less nutritious than fully ripe berries. They have less vitamin C, less quercetin, and only 60 percent as many anthocyanins. A shipping solution that works for the strawberry industry is shortchanging the sensory pleasure and the health of the American public.

CHOOSING THE MOST FLAVORFUL, NUTRITIOUS STRAWBERRIES IN THE SUPERMARKET

If you buy strawberries from the supermarket and without carefully examining them, you are at risk of bringing home berries that are firm, only partially ripe, devoid of flavor, and relatively low in phytonutrients. Learning how to select the freshest, ripest fruit will greatly increase your chances of enjoying more worthy fruit. First, look for strawberries that are completely red—not red on the bottom and white around the shoulders, which is a telltale sign of an unripe and less nutritious fruit. The freshest strawberries have a bright red gloss. Reject containers that have damaged, leaking, or moldy fruit. If you cannot find ripe and fresh-looking strawberries, consider buying other fruit. The berry industry will find ways to produce higher-quality fruit if consumers stop accepting firm and flavorless strawberries.

Some supermarkets feature locally grown strawberries when they are available. The fruit is picked when red-ripe and arrives in the stores within days. Compared to berries shipped from hundreds or even thousands of miles away, they are redder, more aromatic, more intensely flavored, and better for your health. Buying local strawberries in season is like stepping back in time one hundred years.

Buying organically produced local strawberries is even better. Year after year, strawberries are near the top of the lists of the most contaminated fruits and vegetables in the United States. This is partly a result of the chemicals that growers use to rid the soil of fungus, but they use a raft of other compounds as well. Traces of sixty different agricultural chemicals have been found on conventionally raised strawberries. Organic strawberries are not only cleaner, they may also offer you more protection against cancer. A 2007 Swedish study that compared organic and conventionally raised strawberries found that the organic fruit had significantly more vitamin C and was also more effective at killing cancer cells. If you buy nonorganic berries, rinse them thoroughly just before you eat them.

When you bring your strawberries home or harvest them from your garden, eat them within a day or two for the best flavor. If you're going to store them for two or three days, you can either put them in your refrigerator or leave them out on the kitchen counter. At room temperature, the strawberries won't become any riper, but they will become more aromatic and flavorful. Surprisingly, they will also become *richer* in antioxidant activity, a phenomenon that occurs in a few other fruits as well. If you plan to freeze the strawberries, you will preserve more nutrients if you dust them with sugar, powdered pectin, powdered vitamin C, or a combination of these three ingredients before freezing. Thaw them in the microwave for the best retention of anthocyanins and vitamin C.

BEYOND THE SUPERMARKET

You'll get the freshest and ripest berries when you buy them from farmers markets, U-pick berry farms, and specialty produce stores. In these venues, you will also be able to shop by variety. Extra-nutritious varieties include Camarosa, Chandler, Latestar, Ovation, and Sweet Charlie. Ovation was released in 2003 by the USDA's Agricultural Research Service. A June-bearing strawberry, it is higher in antioxidants, anthocyanins, and sugar than most other varieties. It is also a relatively large berry. (See pages 271–72 for other recommended varieties.)

Consider growing your own strawberries. Strawberries come back year after year, more than repaying you for your initial investment. If you plant them in the early fall, they will develop strong roots before winter sets in and produce a good crop the first spring. The ripe berries are a red beacon for birds, squirrels, and chipmunks, however, so depending on where you live, you may need to protect them with netting *before* they begin to ripen.

Wild strawberries, with their bright red runners, make an excellent ground cover. You'll have the best luck finding them in nurseries that specialize in native plants. If you protect the ripening berries from birds and beasts, you can *eat* your landscape as well. For the best flavor and nutrition, look for *Fragaria virginiana*.

CRANBERRIES

Cranberries (*Vaccinium macrocarpon*) are native to North America. The Lenni-Lenape tribe of the Delaware Nation called them pakim, which means "noisy berry," a comment on the "pop" you hear when you bite into them. The berries were gathered after the first frost because cold temperatures concentrate their natural sugars. Some Canadian tribes sweetened the bitter berries, but they used maple syrup rather than concentrated white grape juice or high-fructose corn syrup, as we do today.

Cranberries were domesticated late in the game. In 1816, a Revolutionary War veteran named Henry Hull began cultivating the wild "crane berries" that grew in the marshes near Dennis, Massachusetts. (The Pilgrims called the berries crane berries because the stalks of the bushes look like the long neck of a crane.) Cranberries have changed little since that time. They are still exceedingly tart and disarmingly red. What has changed is that we now know how good they are for us. Their red color comes from anthocyanins, which boost their antioxidant levels into the stratosphere, putting them on a par with acai berries, aronia berries, and black raspberries.

Cranberries have been used as a folk remedy to prevent and treat bladder infections, a health benefit that has now been confirmed by several studies. Eating as little as one serving per week, according to a 2009 study, can lower the risk of a bladder infection by more than 50 percent. A more recent study found that cranberries also defeat a number of food-borne bacteria, including staphylococcus, listeria, and E. coli. Their anticancer properties have become another active area of research.

We are now eating more dried cranberries than fresh cranberries. Unfortunately, the dried berries have only 20 percent of the antioxidant value of fresh berries. The berries are so rich in nutrients, however, that even when dried and infused with syrup they can still provide health benefits. In a 2005 study, women diagnosed with bladder infections consumed either a small box of raisins or a similar quantity of sweetened dried cranberries. Tests taken on the cranberry eaters just a few hours later showed that the bacteria in their urine were less able to attach to cell walls, a necessary condition for an infection to develop and persist. The raisins had no such effect.

Cranberry juice has about half the phytonutrients of whole cranberries, but it, too, has been shown to fight bacteria, including

Helicobacter pylori, which is linked with stomach ulcers. Drinking cranberry juice makes it more difficult for the bacteria to attach to the mucous membranes that line the gastrointestinal tract.

STORING CRANBERRIES

Fresh whole cranberries will stay fresh for a week if you store them in the crisper drawer of your refrigerator and keep them in the perforated bag they came in. The berries are usually sold at a reduced price during the weeks leading up to Thanksgiving and Christmas; stock up and keep a supply in your freezer.

Look for ways to eat more cranberries. Add fresh or frozen cranberries to an apple pie or fruit crisp, or to a standard muffin recipe. Cranberry sauces, jellies, and relish make a tangy counterpoint to fatty cuts of meat and to bland-tasting chicken, pork, and turkey. They are especially good with ham, fried chicken, turkey, and barbecued ribs. Add dried cranberries to green salads, trail mix, oatmeal cookies, muffins, quick breads, pastries, and bread puddings. Drink cranberry juice. Unsweetened cranberry juice is quite bitter, but it is a far more concentrated source of phytonutrients than cranberry juice cocktail and cranberry juice blends.

The following recipe for cranberry horseradish relish takes only fifteen minutes to prepare. The red cranberries and green scallions give it a festive look. For a milder-flavored creamy relish, add the optional sour cream or yogurt.

CRANBERRY HORSERADISH RELISH

TOTAL TIME: 15 MINUTES YIELD: 1¾ CUPS

8 ounces whole fresh cranberries (about 2¼ cups)
¼ cup thinly sliced scallions (including white and green parts)
3 tablespoons granulated sugar or warm honey
1 tablespoon prepared horseradish
2 tablespoons currants, chopped raisins, or dried cranberries
2 tablespoons sour cream or yogurt (optional)

Chop the fresh cranberries until they are finely minced, or put them into the bowl of a food processor and pulse about 5–10 times. Transfer the chopped cranberries to a small mixing bowl and stir in the remaining ingredients. Let rest for about fifteen minutes before serving to allow the flavors to meld and the dried fruit to plump up in the cranberry liquid. Store in the refrigerator.

RASPBERRIES

RED RASPBERRIES

Wild red raspberries grow in all temperate regions of Europe, Asia, North America, and China. They were domesticated more than eighteen hundred years ago, according to Palladius, a fifth-century Roman farmer. Raspberry seeds have been found in a number of ancient Roman forts in England, testimony to the high value that Roman soldiers placed on the berries: they didn't leave home without them. The British developed new varieties throughout the Middle Ages and were exporting plants to New York by the early 1700s.

A significant amount of phytonutrients were lost along the way. *Rubus caucasicus,* a dark red variety of wild raspberries, has two and a half times more antioxidants than the modern cultivar Glen Lyon. Yellow varieties such as Anne have less than the Glen Lyon. To create the novel yellow color, breeders had to "silence" the gene that produces anthocyanins—akin to removing the active ingredient from a prescription drug. The most nutritious of our present-day varieties include Heritage Red, Tulameen, and Caroline.

Raspberries, like blackberries, are composite berries made up of scores of tiny plump fruits called drupelets. Each drupelet contains one small seed. This complex structure gives them a surprisingly high amount of soluble fiber—six grams of fiber per half-cup serving, which is more than most other fruits and vegetables.

Raspberries are valued for their soft, velvety texture, but this makes them exceedingly difficult to ship. They also spoil in a matter of days, so they cannot while away their time in a warehouse. A few large-scale berry producers now specialize in shipping raspberries within a few hours of harvest and getting them to their destinations within one or two days. Understandably, this special care commands a premium price. Whether you are considering buying the deluxe or less coddled berries, look them over and choose the freshest fruits. Fresh raspberries retain their shape and have no signs of leaking juice. If raspberries are not in season or you cannot find berries of high enough quality, buy frozen raspberries, which are almost as nutritious. If you buy them in two-gallon bags, they cost less per pound, and you will have enough on hand to make raspberry smoothies, add the berries to fruit salads, and make a raspberry pastry for Sunday breakfast.

Start your own raspberry patch and you will have an abundant supply in your backyard. The canes produce so many offshoots that you will be able to dig them up and share them with your friends and neighbors. My two rows of bushes have spawned berry patches for many friends.

BLACK RASPBERRIES

Black raspberries, or blackcaps, are native to North America. The good news is that our modern varieties are almost as nutritious as their wild ancestor, *Rubus occidentalis*. They also have almost three times more antioxidant activity than the marionberry, which is one of our most nutritious blackberry hybrids. The anticancer properties of black raspberries have been under investigation for more than a decade, primarily in test-tube and animal studies. Extracts of the berries have prevented colon cancer and esophageal cancer in rodents. These findings may apply to humans as well. The most promising human studies to date have come from Ohio State University. Gary Stoner, PhD, was the lead investigator in a 2007 research project that involved twenty-five patients with newly diagnosed colorectal cancer. During the weeks leading up to their scheduled surgeries, the volunteers consumed a daily dose of sixty grams of freeze-dried black raspberry powder. When the patients' tumors were removed, the researchers discovered that consuming the berries had slowed the growth rate of the cancer cells and the blood vessels that were supplying them. The fact that the patients had been consuming the berry extract for only two to four weeks makes the findings all the more remarkable.

In 2011, Stoner and his colleagues tested the black raspberry extract in a phase 1 clinical trial, which is the second stage of study involved in the approval process for new medications. They got equally good results. The team's long-term goal is to develop a nontoxic therapy that reduces the risk of colon cancer and also increases the effectiveness of conventional forms of treatment. The fact that a great-tasting berry might help fend off colon cancer—our third-most-common cancer—is good news indeed. Stoner does not make claims for the berries that go beyond his limited data, but he does recommend that people eat a serving of berries every day.

At the present time, black raspberries are difficult to find. In Oregon, the state that produces the most berries, the fruit is available from early July to mid-August. Frozen berries and freeze-dried black raspberry powder are also available. (Search for them on the Internet.) The freeze-dried extract is the most effective, because you get far more of the nutrients than you would in capsule form. If you live in a temperate climate zone, consider raising your own black raspberries. A word of warning from one who knows: prune the canes aggressively, or they will grow up to twenty feet long.

RECOMMENDED VARIETIES OF STRAWBERRIES

IN THE SUPERMARKET	
TYPE	COMMENTS
Fresh	Choose strawberries that are fresh and fully ripe. Some stores feature local strawberries during the peak season. Take advantage of the opportunity and buy enough to freeze.
Frozen	Frozen strawberries are almost as nutritious as fresh ones and are available year-round. Thaw in the microwave to retain the most nutrients.

FARMERS MARKETS, SPECIALTY STORES, U-PICK FARMS, AND SEED CATALOGS		
VARIETY	DESCRIPTION	INFORMATION FOR GARDENERS
Bounty	Medium-size, glossy, dark red heart-shaped berries with excellent flavor. Softer than some varieties. Rich in phytonutrients. Developed in Canada in the early 1970s.	Best for zones 4–10. Cold-hardy. Resistant to several common diseases. Heavy producer. Recommended for northern states.

VARIETY	DESCRIPTION	INFORMATION FOR GARDENERS
Camarosa	Large, firm, conical fruit with bright red color and good flavor that is gaining popularity as a U-pick variety. Very high in phytonutrients and ORAC value.	Best for zones 7–9. Early-season berry. Released in 1993.
Chandler	Large berry that is higher in phytonutrients than most other varieties. Excellent flavor and a brilliant red color. Freezes well. Released in 1983.	Best for zones 5–8. Cold-hardy. Grows best on the West Coast and in the Southeast.
Earliglow	Sweet, good flavor, glossy, and firm. Uniformly deep red. Recommended for freezing, desserts, and preserves. Developed by the USDA in 1975.	Best for zones 4–8. Bears fruit in early June. Cold-hardy. A vigorous grower that is resistant to disease.
Honeoye	Intense strawberry flavor. Conical berries. Relatively high in antioxidants and anthocyanins.	Best for zones 3–8. Bears fruit in June. Winter-hardy. Very productive. Highly resistant to berry rot.
Late Star (also Latestar)	Attractive, firm berry. Pleasant flavor with a touch of tartness. More likely to be found in U-pick berry farms than in stores. Three times more antioxidants than some varieties. Created by the USDA and introduced in 1995. Plants can be hard to find.	Best for zones 5–8. June-bearing. Disease-resistant. High yield.
Ovation	Large, bright red berry with a small core. Aromatic with a mild flavor. High ORAC value.	Best for zones 4–8. Exceptionally late variety. Vigorous grower. Disease-resistant.
Selva	Firm, juicy fruit. Higher in antioxidants than Sweet Charlie.	Best for zones 3–9. Fruits within three months of planting and continues to fruit throughout the summer. Vigorous and able to withstand wet conditions.
Sweet Charlie	A high-sugar, low-acid variety that is orange-red in color. Winner of a number of taste tests. Extracts were found to be more effective in killing human breast cancer cells than all other varieties tested. Released in 1992 by the University of Florida.	Best for zones 7–9. Well suited for the southeastern states, California, Oregon, and Washington. Resistant to crown rot, fruit rot, two-spotted spider mites, and powdery mildew. Highly resistant to anthracnose fruit rot.

RECOMMENDED VARIETIES OF CRANBERRIES

ALL MARKETS	
VARIETIES	COMMENTS
All varieties, fresh or frozen	All varieties are high in phytonutrients and are similar to wild cranberries in nutritional content.

IN THE GARDEN	
Early Black, Howes, and Ben Lear are popular varieties that were selected from the wild. They are higher in antioxidant value than most other varieties. Early Black has slightly more phytonutrients than the other two. Stevens is a hybrid created by the USDA for greater disease resistance and productivity. It is lower in phytonutrients than the varieties mentioned above, but it is a very nutritious berry nonetheless.	Best for zones 2–7. Needs moist to boggy soil that is high in acidity (pH 4.5–6.5). Cranberries require specific growing conditions. You will find more growing advice online.

RECOMMENDED VARIETIES OF RED AND BLACK RASPBERRIES

IN THE SUPERMARKET	
TYPE	COMMENTS
Fresh	Look for fresh berries that have held their shape, or buy frozen raspberries.
Frozen	Frozen raspberries are available year-round and retain much of the nutritional content of the fresh fruit. Defrost in the microwave.

FARMERS MARKETS, SPECIALTY STORES, U-PICK FARMS, AND NURSERIES		
RED RASPBERRIES	DESCRIPTION	INFORMATION FOR GARDENERS
Caroline	Large, great-tasting berries that are firmer than many other varieties. High in antioxidants, and has anticancer properties as well.	Best for zones 4–9. Hardy. Delivers two bumper crops – one in late June and another from August until September.
Heritage Red	Most popular fall-bearing raspberry on the market. Medium-size fruit with good flavor. Rich in antioxidants.	Best for zones 3–11. Late fall-bearing variety that fruits from late August until first frost.
Summit	Large fruit with a mild flavor.	Suitable for zones 3–11, but does best in mild climates. High resistance to root rot.
BLACK RASPBERRIES	DESCRIPTION	INFORMATION FOR GARDENERS
All	All black raspberries are high in antioxidants and have anticancer properties, according to lab tests and animal studies.	Black raspberries should not be planted within 75–100 feet of blackberries or any other type of raspberry because of the likelihood of cross-pollination.
Bristol	Large, black, with attractive glossy skin and firm flesh. Good flavor. Good for canning, baking, freezing, and eating fresh.	Best for zones 5–8. Cold-tolerant. Vigorous, upright canes do not require staking. Ripens in July. Easy to pick. Self-pollinating.
Jewel	Large berries with firm, glossy black fruit. Sweet and rich flavor. Good choice for making jams and jellies.	Best for zones 4–8. Reliable and hardy. Bountiful midseason crop. Tall, vigorous, productive plant. Recommended for both home and market growers.

STRAWBERRIES, CRANBERRIES, AND RASPBERRIES: POINTS TO REMEMBER

1. ***Select red, ripe strawberries.***
   Most strawberries are harvested when they are only three-quarters ripe. They do not ripen beyond this point and are never as sweet and nutritious as field-ripened fruit. For the most flavorful fruit, buy local berries, harvest them at a U-pick farm, or grow them yourself. Choose berries that are a uniform, dark red color. Eat them within a few days. You can increase their antioxidant value by storing them on the counter for two days. If you buy frozen berries, thaw them in the microwave to preserve more nutrients. Before freezing strawberries, dust them with sugar, powdered vitamin C, and/or powdered pectin to preserve their nutrients. You can find commercial "stay-fresh" preparations in the supermarket.

2. ***Eat cranberries throughout the year.***
   Cranberries are very high in antioxidants. Use them in side dishes, sauces, and relishes throughout the year, not just during the holidays. Dried cranberries are less nutritious than fresh cranberries, but they have enough antioxidant value to provide significant health benefits. Cranberry juice has proven health benefits as well. Unsweetened juice offers more benefits than cranberry juice cocktail or cranberry juice blends.

3. ***Raspberries are high in fiber and antioxidants.***
   Dark red raspberries have a rich mix of phytonutrients and are remarkably high in fiber. Black raspberries are even more nutritious than the red varieties, and they have promising anticancer properties as well. Fresh black raspberries are easiest to find in the Pacific Northwest. If you live in other areas, you can buy frozen berries or freeze-dried black raspberry powder in some stores and on the Internet.

CHAPTER 13

STONE FRUITS

TIME FOR A FLAVOR REVIVAL

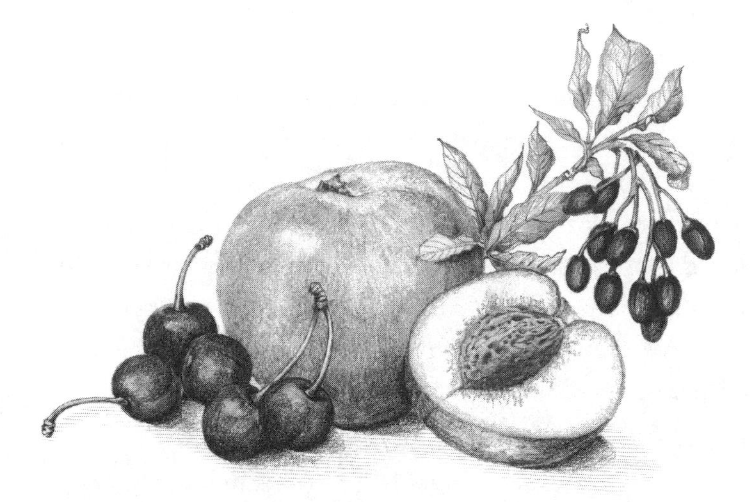

Bing cherries, peach, and wild plum

Stone fruits are a family of soft-fleshed fruits that have a large hard seed, or "stone," instead of individual seeds. Peaches, nectarines, apricots, cherries, and plums are the most popular stone fruits in this country.

Stone fruits are not as well liked as they were just a few decades ago. In fact, some people have stopped buying them altogether because they have been disappointed time and again by the texture and flavor of the fruit sold in conventional supermarkets. Why spend good money on fruit that fails to ripen or is mealy, leathery, or dry? Bananas and oranges are a safer bet. Armed with the information in this chapter, though, you will become an expert in selecting the best-tasting, most nutritious stone fruits available.

PEACHES AND NECTARINES

Peaches and nectarines are identical except for one gene that codes for "fuzziness" and a few other minor traits. Proof of their twinship is that peaches appear spontaneously on nectarine trees and nectarines show up on peach trees. Their common ancestor, according to ancient Chinese manuscripts, is a small, bitter, hairy fruit native to China that was domesticated as early as 4000 BC. Through careful breeding and selection, Chinese fruit growers began to transform the unpleasant fruit into much more palatable varieties. Alexander the Great, the peripatetic fruit lover, tasted some of those peaches during his fourth-century BC campaign against Persia. He found the fruit so desirable that he gathered some of the pits and sent them back to Greece. In Europe, the fruit became known as Persian apples.

One thousand years later, peaches and nectarines were growing throughout Europe and Asia. Records show that peach trees were growing in the royal garden of Edward I at Westminster in 1276. In the late fifteenth century, Spanish explorers brought peaches to what is now the southeastern United States. The trees did so well in their new environment that they became feral and spread up the East Coast. Native Americans harvested large quantities of the fruit. When early English explorers encountered forests of peach trees, they assumed that peaches were native to the New World.

Peaches were very popular during the colonial period. In 1815, Thomas Jefferson wrote to his daughter Martha Randolph, "We abound in the luxury of the peach." This was an understatement. In one year alone, Jefferson ordered the planting of 1,157 peach and nectarine trees in his North Orchard at Monticello. This ambitious undertaking included thirty-eight named varieties and even more unknown varieties that he had grown from pits or received as gifts.

Jefferson and his entourage consumed the peaches in a multitude of ways. Many of the peaches were made into pies, cakes, and tarts. An unsweetened peach pudding was served with savory meat dishes. Some of the fruit was turned into a popular alcoholic drink called mobby punch. When the punch was distilled, it made a fine peach brandy. One year, a severe frost killed most of Jefferson's peach trees, and this led to his discovery that peach trees make excellent firewood as well.

At the turn of the nineteenth century, Americans could choose from hundreds of varieties of peaches. Most of them are now extinct; all that is left is their glowing descriptions. The Lafayette Free peach, according to an old fruit catalog, "is a fine dark crimson next to the sun; flesh very juicy and delicious, and deep stained with crimson throughout. A beautiful variety." The Yellow Red Rareripe had "deep yellow flesh that is rich, sweet, juicy, and of a most delicious flavor. A very first-rate and extraordinary variety."

THE LOSS OF FLAVOR AND JUICINESS

We are less pleased with our peaches and nectarines today—at least those sold in conventional markets. To the dismay of California fruit growers, sales have been flat for more than twenty years. To learn the reasons for the flagging sales, researchers at the University of California asked 1,552 randomly selected consumers to describe their recent experiences with peaches. The researchers got what they asked for. The most common complaints were that supermarket peaches were "too soft," "not sweet," "not ready to eat," "overripe," "mealy," and "stringy." Respondents also complained that the peaches spoiled too quickly and had a lackluster flavor. No wonder sales have been down.

What is the reason for the dismal quality of our supermarket peaches and nectarines? As is true for most soft fruits, stone fruits are picked before they are ripe in order to prolong their shelf life and make them more durable for transport. Like many fruits, they will continue to ripen after harvest—provided they are kept under ideal conditions. The problem is that stone fruits have a unique requirement: their internal temperature must be kept above fifty degrees at all times during transport and storage. If they become chilled, they are vulnerable to a condition called chilling injury, or CI. When stone fruits develop CI, they can become dry, brown, leathery, or mealy—or fail to ripen altogether. CI is common in the stone fruit industry because the temperature inside many warehouses and refrigerated trucks drops below fifty degrees at some point in time. According to a 2002 University of California survey, as many as eight out of every ten peaches are exposed to the conditions that trigger CI. This is the hidden reason that so many of the peaches and nectarines sold in supermarkets fail to live up to our expectations.

CHOOSING THE BEST PEACHES AND NECTARINES IN THE SUPERMARKET

You can reduce the odds of bringing home cold-damaged fruit if you select those that are ripe or nearly ripe. Because they have already begun to soften and ripen, you know that they were not severely damaged by CI. How do you pick ripe fruit? You can't judge by the redness of the skin, unfortunately. Some of the newest varieties have been bred to have a dark red blush when still immature, giving them the illusion of ripeness. To get around this subterfuge, choose peaches and nectarines by their *background* color, not their blush. When white-fleshed peaches and nectarines are ripe, they have a creamy white background with little or no trace of green. Ripe yellow-fleshed varieties have a cream-colored or yellow background, not white or green. Once you have selected fruits with the right background color, press them gently between the palms of your hands to confirm their overall ripeness. Ripe peaches have a slight give.

There are also ways to choose some of the most nutritious peaches and nectarines in the store, even when the varietal names are not mentioned. Simply choose white-fleshed varieties rather than yellow-fleshed varieties—another exception to the shop-by-color rule. Lab studies show that you would have to eat six yellow-fleshed Flavorcrest peaches to get the same antioxidant benefits as in one white-fleshed Snow King. The same is true for nectarines. The white-fleshed nectarine Brite Pearl has six times more antioxidants than the yellow May Glo. The white varieties are sweeter as well. (The added sugar in the sweeter peaches is not enough to cause a significant rise in blood sugar.) If you do nothing more than choose white peaches and nectarines over the yellow varieties, you will gain a nutritional edge.

The skin of peaches and nectarines is the most nutritious part. The skin of a Champagne peach, for example, has three times more phytonutrients per ounce than the flesh. Eat the skins whenever possible. If you dislike eating fuzzy-skinned peaches, wipe the peaches with a damp cloth to remove some of the fuzz, or switch to nectarines.

If you eat the skins, buy organically certified fruit. Year after year, peaches and nectarines are counted among our most contaminated fruits. In a recent survey, 95 percent of randomly selected peaches and nectarines tested positive for pesticide residues. Some individual peaches had traces of up to sixty-seven different chemicals—more than any other fruit or vegetable in the survey. If you choose organic fruit, you will not be exposed to such an onslaught of pesticides. You might get more antioxidant protection as well. An Italian study determined that one variety of peaches that was raised organically had significantly more phytonutrients than the same variety that was raised using conventional methods.

BEYOND THE SUPERMARKET

The best peaches and nectarines of all are locally grown and harvested when ripe. No fruit can develop chilling injury if it remains on the tree until it's ready to eat. Some supermarkets feature locally produced fruit during peak season; take advantage of this opportunity. The stone fruits sold in farmers markets are ripe and freshly harvested, and most of them are organically grown as well. In these venues, you will also be able to shop by variety. Some of the most nutritious varieties include Snow Giant, Snow King, September Sun, Spring Crest, Brite Pearl, Red Jim, and Stark Red Gold. Be on the lookout for peaches with red flesh, which are known as blood peaches. As you can see by the graph below, they are the most nutritious of them all. Turn to the chart on pages 295–96 for additional recommendations.

If you spend half a day picking peaches at a U-pick orchard, you will be able to harvest enough fruit to can or freeze. Freezing preserves more antioxidants than canning. To preserve the most antioxidant activity when freezing, slice the fruit and sprinkle it with sugar, powdered vitamin C, powdered pectin, or a combination of all three. You will also find commercial "stay-fresh" products in the supermarket. Thaw the frozen fruit in the microwave to retain the most nutrients.

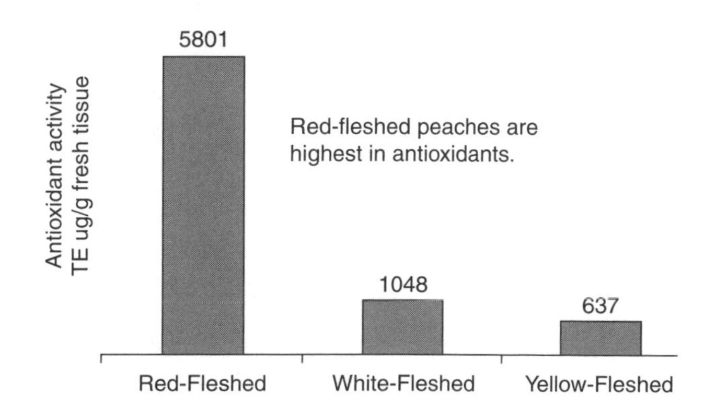

APRICOTS

Apricots (*Prunus armeniaca*) are native to western China, according to most botanists. The wild fruits, which still grow in that region, are about half the size of our modern varieties. They are also less juicy, less sweet, and more acidic. In remote, high-altitude regions of India, villagers still harvest them. They eat some of the apricots fresh and dry the rest to eat throughout the year. One traditional drying method is to place the fruit on top of the thatched roofs. The sun dries the apricots in less than a week. Once the fruit is dried, villagers sometimes boil it in a small amount of water and add a little jaggery, or raw sugar. The apricots are left to soak overnight. In the morning, the fruit mash—a low-sugar version of our apricot jam—is spread on fresh bread.

Some of the wild apricots gathered in India have bitter or poisonous kernels. Others have sweet and edible kernels. The villagers eat the sweet kernels as they would almonds and press the oil to use in cooking. (The kernels of our supermarket apricots are not edible, as they contain measurable amounts of cyanide.)

Apricots were first cultivated several thousand years ago. In the centuries that followed, generations of clever farmers developed new varieties that were larger and more pleasing to eat. Alexander the Great became acquainted with these "improved" apricots while traveling in Persia. He brought apricot pits back to Greece to plant in his own orchard. Within a few centuries, apricots had spread throughout southern Europe.

Apricots were one of the most popular fruits growing in the Mediterranean "pleasure gardens" that began to appear in the homes of the wealthy during the first few centuries AD. These walled gardens had sunken paths and shaded areas with marble benches. Fountains and statuary were interspersed between fruit and nut trees. The fruit could be harvested year-round, thanks to the warm Mediterranean climate. During hot, cloudless summers, the pleasure gardens were a cool, green oasis; ripe, orange apricots completed the picture.

In 1542, a French priest and gardener to King Henry VIII toured the continent in search of the most delectable fruit to grow in the king's garden. The priest sampled apricots in Italy and decided they were worthy enough for the king's table. About two hundred years later, apricots were brought to North America. People soon realized that the trees were ideally suited for California's Mediterranean climate.

MODERN VARIETIES OF APRICOTS

Today, 95 percent of US apricots are grown in California's central valleys. They have retained far more nutrients than most people realize. As a rule, apricots have from three to eight times more phytonutrients than peaches or nectarines. Like all stone fruits, however, they are picked when semiripe so they can be handled with minimal damage and spoilage. If all goes well, the fruit ripens in the warehouse, grocery store, or on your kitchen counter. But if apricots are chilled before they are ripe, they, too, are vulnerable to chilling injury.

Some of the new varieties have been bred to meet the needs of large-scale producers more than consumers. Apricots bruise very easily, so new extra firm cultivars have been developed that are less prone to damage. They are also less juicy. Some varieties have been bred to ripen early in the year so they can be sold before other varieties reach the market. These early bloomers tend to be much less nutritious than varieties that ripen weeks later. A 2010 study of twenty-seven varieties of apricots revealed that varieties that ripen in May have, on average, only one-fifth the amount of antioxidants as varieties that mature in August. "Slow growing" deserves to be an important part of the slow food movement.

CHOOSING THE BEST APRICOTS IN THE SUPERMARKET AND FARMERS MARKETS

You can revel in the most delicious and nutritious apricots by making wise choices in the food markets. First, if you wait until midsummer to buy apricots, they are likely to be riper and more nutritious than those that are available earlier in the year. In addition, make sure that the apricots are ripe; this way you won't be stuck with semiripe apricots that fail to ripen when you bring them home. A ripe apricot is plump and tight-skinned. Its skin is yellow or orange, with only minimal amounts of pale yellow. Finally, it gives a little when you touch it gently in the middle.

At farmers markets, specialty produce stores, and local orchards, you will be able to shop by variety. One variety to look for is the Royal Blenheim, or simply Blenheim. It is a venerable fruit that has been grown for its rich flavor and delicate texture for more than sixteen generations. We now know that it is also richer in beta-carotene than most other varieties. For more suggestions, see the list of varieties on page 297.

DRIED APRICOTS

In the United States, we eat three times more dried apricots than fresh apricots. Apricots destined for drying are picked when they are fully ripe and most flavorful, which is a point in their favor. Unfortunately, drying them in the sun destroys many of their nutrients. As the fruit dries, enzymes begin to degrade its beneficial compounds. The longer the fruit takes to dry, the less nutritious it becomes. Sun-dried apricots have about half the phytonutrient content of the fresh-picked fruit. For greater retention of nutrients, purchase apricots that have been "tunnel-dried" or "hot-air dried," which is a speedier process. Tunnel-dried apricots have 75 percent more antioxidants than sun-dried fruit.

Typically, apricots in this country are treated with sulfur dioxide before they are dried, a practice that began early in the twentieth century. The sulfur kills microbes and prevents the fruit from turning brown. It wasn't until 2007 that tests showed that sulfured apricots have far *more* antioxidants than dark-colored, untreated apricots. The reason is that the sulfur slows down the activity of the antioxidant-destroying enzymes. What about the negative effects of sulfur? Some people are allergic to high concentrations of sulfites and should avoid all sulfured products. The FDA removed sulfured fruit from its Generally Recognized as Safe (GRAS) list for this reason. Most people have no ill effects, however. Nonetheless, many people have stopped buying sulfur-treated fruit whether it harms them or not. The fewer chemicals the better, according to their point of view.

For a chemical-free alternative, you can dry apricots at home in a food dehydrator. Select ripe, deep orange apricots. The faster you dry them, the more antioxidants they retain. The standard temperature setting for home-dried fruit is 120–130 degrees Fahrenheit. If you raise the temperature to 190 degrees, you will create a more nutritious product. At the higher temperature, you will need to monitor the apricots more closely to prevent them from becoming too dry. You can find more detailed information on drying fruit on numerous websites.

If you buy sulfur-treated apricots, you can choose them on the basis of color, because sulfured fruit retains its original hue. Most of the varieties of apricots grown in Turkey are yellow or yellow-orange in color. They are lower in beta-carotene than most American varieties and less sweet as well. The most nutritious sulfured apricots are deep orange or red-orange. Dried Blenheim apricots are red-orange and have a superb flavor and soft texture. If you cannot find them in a store, you can order them on the Internet.

CHERRIES

The *Prunus virginiana* wild cherry tree is native to the United States. Two hundred years ago, it was growing in every region of the country except the Southeast. The common name for the fruit is chokecherry. You wouldn't choke if you ate them, but you would probably spit them out.

Despite their bitterness, the fruit was consumed by many North

American tribes. Daniel Moerman, a leading authority on the diet of Native Americans, lists more tribal uses for chokecherries than any other plant. Chokecherries, it's been discovered in recent years, are extremely high in phytonutrients, surpassing all other wild fruits, including wild blueberries. They have a remarkable twenty times more antioxidants than our modern cherries. It does not matter how nutritious a food is for you, though, if it is too bitter to enjoy. Chokecherries fall into that category.

Our modern cherries come from a different part of the world and from a different species altogether. Sweet cherries come from a wild species called *Prunus avium,* and sour cherries come from the species *Prunus cerasus.* Both are native to western Asia. Wild sweet cherries are small, dark-colored, and either sweet or bitter, but never sour. Sour cherries are, as you might suppose, quite sour. Sweet and sour cherries were domesticated more than two thousand years ago. Pliny the Elder, writing in the first century AD, mentioned eight different varieties of cherries, all of them clones of select trees. He reported that cherries were highly favored in Rome and that they were growing as far away as Great Britain.

Cherries were one of the first Old World fruits to be grown in this country. French settlers in New York planted thousands of cherry pits from their best French varieties, creating vast cherry orchards along the Saint Lawrence River. There was great demand for this fruit, given the fact that most European expats found the North American wild cherries inedible. Massachusetts colonist William Wood, writing in 1629, did not mince words. "The [wild] Cherry trees yield great store of cherries which grow in clusters like grapes; they be much smaller than our English cherry. . . .They so furre the mouth that the tongue will cleave to the roof and the throat wax hoarse with swallowing those red Bullies (as I may call them)." Not surprisingly, no attempt was made to domesticate the wild North American cherries when superior fruit trees could be imported from Europe.

It wasn't long before American farmers began crafting their own varieties of the European fruit. They planted the pits, let the trees grow to maturity, and then sampled the fruit. The trees that produced the most promising cherries were propagated by grafting. Our most popular cherry, the Bing cherry, was created by a determined nurseryman from Iowa named Henderson Luelling. In 1847, forty-year-old Luelling gathered up his wife, eight children, and seven hundred select varieties of young trees and shrubs and transported them all by ox-driven wagon train over the Oregon Trail from Missouri to Milwaukie, Oregon, a distance of seventeen hundred miles. His sturdiest wagon carried the traveling nursery. Along the way, people tried to persuade him to leave the heavy wagon behind, warning him that he was jeopardizing his oxen and his family by hauling it. Luelling would have no part of it. He and his family arrived safely in Milwaukie that fall, and he went to work planting his orchard and propagating new trees. Just six years later, he had one hundred thousand trees for sale, which he sold for between one dollar and a dollar and a half apiece—a small fortune at the time.

The Bing cherry grew from a pit of one of those trees. The tree produced such sweet and attractive fruit that Luelling cloned it and named it after one of his Chinese workers. All the Bing cherries grown today can be traced back to that one tree. Another popular variety, the Lambert, a dark red heart-shaped fruit, also came from his orchard. The Bing and the Lambert are two of the most widely grown sweet cherries today.

CHOOSING THE BEST CHERRIES IN THE SUPERMARKET

Sweet cherries and sour, or "pie," cherries are sold in most supermarkets. Sweet cherries are usually eaten fresh. The sour cherries are made into pies, cobblers, and other desserts. Some varieties are much more nutritious than others. Fortunately, most supermarkets display the varietal names of their cherries, so it is easy to select the best ones. Luelling's Bing cherries are an excellent choice. You will find them in most supermarkets from early May to late June. They are tops in anthocyanins and have been shown to calm inflammation and reduce the levels of several compounds that are linked with arthritis and gout. They have an excellent flavor as well. Brooks cherries are also nutritious and tasty.

The Rainier variety is a supersweet cherry that was introduced in 1952. It has one-fourth the antioxidant value of the Bing. People who love Rainiers, however, are likely to keep buying them nonetheless. They are so sweet that people are willing to pay as much as five to six dollars a pound for them. Recently, they sold for more than one dollar *apiece* in Japan. Royal Anne (also known as Queen Anne) cherries resemble Rainiers, but they are not as sweet and are considerably higher in phytonutrients. You'll find information about other varieties on pages 298–99.

BEYOND THE SUPERMARKET

When you shop in farmers markets and specialty stores, you will find a larger variety of cherries than you will find in the supermarket. The most popular sour cherry is the Montmorency. Studies show that Montmorency cherries can reduce pain and inflammation, including pain caused by strenuous exercise. In 2009, a group of fifty-seven male and female runners took part in a study conducted by the Oregon Health and Science University School of Medicine. The participants were scheduled to compete in Oregon's Hood to Coast Relay race, a challenging two-hundred-mile course that traverses two mountain ranges. The runners in one group drank two glasses of Montmorency cherry juice—one before the race began and one during the race. The volunteers in the other group consumed an equal amount of a cherry-flavored drink. When the race was over, the runners who drank the real cherry juice reported significantly less pain. A similar study showed that tart cherries can speed muscle recovery after exercise.

Another sour cherry to look for is Balaton. Although not quite as rich in phytonutrients as the Montmorency, it is still more nutritious than most other cherries. It, too, has proven anti-inflammatory properties. The Balaton was developed in Hungary, where it continues to be a highly sought-after fruit. Hungarians eat it raw, enjoying its tart flavor.

At the present time, it is easier to buy products made from tart cherries than the actual cherries themselves. You can find these products in natural-food stores, dietary-supplement stores, and on the Internet. Both the juice and the dried fruit retain a significant amount of the cherries' antioxidant properties. Tart cherries that are dried without added sugar have more antioxidant value than those dried with sugar. (Dried Bing cherries, although sweet, are also rich in phytonutrients.) The interest in the health benefits of tart cherries is growing, so expect to see a larger crop of them in the coming years. If you have room, grow a tree of your own. You don't have to grow the enormous cherry trees of the past. You can plant dwarf or semidwarf trees, which makes it much easier to harvest the fruit and safeguard it from birds. Toss bird netting over the trees when the cherries are almost ripe, and most of the crop will make it into your kitchen. See pages 298–99 for recommendations of specific varieties.

EAT CHERRIES — DON'T STORE THEM

All cherries have a rapid respiration rate that starts to deplete the fruit's antioxidants as soon as it is picked. Buy the freshest cherries you can find. Fresh cherries are firm, shiny, and free of dents, bruises, and tiny pits. The best indicator of freshness, however, is the color and flexibility of the stem. The stems respire fifteen times faster than the fruit itself, so they are the first to show their true age. Fresh cherries have bright green stems that are supple but firm. If the stems are withered or turning brown, the cherries were harvested long ago. Don't buy them.

Choosing the freshest cherries could make a significant difference in your health. A 2004 lab study showed that freshly harvested cherries can slow the oxidation of LDL cholesterol. Oxidized cholesterol is most likely to clog your arteries and trigger a heart attack or stroke. In the study, cherries that had been picked just a few days earlier had lost this protective property. Look for those bright green stems!

US cherries have three times more pesticides than imported cherries, according to data from the FDA and the Environmental Protection Agency, which is the opposite of what some people would think. As many as sixteen different pesticides have been found on a single batch of US cherries. In a recent year, only 2 percent of imported cherries had been sprayed with more than one pesticide. Buy organic cherries to reduce your exposure to these noxious chemicals.

When you harvest cherries or bring them home from the store, refrigerate them right away. Place them in a microperforated plastic bag to allow a slow exchange of gases. Store the fruit in the crisper drawer of your refrigerator and eat it as soon as possible.

It Doesn't Get Any Fresher Than This!

Lord Ludovico Sforza, the Duke of Milan from 1489 through 1508, is best known for commissioning *The Last Supper,* Leonardo da Vinci's world-famous painting.

Although Sforza's taste in art is renowned, few know about his love of great food. The duke ordered the creation of extensive fruit and vegetable gardens in the area surrounding his Milan castle. The gardens were so productive that they supplied much of the fresh produce for the castle and nearby households.

The fruit that was served to Sforza and his intimates, however, came from a more rarefied source. The duke had a private garden of fruit trees and bushes that were planted in large wheeled carts. When the duke wanted to eat some fruit, his movable feast was brought to his private chamber or the dining table so he could reach out and pluck a perfect specimen from a living plant.

Chronicle of America: A New History for a New World, volume 12, by Gonzalo Fernández de Oviedo y Valdés (1478–1557)

PLUMS AND PRUNES

The wild Indian plum (*Osmaronia cerasiformis*) grows west of the Cascade mountain range from Northern California to British Columbia. The fruit is remarkably sweet, but it is so small that it is more stone than fruit. Native Americans gathered the plums despite their small size because of their high sugar content. The Tolowa tribe of Northern California gathered large quantities of the fruit, but they had one complaint. The trees bloomed in February, which raised their hopes of an early feast, but the plums didn't ripen until summer, long after other fruits had been harvested. The Tolowa considered this to be false advertising. Their name for wild plum trees means "the tree that lies."

The Indian plum and all other wild plums are highly nutritious. The Australian Kakadu plum has more vitamin C than any other food analyzed to date—three thousand milligrams per serving, which is fifty times more than is contained in one serving of oranges. The Kakadu has five times more antioxidants than the typical blueberry.

SHOPPING FOR PLUMS IN THE SUPERMARKET

Our modern varieties of plums cannot match the phytonutrient content of wild plums, but some varieties are very nutritious. Red, purple, blue, or black plums are your best choices. Some of these deeply pigmented fruits have even more phytonutrients than red cabbage, spinach, onions, or leeks. Plums with yellow, rose, or green skins are less nutritious because they are lower in anthocyanins.

Plums, like all stone fruits, are vulnerable to chilling injury. You can minimize this problem by buying ripe plums. Press them between your palms; ripe plums have a slight give. If you wait until July to buy plums, they are likely to be riper and more flavorful than those harvested earlier in the year. For the best quality and nutritional value, buy tree-ripened fruit from local orchards or farmers markets.

When shopping in farmers markets or buying a plum tree for your yard, look for the recommended varieties on pages 299–301. Cacak's Best, French Damson, Italian Prune, and Stanley are among the most nutritious.

How Do Prunes "Work"?

Why do prunes and prune juice help people stay regular?

The main reason is that they are high in soluble and insoluble fiber. The soluble fiber softens the stool, and the insoluble fiber speeds it on its way.

Prunes also contain a sugar called sorbitol, which promotes the growth of microorganisms in the colon, which in turn promotes regularity.

DRIED PLUMS

Dried plums, formerly known as prunes, are making a comeback. In previous decades, they were best known for their laxative properties and were associated with constipated, "prune-faced" adults. In 2000, after ten years of declining sales, the California Prune Board decided it was time to upgrade the fruit's image. The board commissioned a consumer survey and discovered that 90 percent of the participants would be more likely to buy prunes if they were renamed dried plums. Armed with this information, the board persuaded the FDA to approve the name change. With the new alias, prune sales began to climb. The French D'Agen plum is the most popular variety for drying. Perhaps the California Prune Board—now called the California Dried Plum Board—should consider another name change: "dried *French* plums" might set off a buying frenzy.

It's more than the name change that is boosting sales, however. Prunes are proving to be higher in antioxidants than many other nutritious fruits, including most varieties of blueberries and strawberries. A new finding is that they can also strengthen bones. In a yearlong British study, 160 postmenopausal women with low bone density (osteopenia) took part in a fruit-eating experiment. For a year, each volunteer consumed a daily serving of dried apples or dried plums. Measurements taken during and after the study showed that the consumption of both dried fruits led to an increase in bone density, but the women eating the prunes showed the greatest improvement. The reason that prunes help build bone, the researchers believe, is that they reduce the inflammation that contributes to bone loss. Prunes are also a good source of the mineral boron, which can speed bone development.

Once upon a time, all plums were sun-dried. Today, most of them are dried in hot-air tunnels that dehydrate them more rapidly, thus preserving more antioxidants. The plums do not need to be treated with sulfur to prevent them from browning, because they are dark-colored to begin with. Dried plums are an overlooked, inexpensive superfood. Although they are high in natural sugars, they are rich enough in antioxidants to reduce most of the negative effects of the sugar.

In today's supermarkets, you will find two kinds of dried plums—plums that have been soaked in juice or syrup to make them sweeter and softer, and plums that have been dried without any additional ingredients. The ones that have not been soaked in liquid can be quite firm and chewy. In the past, people soaked dried prunes in water or stewed them to soften them. To stew prunes, put them in a saucepan with enough water to cover. Bring to a boil, lower the heat, and simmer for twenty minutes. Add a slice of lemon or a little sugar for more flavor.

SAVORY PLUM SAUCE

PREP TIME: 5 MINUTES
COOKING TIME: 30 MINUTES
TOTAL TIME: 35 MINUTES YIELD: 1½ CUPS

1 clove garlic
12 red, blue, or black plums, pitted and cut in half
½ cup red wine
1 tablespoon unsalted butter
⅛ teaspoon salt
⅛ teaspoon ground cloves
½ teaspoon ground cinnamon
1 tablespoon honey or firmly packed light or dark brown sugar

Push the garlic through a garlic press and set aside. Combine the plums and red wine in a medium saucepan and simmer, uncovered, for 10 minutes. Cover and simmer for an additional 10 minutes.

Add the reserved garlic and the remaining ingredients, cover, and simmer for another 10 minutes. Add a tablespoon or two of water if needed to maintain a pourable consistency. Spoon into the bowl of a food processor or blender and pulse ten times, or until the peels are finely chopped. Serve warm over beef, pork, poultry, or lamb.

RECOMMENDED VARIETIES OF PEACHES AND NECTARINES

IN THE SUPERMARKET	
TYPE	COMMENTS
White-fleshed	White-fleshed peaches and nectarines are higher in phytonutrients than yellow-fleshed varieties. The skin is the most nutritious part of the fruit. Peaches and nectarines are sprayed with a significant amount of pesticides. Buy organic fruit to lower your exposure to these unwanted chemicals.

FARMERS MARKETS, SPECIALTY STORES, U-PICK FARMS, AND NURSERIES		
PEACHES	DESCRIPTION	INFORMATION FOR GARDENERS
Champagne	Large, white-fleshed, freestone peach. Light-colored blush over cream-colored skin. Juicy, sweet, and low in acid. Fine-textured. High in antioxidants, especially in the skin. Released in 1982.	Best for zones 7–9. Peaches ripen in mid-August. Vigorous, productive tree.
Indian Blood Cling	A large clingstone peach with red skin and white flesh streaked with red. Aromatic when ripe. Uncommon. High in anthocyanins and overall antioxidants. Heirloom from the 1700s.	Best for zones 4–8. Ripens in mid-September. A heavy producer. Does best with a pollinator.
O'Henry	Large, firm peach with yellow flesh that is streaked with red. Great flavor. Heirloom variety. Higher in antioxidants than most other yellow-fleshed varieties.	Best for zones 6–9. Midseason harvest. Strong, vigorous, heavy-bearing, and self-pollinating.

PEACHES	DESCRIPTION	INFORMATION FOR GARDENERS
September Sun	Juicy, firm, yellow-fleshed freestone peach. Very high in antioxidant value for a yellow-fleshed variety.	Best for zones 5–9. Late-season peach that ripens from late August to early September.
Snow Giant	White-fleshed freestone peach. Very large, firm, and sweet with low acidity. Red blush over creamy white skin. Slightly lower in phytonutrients than Snow King.	Best for zones 4B–8B. Late August harvest.
Snow King	Large, red-skinned, sweet-flavored peach with white flesh. Has the highest antioxidant content of all the varieties of peaches recommended in this chart. Introduced in 1993.	Best for zones 5–9. August harvest. Self-pollinating.
Spring Crest (also called Springcrest)	Medium-size peach with little fuzz. Firm, yellow flesh with skin that blushes red. In one study, second highest in nutritional content of 11 varieties tested.	Best for zones 5–9. Early-season variety. Ripens from late May through mid-June.
NECTARINES	DESCRIPTION	INFORMATION FOR GARDENERS
Arctic Snow	White-fleshed freestone nectarine. Low-acid, sweet fruit that is rich in phytonutrients.	Best for zones 5–9. Late-harvest variety. Ripens from the last week of August to the first week in September.
Brite Pearl (also called Bright Pearl)	White-fleshed nectarine that is very high in antioxidants. The skin is much richer in phytonutrients than the flesh.	Best for zones 5–9. Not cold-hardy.
Crimson Gold	Yellow-fleshed freestone nectarine with a bright red blush over golden skin.	Best for zones 5–9. Ripens in July.
John Boy II	Yellow-fleshed freestone nectarine. Sweet and tart.	Best for Zones 5–9. Vigorous grower. Earliest-ripening nectarine.
Red Jim	Red-fleshed clingstone nectarine. Rich in anthocyanins.	Best for zones 5A–9B.
Zee Fire	Yellow-fleshed clingstone nectarine. Skin has a red blush over yellow skin. Supersweet, low in acid, and quite firm. Among the highest in phytonutrients.	Best for zones 5–9. Ripens in May. Productive. Good for warm climates, as it does not require long, cool winters to bear fruit.

RECOMMENDED VARIETIES OF APRICOTS

IN THE SUPERMARKET	
VARIETY	COMMENTS
All varieties	Apricots are more nutritious than peaches and nectarines. For the most phytonutrients, choose apricots with dark orange or red-orange skin and flesh. Ask the produce manager to cut one open for you.

FARMERS MARKETS, SPECIALTY STORES, U-PICK FARMS, AND NURSERIES		
VARIETY	DESCRIPTION	INFORMATION FOR GARDENERS
Blenheim	Firm, light orange flesh with a very good, intense flavor. Medium-to-large-size fruit. Thirty percent of apricots grown in California are Blenheims.	Best for zones 4–8. Ripens from June to early July. Self-pollinating.
Goldstrike	Large, firm fruit. Light orange flesh and slightly glossy skin. Firm, meaty, and moderately juicy. Excellent flavor and texture.	Best for zones 4–8. Ripens in early July. Rapid-growing tree. Requires a pollinator.
Hargrand	Very large, sweet, and juicy apricot with deep orange skin and flesh. Very high ORAC value – twice as high as many varieties of red grapes. Freestone. Released in 1980.	Best for zones 4–8. Winter-hardy. Fruits in mid-to-late July. Self-pollinating and disease-resistant.
Harogem	Medium-size fruit with a bright red glossy blush over orange background. Ten times higher in beta-carotene than the average peach. Released in 1979.	Best for zones 4–8. Very cold-hardy. Fruits from June through July. Resistant to brown rot and perennial canker.
Robada	Large, juicy, with a good balance between sweet and acid. Attractive skin color with a red blush. Deep orange flesh.	Best for zones 5–8. Fruits from late May to mid-June. Vigorous and productive variety.
Wilson Delicious	Golden orange fruit with a rich, distinctive flavor. Third highest in antioxidants in a survey of 22 varieties.	Best for zones 5–8. Ripens in early July. Heavy bearer. Self-pollinating.

RECOMMENDED VARIETIES OF CHERRIES

IN THE SUPERMARKET	
VARIETY	COMMENTS
Bing	Very common sweet cherry with skin that ranges from dark red to almost black. One of the most nutritious varieties. Fresh cherries have bright green, flexible stems.
Hartland	Sweet, firm, glossy purple cherry. Highest in antioxidants of sweet cherries in a recent survey.
Royal Anne (also called Queen Anne)	Sweet, large, firm cherries with yellow skin and a red blush. Twice as high in phytonutrients as Rainier cherries, which they closely resemble.

FARMERS MARKETS, SPECIALTY STORES, U-PICK FARMS, AND NURSERIES		
VARIETY	DESCRIPTION	INFORMATION FOR GARDENERS
Balaton	Tangy, large, firm cherry with red juicy flesh. Hungarian heirloom.	Best for zones 5–8. July harvest. Vigorous trees.
Bing	Very common sweet cherry with dark red to almost black skin. One of the most nutritious varieties. Rich in anthocyanins. US heirloom.	Best for zones 5–9. Requires a pollinator.
Early Black (also called Knight's Early Black)	Skin a dark, dull red; almost black when fully ripe. Significantly higher in anthocyanins than most other varieties. Heirloom variety from 1810. Rare.	Best for zones 5–8. Ripens in mid-June. Crack-resistant and hardy.
Hartland	Sweet, firm, glossy purple cherries. Less sweet than some sweet cherries but ranks high in flavor nonetheless. Highest in antioxidants of sweet cherries in a recent survey.	Best for zones 5–9. Midseason producer. Requires a pollinator. Winter-hardy. Heavy-bearing. Disease-resistant and resistant to cracking and rot.

VARIETY	DESCRIPTION	INFORMATION FOR GARDENERS
Montmorency	Tangy, medium-large, bright red sour cherry. Great in cherry pies. Proven anti-inflammatory properties.	Best for zones 4–9. Ripens in June. Upright tree with an abundance of cherries.
Royal Anne (also Queen Anne)	Sweet, large, firm cherries with yellow skin and a red blush. Twice as high in antioxidants as Rainier cherries, which are similar in appearance.	Best for zones 4–9. Ripens in late May and early June. Partially self-fertile but benefits from having a pollinator.
Summit	Sweet, crisp, and juicy. Very large, heart-shaped, dark red fruit with light pink flesh. Moderately firm, with a small stone.	Best for zones 5–8. Early-season cherry ripens in mid-June. Requires a pollinator. Fairly resistant to cracking.

RECOMMENDED VARIETIES OF PLUMS

IN THE SUPERMARKET	
TYPE	COMMENTS
Red, dark blue, and black	Plums with red, dark blue, and black skins are more nutritious than yellow- or green-skinned varieties.

FARMERS MARKETS, SPECIALTY STORES, U-PICK FARMS, AND NURSERIES		
VARIETY	DESCRIPTION	INFORMATION FOR GARDENERS
Angeleno (also called Angelina)	Large, purple-skinned fruit. One of the top 10 varieties produced in California. Highest in antioxidants in a survey of 5 varieties.	Late-season variety. Ripens in mid-September. Very good producer.

VARIETY	DESCRIPTION	INFORMATION FOR GARDENERS
Autumn Sweet	Very sweet clingstone plum. Second highest in antioxidants of 11 varieties. New release. Similar to Italian Prune plum, but larger.	Best for zones 5–8. Late-season variety. Winter-hardy. Heavy-bearing.
Black Beaut	Large, dark purple fruit with gorgeous red flesh. Juicy and moderately sweet. Second highest in antioxidants in a survey of 5 varieties. One of the first plums to ripen in the summer.	Best in zones 5–9. Ripens in early June. Once popular in California, but no longer so.
Black Diamond	Hard-to-find, highly nutritious plum. Very high ORAC value of 7,581, which is higher than artichokes and black beans.	Best in zones 5–9. Early-to-midseason variety.
Cacak's Best	Large, blue-black plum with pale yellow flesh from Yugoslavia. Freestone. One of the 3 most nutritious plums in a 2003 study.	Best in zones 5–8. Midseason variety. Requires pollinator. Good resistance to the plum pox virus. A healthy tree with an open crown.
Castleton	High-quality, medium-size, blue-skinned fruit that resembles the Stanley variety. Released in 1993.	Best in zones 4–7. Tolerates cold winters. Ripens in August. Self-pollinating. Good bearer.
French Damson (also called Damson)	Small, round plum with blue skin and green flesh. Flavor can be too intense and tart for some people. One of the 3 most nutritious plums in a 2003 study.	Best in zones 5–9. Ripens in mid-September. Pest- and disease-resistant.
Italian Prune	Medium-to-large fruit with dark purple skin and yellow-green fruit. The plum that's most commonly made into prunes. Very sweet, but with a hint of lemon.	Best for zones 5–9. Heavy bearer. Self-pollinating.
Longjohn (also called Long John)	Blue-colored plum with an elongated teardrop shape. Freestone. Third highest in antioxidants in a study of 11 varieties. Developed in 1993.	Best for zones 5–9. Upright tree, somewhat willowy in shape. Partially self-pollinating, but does better with another pollinator.

VARIETY	DESCRIPTION	INFORMATION FOR GARDENERS
Red Beaut (also called Red Beauty)	Pleasantly sweet with a fairly tart skin. Medium-size, with a bright red skin that turns purple when ripe.	Best for zones 5–9. Early-season variety. Ripens in late May. Requires a pollinator.
Stanley	Firm, tender, large plum with dark blue skin. Sweet. Common.	Best for zones 5–9. Late-summer harvest. Late-blooming. Self-pollinating, but does best with another pollinator. Large, reliable crop.

STONE FRUITS: POINTS TO REMEMBER

1. ***Buy ripe or nearly ripe stone fruits.***
   Stone fruits that are exposed to cold temperatures when they are immature may never fully ripen, or their flesh may turn brown, dry, or leathery. If you buy nearly ripe or ripe fruit, you increase the odds that the fruit will be of reasonable quality.

2. ***Choose peaches and nectarines with care.***
   When buying peaches and nectarines in the supermarket, look for ripe fruit that has a creamy yellow or white background with only traces of green. The fruit should be free of dents and bruises and have a slight give when you press it gently between your palms. As a rule, white-fleshed peaches and nectarines are richer in phytonutrients than yellow-fleshed varieties.

3. ***Eat the skins.***
   When you eat the skin of stone fruits, you are getting all the health benefits they have to offer. If you don't like to eat peach fuzz, you can "defuzz" a peach by wiping it gently with a damp cloth. You can also switch to nectarines, which are the same species. Buy organic fruit to limit your exposure to pesticides, which are most concentrated in the skin.

4. ***Shop for dried apricots by color.***
   Most conventionally raised apricots are treated with sulfur dioxide before they are dried to kill bacteria and fungus and maintain a light color. This process also retains more of their phytonutrients. Some people are acutely sensitive to products containing sulfur dioxide, but most experience no ill effects. Dried apricots made from deep orange or orange-red fruits are more nutritious than those made from yellow or light-orange fruits.
5. ***Choose the most nutritious cherries.***
   Bing cherries, the most common sweet variety, are rich in phytonutrients. Tart cherries, such as Montmorency and Balaton, help calm inflammation. All cherries are best when freshly picked. Bright green, flexible stems are the best indicator of freshness. Grow your own dwarf or semidwarf cherry tree and you can harvest the cherries of your choice from your own backyard.
6. ***Blue, black, and red plums are higher in antioxidants than yellow and green varieties.***
   The darker the color of the skin and flesh of a plum, the more anthocyanins it contains. As a general rule, varieties that mature in the summer are sweeter and less acidic than those that ripen earlier in the year. Buy ripe or nearly ripe plums to be assured of the best quality. Dried plums (formerly called prunes) are among the most nutritious foods in the grocery store.

CHAPTER 14

GRAPES AND RAISINS

FROM MUSCADINES TO THOMPSON SEEDLESS

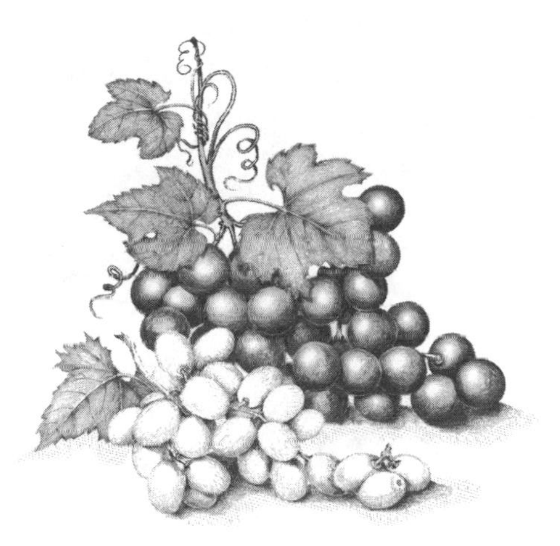

Wild and Thompson grapes

Wild muscadine grapes are round, large, dark purple fruits that grow on unruly vines. Native to the southeastern United States, they once extended from Florida to Delaware and then west to Texas. Sixteenth-century explorers were awe-struck by their wild and rampant nature. In 1584, Sir Walter Raleigh, the English explorer, spy, and courtier, described them as being "on the sand and on the green soil, on the hills as on the plains, as well as on every little shrub . . . also climbing towards the tops of tall cedars . . . in all the world the like abundance is not to be found." Raleigh was exploring Roanoke Island, off the coast of present-day North Carolina, in 1585 when he came across a monster muscadine vine. He reported that it was two feet thick at the base and sprawled over a half acre of land. The vines were wrapping around trees for support and setting fruit sixty feet above the ground. Kudzu seems tame by comparison.

The grapes were as tasty as they were prolific. Thomas Hariot, a naturalist on the Raleigh expedition, described them as "luscious sweet." The English were accustomed to the tart wine grapes of Europe, so the New World fruit seemed as sweet as candy. They are sweet by our present-day standards as well. Muscadines are almost 30 percent sugar—25 percent sweeter than most of our table grapes.

Native Americans feasted on the grapes, eating them fresh or making them into juice, raisins, and fruit leather. Italian explorer Giovanni da Verrazano explored the Cape Fear region of North Carolina in 1525 and noted that the native people "carefully remove shrubbery from around them, wherever they grow, to allow the fruit to ripen better." He also commented on the health of the Native Americans. He described them as "well featured in their limbs, of average stature, and commonly somewhat bigger than we; broad breasted, strong arms, their legs and other parts of their bodies well fashioned. . . .They are sharp-witted, nimble and great runners, as far as we could learn by experience."

Could the grapes have been contributing to their good health? Perhaps so. Muscadines are rich in fiber, zinc, manganese, iron, and calcium. The skins contain high amounts of ellagic acid, a phytonutrient with anticancer properties. In addition, muscadines have more overall antioxidant value than any of our table grapes. They even surpass pomegranates and blueberries, the new superfruits.

When the Spaniards first settled in the area they named Florida, they used their Old World wine-making skills to make muscadine wine, the first wine produced in this country. It was the most popular wine in America for 350 years. Thomas Jefferson proclaimed that it "would be distinguished on the best tables in Europe for its fine aroma and crystalline transparence." In 1920, when Prohibition put an end to the commercial production of wine, southerners weathered the dry spell by making muscadine moonshine.

Memories of Muscadines

In places the wild muscadine vines stretched from tree to tree, making arbors which were always full of butterflies and buzzing insects.

It was delightful to lose ourselves in the green hollows of that tangled wood in the late afternoon, and to smell the cool, delicious odors that came up from the earth at the close of the day.

—Helen Keller, 1903

Muscadine grapes continue to run wild in remote areas of the Southeast, but most people prefer the hybrid varieties that grow in constrained rows in commercial vineyards. The hybrids have bronze, red, or black skins. The red and black varieties are the most nutritious. Both the wild and the man-made varieties are highly resistant to disease and require little chemical intervention to fend off bacteria, mold, fungus, and insects.

Although muscadine grapes are sweet and hardy and more American than apple pie, even the new hybrids have a small following. Most people are not fond of their thick skins and many seeds, traits that have been bred out of most other grapes. The grapes have a musky flavor as well, which betrays their wild origins. A final demerit is that the fruit drops off the vine as it ripens, making it more difficult—and costly—to harvest.

Although it is difficult to find fresh muscadine grapes outside the southeastern United States, several companies are now producing muscadine extracts, powders, juices, and wine. (The processing steps involved in the manufacture of the individual products determine how many of the original nutrients are retained.) A grape that once blanketed the South has a new though more limited life as a high-priced nutraceutical. You'll find muscadine products on the Internet and in health-food stores.

DOUBLE-MUTANT THOMPSON SEEDLESS GRAPES

Our most popular grape, the Thompson seedless, outsells muscadines by a thousand to one. These pale green grapes have none of the shortcomings of the wild fruit. They have thin skins, no seeds, and not a whiff of mustiness. Although Thompson grapes look like a made-for-industry hybrid, they are an ancient heirloom that was discovered centuries ago in the Ottoman Empire, where they were known as sultaninas or sultanas. Sultaninas were different from other grapes that grew in the region because they were so light-colored. They were also free of seeds. Both these characteristics came about because of spontaneous mutations. One mutation blocked the grape's ability to produce anthocyanins, the phytonutrients that give other grapes their vibrant color and many health benefits. A second mutation eliminated their seeds, a change that made them very popular. Then, as now, people liked to eat grapes without having to spit out the seeds. Just as important, a seedless grape could be made into raisins without having to remove any seeds, which is a time-consuming process. Sultaninas were brought to California in 1863 by William Thompson, an English vintner who lent them his name.

The low phytonutrient content of Thompson seedless grapes was revealed in a 2010 study. They have only one-third to one-fourth the antioxidant activity of the red and black varieties sold in our stores. Once again, a lightweight in terms of nutrition is a heavyweight in terms of sales.

Not satisfied with nature's changes, we humans have been making our own alterations to the Thompson seedless grape. Since the 1960s, most US grape producers have been spraying them with a

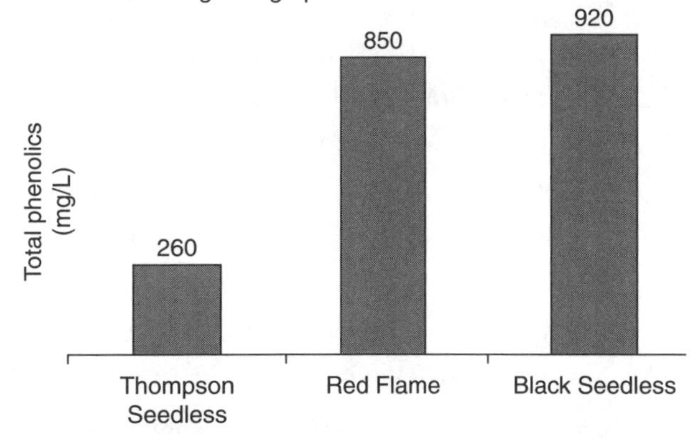

plant hormone called gibberellic acid. The hormone elongates them, which increases their overall size by as much as 75 percent. Virtually all the Thompson seedless grapes sold in the United States have been "gibbed."

To extend the market season and make the fruit easier to ship and store, they are also being harvested before they are ripe. Grapes, unlike many fruits, do not ripen once they've been harvested. If picked before their time, they remain firm and tart until they spoil. There is a marked visual and gustatory difference between Thompson seedless grapes that have been gibbed and harvested prematurely and those that have not been gibbed and allowed to ripen on the vine. The more natural grapes are smaller, rounder, more golden, less crisp, and have a sweeter and more complex flavor. Buy vine-ripened, organic Thompson seedless grapes for the best flavor and texture and to reduce your exposure to unwanted chemicals.

CONCORD GRAPES AND WELCH'S GRAPE JUICE

Concord grapes (*Vitis labrusca*), like muscadines, were born and raised in the USA. In the 1840s, a determined Massachusetts plant breeder named Ephraim Bull created the iconic variety by cross-breeding wild fox grape plants, which are native to the East Coast. He wasn't satisfied with his efforts until he had mixed and matched more than twenty-two thousand individual plants. His final creation, the Concord grape, won first place in the 1853 Massachusetts Horticultural Society exhibition. The grapes continue to gain recognition today, only now for their health benefits as well as their flavor.

Concord grape juice is the consummate all-American drink. In 1869, Dr. Thomas Bramwell Welch, a steward at a Wesleyan church in Vineland, New Jersey, began searching for a nonalcoholic beverage to serve during communion. When grapes are pressed into juice, the juice begins to ferment and turns into wine in a matter of days. Welch wanted to find a way to stop the natural fermentation process and thereby preserve the sobriety of the congregation. He developed a novel pasteurization technique that did the job. He named his juice Dr. Welch's Unfermented Wine. We now know it as Welch's grape juice.

Welch's grape juice was especially popular in the 1950s. To get children to drink more of it, marketers aired persuasive commercials on children's TV shows, including *The Howdy Doody Show,* the first program to run advertisements aimed at children. To tie the bottled juice into the show, a picture of Howdy Doody was added to the label along with the caption "My favorite juice!" Now that the fans of Howdy Doody, Buffalo Bob, and Clarabell the Clown are beginning to draw Social Security benefits, it's time to take a closer look at the health properties of the drink. In a 2008 University of California survey of a variety of types and brands of fruit juice, lab tests showed that Welch's Concord grape juice had a higher ORAC value than all the other juices tested, including acai juice, a Brazilian interloper that can cost a hefty six dollars more per quart.

A few small studies suggest that the juice might slow the memory loss that accompanies old age. In a 2012 dietary study, British researchers enrolled twenty-one adults who were showing early signs of memory loss. Each day for four months, half the participants drank two cups of Concord grape juice, and the other half consumed an equal amount of a nonnutritious drink. The participants were given brain scans at the beginning and end of the study to measure the activity in the regions of the brain devoted to learning and memory. The people who had been drinking the grape juice showed a marked increase in activity. The other participants showed little change. More studies are under way. Another study, this one published in the *American Journal of Cardiology,* determined that Concord grape juice could make people's arteries more flexible and lower their blood pressure.

Other research has shown that the juice can thin the blood, reducing the risk of blood clots that can trigger a heart attack or stroke. The juice also slows the oxidation of LDL cholesterol, which keeps it from invading your artery linings. In test-tube studies, Concord grape juice has protected normal breast cells from toxic chemicals that can damage the cells' DNA. DNA damage is often the first step in the deadly progression to cancer. The fact that Concord grape juice is inexpensive, tasty, all-American, and available in supermarkets everywhere makes this research all the more exciting. We have gained a great deal from the diligent breeding efforts of Ephraim Bull.

SHOPPING FOR GRAPES

People living on the East Coast have the best chance of finding fresh Concord grapes. In other markets, they've been squeezed out by the new generation of seedless grapes. Several other varieties offer similar benefits, however, and they are widely available. Black and red grapes are the most nutritious of all, and they are now available in seedless and seeded varieties. Autumn Royal, a new seedless variety, was released by the Agricultural Research Service in 1996. It is a sweet, crisp grape that ripens in October, when most other varieties have been harvested. Other recommended varieties include Crimson Seedless, Flame Seedless, Red Globe, and Sheridan. You will find additional suggestions on pages 314–15.

SELECTING THE FRESHEST GRAPES

Some of the table grapes sold in conventional supermarkets have been stored in warehouses for up to eight weeks. Typically, they have also been treated with sulfur dioxide to prevent rot and preserve the appearance of freshness. A common practice in California, which produces 90 percent of our grapes, is to fumigate the fruit with sulfur dioxide gas as soon as it is packed and then dose it again once a week until it is shipped. The use of sulfur dioxide is not mentioned on grapes sold without wrappers, but you will find a disclosure on the labels of some packaged grapes. Whether the sulfur dioxide use is noted or not, it is safe to assume that most conventionally raised grapes have been fumigated.

To choose the freshest grapes available in the supermarket, look for those that are plump and firm. Pick up a bunch by the stem and give it a gentle shake. The grapes should stay on the vine. As is true for cherries, the stems are your most reliable guide to freshness. The stems should be bright green, flexible, and show no signs of withering. When grapes are sold in plastic bags, it can be difficult to judge their freshness and quality. Peer through the plastic the best you can. Reject bags of grapes that are sticky or moist or contain loose grapes—all indicators that the fruit is past its prime.

Grapes are among the most heavily sprayed of all our fruits and vegetables. In 2011, the USDA reported that 97 percent of all the grapes tested had residues from at least one type of pesticide. The same year, the Environmental Working Group ranked grapes seventh on the "Dirty Dozen," their annual list of the twelve most contaminated fruits and vegetables. The group detected fourteen separate chemicals on one sample of imported grapes. Our domestic grapes fared little better: traces of thirteen different pesticides were detected on one sample. Buy organic grapes to reduce your exposure to agricultural chemicals.

Once you harvest or buy your grapes, cool them as quickly as possible. Rapid chilling slows the loss of antioxidants and preserves their juiciness and flavor. Do not rinse the grapes before storing, because the added surface moisture will promote decay. Place them in a sealed plastic bag that you have pricked with about twenty tiny holes to allow a slow exchange of gas. Store in the coldest part of your refrigerator. (They do best between thirty and forty degrees, which is colder than most refrigerators.) When you are ready to eat the grapes, clip off the amount you plan to use and leave the rest in the refrigerator, where they will stay cool and moist. Rinse the grapes just before eating.

EAT MORE FRESH GRAPES

Grapes make excellent snacks and hors d’oeuvres, and they are a favorite addition to fruit salads. Experiment with adding them to green salads as well. If you cut red or black grapes in half, they will stand out like jewels against green and red lettuce. For a simple hors d’oeuvre, skewer a fresh grape and a chunk of cheese on a toothpick. Wine experts suggest that you pair goat cheese with Concord grapes and Roquefort with black or red seedless grapes, but combining any type of grape with any type of cheese will work. My preference is for black grapes with feta, festooned with a small leaf of fresh mint. The recipe below combines these three ingredients in a refreshing salad that you will want to make again and again.

GRAPE, MINT, AND FETA SALAD

PREP TIME: 20 MINUTES
RESTING TIME: 30 MINUTES
TOTAL TIME: 50 MINUTES YIELD: 4 SERVINGS

3 cups (about 1¼ pounds) black or red seedless grape halves
½ cup crumbled feta cheese
¼ cup chopped walnuts or pecans
2 tablespoons chopped fresh mint or 2 teaspoons dried mint
1 tablespoon freshly squeezed lemon juice
2 tablespoons extra virgin olive oil, preferably unfiltered

Combine the grape halves, feta cheese, nuts, and mint in a medium bowl.

In a small bowl, whisk together the lemon juice and olive oil. Pour the dressing over the fruit and toss until combined. Let rest at room temperature for 30 minutes before serving.

RAISINS

When hunter-gatherers foraged for grapes late in the season, they would come upon fruit that had withered on the vine. These dried tidbits, they quickly discovered, were sweeter than fresh grapes and kept for months without spoiling. Eventually, they began picking ripe grapes and drying them in the sun or over a fire to amass a year-round supply of concentrated energy.

Today, sun-dried raisins are our most popular dried fruit. But 95 percent of the raisins sold in US markets are made from Thompson grapes, the least nutritious variety. Conventional drying methods further reduce their antioxidant levels. The customary way to dry the light-colored grapes is to spread them out on paper trays that are placed between the rows of vines. In two or three weeks, the grapes are fully dried. Meanwhile, the polyphenol oxidase enzymes have had ample time to use up many of the grapes' phytonutrients and also turn the raisins a dark brown color.

Golden raisins are made from the same Thompson seedless variety as dark-colored raisins, but they have been treated with sulfur dioxide to speed up the drying process, prevent the formation of mold and mildew, and to keep the fruit from browning. As is true for apricots, the sulfur also blocks the action of the enzymes that destroy the grape's phytonutrients. As a result, golden raisins have a much higher ORAC value than dark brown raisins (see the graph below). Golden raisins do contain faint traces of sulfur dioxide, however, which some people cannot tolerate and others choose to avoid.

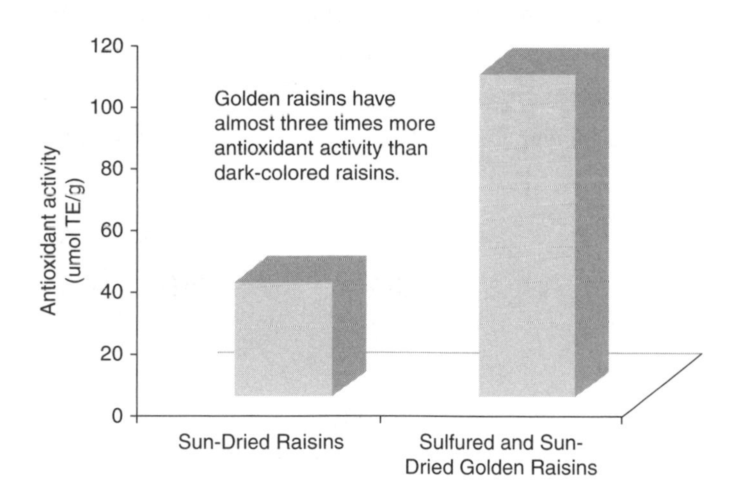

CURRANTS

In 75 AD, Pliny the Elder described a tiny, thin-skinned, seedless grape from Corinth, Greece, that was juicy and sweet. Only small amounts of these grapes, known as Black Corinth grapes today, are grown in this country, and most of them are dried and sold as "Zante currants" or "black currants." (Even though they are called currants, they belong to the grape species, *Vitis vinifera*.) Currants comprise only 1 percent of the US raisin market, but they are available in most supermarkets. We should eat more of them. They have more phytonutrients than most dried fruits, including golden raisins. They are tart and sweet, giving them a livelier flavor than Thompson seedless raisins. I consider them one of the hidden treasures in the grocery store. Look for them in the dried-fruit section. If your supermarket or specialty store sells dried fruit in bulk, compare the price of currants to the price of raisins. In most stores, the currants are less expensive.

In Europe, currants are an essential ingredient in many traditional breads, pastries, coffee cakes, and even meat dishes. Substitute currants for raisins in some of your recipes. Add them to granola and to cooked or dry cereal. They make a delightful addition to scones, pancakes, waffles, cinnamon rolls, and muffins. Add them to trail mix for extra antioxidant protection. Add a half cup or more to banana bread, apple pie, carrot cake, or apple cake. Carry them in the car for a nutritious and convenient snack.

RECOMMENDED VARIETIES OF GRAPES

IN THE SUPERMARKET	
TYPE	COMMENTS
Red, purple, or black	Many supermarkets list the varietal names of their grapes. If the names are not listed, look for blue-, red-, and black-skinned varieties. Thompson seedless is the lowest in nutritive value. If the varietal names are listed, look for the varieties mentioned below.

FARMERS MARKETS, SPECIALTY STORES, U-PICK FARMS, AND SEED CATALOGS		
VARIETY	DESCRIPTION	INFORMATION FOR GARDENERS
Autumn Royal	A crisp, sweet-tasting, seedless grape with black or purplish-black skin. High in phytonutrients.	Best in zones 7–8. Does not require a pollinator.
Concord	Large, blue-black grapes with seeds. Most common on the East Coast. A new seedless variety is now available.	Best for zones 4–9. Ripens in September. Self-pollinating. Can withstand cooler temperatures than many other varieties. Hardy and productive.
Crimson Seedless (also called Red Crimson Seedless)	Very sweet, medium-size seedless grapes with red skin.	Best for zones 6–10. Ripens from late September through October. Large triangular clusters.
Glenora	Sweet, seedless, extra-juicy, blue-black grape with a spicy finish and thin skin. Developed by Cornell University in 1952 by crossing a Russian seedless black grape with a Western variety.	Best for zones 5–8. A vigorous, highly productive, disease-resistant grape. Resistant to phylloxera and mildew. Self-pollinating. Begins to bear after 2 years.
Noble	Highest in antioxidants of all the cultivated varieties of muscadines. Very good quality medium-size fruit that is 16 percent sugar.	Best for zones 7–9. Ripens from early to midseason.
Red Flame Seedless (also called Flame Seedless)	Ranges in color from red to dark purple. Crisp fruit has excellent flavor. Second-most-popular grape in the United States. Highest antioxidant content in a survey of 7 varieties of table grapes. Introduced in the 1970s.	Best for zones 7–9. Vigorous, heavy-bearing vines that require a long growing season. Self-pollinating. Firm, large clusters of medium-large grapes.
Red Globe	Very large, seeded red grapes with firm flesh. Second to Red Flame. High antioxidant levels.	Best for zones 7–11. Harvest from September to October.
Ribier	Large, round, black grapes with seeds. Originated in France.	Best for zones 7–10. Ripens from August through October.

GRAPES AND RAISINS: POINTS TO REMEMBER

1. ***Red, purple, and black grapes are best for your health.***
   Thompson seedless grapes and other pale green grapes have little or no anthocyanin, the phytonutrient that provides most of the health benefits of grapes. Muscadine and Concord grapes are especially high in anthocyanins, as are other red, purple, and black varieties. Concord grape juice is an inexpensive, widely available, low-cost beverage that has more phytonutrients than much more expensive juices.
2. ***Look for the freshest grapes.***
   Some grapes sold in supermarkets have been stored for weeks before going on display, and this compromises their flavor and health benefits. Look for grapes that are plump and firmly attached to the vine. Their stems should be bright green and flexible. Reject bags of grapes that are sticky, moist, or contain loose fruit.
3. ***Store grapes properly to preserve their freshness and flavor.***
   Chill grapes as soon as you get them home to slow their rate of decay and preserve their flavor and phytonutrient content. Place them in a sealed plastic bag pricked with about twenty tiny holes and store them in your crisper drawer. Clip off the quantity of grapes you intend to use and leave the rest of the bunch in the refrigerator.
4. ***Buy organic grapes to reduce your exposure to pesticides.***
   Grapes have more pesticide residues than most other fruits. To reduce your exposure to the chemicals, rinse them thoroughly or buy organic grapes.
5. ***Golden raisins have more phytonutrients than conventional black raisins.***
   Most of the raisins in this country are made from pale Thompson seedless grapes. Drying them in the sun darkens their color

and destroys phytonutrients. Golden raisins are made from the same grapes, but are treated with sulfur dioxide to prevent browning. This treatment preserves more of the antioxidants, making them the more nutritious choice. Avoid golden raisins if you are sensitive to sulfur dioxide.

6. ***Eat more currants.***
   Currants are made from Black Corinth grapes, a variety with very small fruit. Currants have more antioxidants than traditional raisins or golden raisins. They are aromatic and a lively blend of sweet and tart. Use them in place of raisins in many of your recipes. If you buy them in bulk, they are likely to be less expensive than raisins.

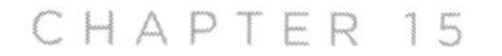

CHAPTER 15

CITRUS FRUITS

BEYOND VITAMIN C

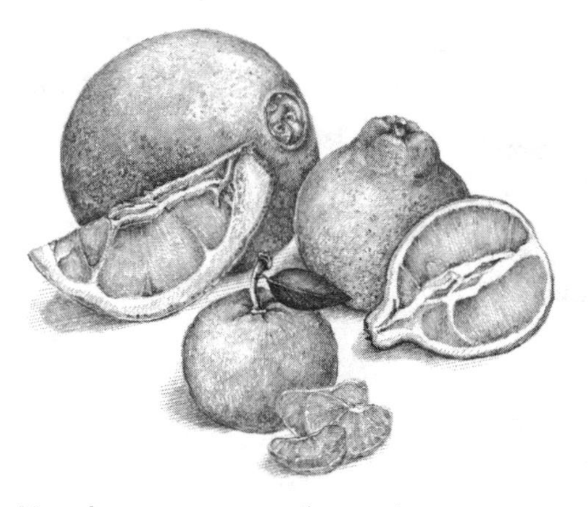

Navel orange, tangelo, and tangerine

Tang, an artificially flavored and colored breakfast drink, first appeared on American breakfast tables in 1959. The drink was a chemist's concoction of water, sucrose, citric acid, orange food dye, and artificial flavorings. At the time, vitamin C was the only nutrient in oranges that was deemed important for health. A decision was made to add vitamin C powder to the drink to make it seem nutritionally equivalent to orange juice.

Sales were slow until the mid-1960s, when NASA sent Tang into space on John Glenn's Mercury flight and then on the 1965 Gemini mission. The General Foods Corporation began exploiting the NASA connection immediately, including designing new ads targeted at children. A TV commercial that aired on *The Howdy Doody Show* featured a brief clip of a rocket ship blasting into space with the following voice-over: "The astronauts do some of the same things *you* do. In space, they drink Tang, but they have to use a zero-gravity pouch. . . .Tang tastes orangey! It tastes great! Has lots of vitamins C and A! Have a blast! Have some Tang!" Years later it was revealed that the only reason NASA sent the powdered drink into space was to disguise the unpleasant taste and odor of the ship's recycled drinking water.

Tang, now owned by Kraft Foods, comes in dozens of varieties. Some of the newest drinks are supplemented with vitamin C, calcium, vitamin E, and three of the B vitamins. In some of the products, half the sugar has been replaced with artificial sweeteners. Tang is now a multivitamin powder afloat in artificially dyed, flavored, and sweetened water.

No matter how many vitamins and minerals the food designers add to Tang, however, the drink will never approach the wholesomeness of oranges. Oranges, food scientists have discovered in recent years, contain more than 170 individual phytonutrients. Together, these compounds provide more antioxidant protection than vitamin C itself. In fact, more than 76 percent of the antioxidant value of oranges comes from these newly identified compounds.

In the future, it is likely that food chemists will create a new "high-antioxidant" Tang, but even if they add a dozen phytonutrients, more than a hundred will still be missing. One bionutrient that they might not include is hesperidin, a compound that has yet to become a household word. Animal studies show that hesperidin has the potential to relieve depression, calm inflammation, protect DNA from radiation damage, and slow the growth of several types of cancer. If we want these potential benefits, we need to eat the whole fruit.

THE WILD ROOTS OF CITRUS FRUITS

The wild ancestors of our citrus fruits are native to Southeast Asia. By 500 BC, the fruits had spread to Greece and the Mediterranean region. Most of the early species were very bitter—so bitter, in fact, that anthropologists speculate they were used for medicine, beauty treatments, cleansers, and embalming fluid, not for food. Sour oranges and citron were among the first truly edible varieties. Citron is a large, bitter, bumpy fruit with little flesh and lots of rind. Historical accounts suggest that it was an effective antidote for poison. According to the Greek philosopher Democritus, born in 460 BC, it could even neutralize snake venom. While traveling in Egypt, Democritus heard about a number of Egyptian prisoners who had been condemned to die by being thrown into a pit of venomous snakes. Just before they were tossed to the vipers, according to the story, a street vendor gave the men some citron to eat. Although the men were savaged by the snakes, they were not poisoned by the venom.

In the thirteenth century, sweet oranges appeared in the Mediterranean, most likely the result of a spontaneous mutation of a sour orange. Two centuries later, Christopher Columbus packed a bag of the orange seeds aboard the *Santa Maria* and sailed off to the New World, introducing the tasty fruit to a new and appreciative audience.

Around the world, wherever citrus fruits happened to be growing, new varieties would appear spontaneously—not just from natural mutations but from spontaneous crossbreeding as well. Citrus fruits interbreed very readily. Whenever the pollen of one tree pollinates the flowers of another species of citrus, there is the possibility of creating a hybrid offspring. This happens so often that it takes a DNA expert to figure out which fruits commingled to produce each kind of fruit. The best guess is that our modern sweet oranges are a cross between a tangerine and a larger fruit called a pomelo (*Citrus grandis*). Pomelos are the likely ancestors of our modern grapefruits as well. Popular in Asian countries, pomelos look like extra-large grapefruits. The flesh is green when the fruit is immature, but mellows to a pale yellow when ripe.

Fruit Ripening

These fruits are best picked when fully ripe, because they do not ripen after harvest:

Citrus fruits
Berries
Cherries
Grapes
Pineapples
Pomegranates

These fruits can be picked when semiripe, because they can ripen after harvest:

Apples
Apricots
Avocados
Bananas
Guavas
Kiwifruits
Mangoes
Nectarines
Peaches
Pears
Plums
Tomatoes

SWEET ORANGES

THE WASHINGTON NAVEL

Sweet oranges are the most popular citrus fruits in the United States. US citrus growers produce more than eleven million tons a year—three times more than all other citrus fruits combined. The best known orange is the Washington navel, which is commonly known as the navel orange. You can identify it by its belly button. On the blossom end of each fruit is a circle filled with an orange bulge. This bulge is an undeveloped second orange; think of it as a twin that failed to thrive. Break the orange into segments and you will get a better view of the half-formed twin. This curious appendage is coded into the genes of every navel orange, making it the botanical equivalent of a registered trademark.

The Washington navel orange is believed to have originated in Bahia, Brazil, prior to 1870. Like so many of our most popular varieties of fruits and vegetables, it, too, was the result of a spontaneous mutation. An unknown eagle-eyed Brazilian farmer spotted the fruit growing on the limb of a conventional orange tree. Compared with the original fruit, it was bigger, sweeter, easier to peel, and seedless—a bundle of benefits that were the result of a minor tweaking of its genome. The Brazilians called it laranja de umbigo: "the orange with a navel," a name that persists to this day.

The US commissioner of agriculture heard about these intriguing fruits in 1871 and imported a number of young sapling trees to plant in Florida. The trees had a difficult time adapting to the hot, humid climate. None of them produced fruit, and most of them died. Three of the surviving trees were shipped to California in hopes they would do better in a cooler, drier environment. The trees came under the care of Eliza Tibbets, a friend of the commissioner, who was living in Riverside, California. The trees thrived under her watchful eye. Rumor has it that Mr. Tibbets refused to pay to pipe fresh water to the trees, so Eliza had to water them with buckets of dishwater.

When the trees bore fruit, the oranges were judged to be superior to all other varieties in the region. Local nurserymen lined up to buy budwood from Mrs. Tibbets's trees. The nurserymen grafted the buds onto other varieties of oranges, creating the first clones of the South American mutant. These initial clones would be multiplied thousands of times, until they filled hundreds of orange groves, and then many more times, until they were growing all around the world. All these Washington navel trees can trace their lineage back to one of Mrs. Tibbets's trees. If she had been less diligent with her watering, the multibillion-dollar navel orange industry might never have gotten off the ground.

Incredibly, one of Mrs. Tibbets's original trees survives to this day. In 1902, it was moved to a park on the corner of Arlington and Magnolia Avenues in Riverside. By then, navel oranges had become a nationwide phenomenon. Moving the tree was such a newsworthy event that President Theodore Roosevelt took part in the ceremony. As of this writing, that original tree is still capable of bearing heavy crops of fruit. Fruit enthusiasts, not insects or disease, are the main threat to its survival. Hundreds of people have attempted to lop off buds and branches to make their own clones of the world-famous tree. Sturdy bars had to be erected to keep them away.

Today we know that the Washington navel is not only large, sweet, and seedless, it has more phytonutrients per serving than many other nutritious fruits and vegetables, such as red grapes, asparagus, yellow onions, and broccoli raab. It is also an excellent source of vitamin C, a good source of fiber (more than three grams per orange), and it does not cause a spike in your blood sugar. One medium-size fruit has only eighty calories, which makes it a nutrient-dense food as well. Although the navel is not as nutritious as some of the other oranges I describe later on, it is a very good choice all the same.

THE "DEGREENING" OF ORANGES

In the nineteenth century, people were able to identify a ripe orange with ease. A ripe orange was orange, and an unripe orange was green. Choosing ripe oranges became much more difficult in the early 1900s, when the citrus industry began to "degreen" immature oranges to give them the semblance of ripeness. This was deemed necessary because oranges met the minimal definition of maturity while their skins were still green. Citrus growers discovered that if they dipped green-skinned oranges in orange dye, people were much more likely to buy them. (At the time, no notification about the use of dye was required.) This practice continued until 1955, when the dye used by the citrus industry, Red 32, proved to be toxic. The Supreme Court quickly outlawed the practice.

Without the use of the dye, the orange industry had to develop another way to disguise the immaturity of the oranges. The most effective method—and the one still in use today—was to harvest oranges before they were ripe, ship them to warehouses, and then expose the fruit to precise amounts of ethylene gas, which triggers the ripening process in many fruits. With the right temperature, humidity, and concentration of gases, the oranges turned the requisite color in a matter of days. This is similar to the process now used to ripen green tomatoes. But ethylene exposure does not ripen the *flesh* of oranges, as it does with tomatoes; it simply alters the color of their skins. The oranges may look ripe, but they are more acidic, less sweet, and have fewer bionutrients than fully ripened fruit.

HOW TO IDENTIFY TRULY RIPE ORANGES

Today, the FDA approves the degreening of oranges and does not require any notification on the fruit. This makes it difficult—though not impossible—to select the ripest and most flavorful fruit. First, survey all the oranges in a given display. If the skin of the oranges ranges in color from yellow to deep orange, then you know they have not been degreened. (If they had been degreened, they would all be the same color of orange.) In this case, simply choose the orangest oranges you see.

But if the oranges are all a deep orange color, you can't tell if they got their color honestly or under the influence of ethylene gas. In that case, when all the oranges are the same color, you can increase your odds of bringing home ripe fruit by selecting the largest fruit in the display. Like most fruits, oranges grow larger as they ripen, so a large orange has been on the tree for a longer period of time than a smaller one and is likely to be riper as a result.

You can also wait to buy navel oranges until they are in peak season. The first crop of US oranges arrives in the supermarkets in October. At this time of year, most of them are not fully ripe, but they have enough sugar to meet minimal harvest standards. These early fruits are the ones that are most likely to be degreened. If you wait until December to buy them, however, the fruit is more likely to be ripe, sweet, low in acid, and more nutritious. The fact that most fruits and vegetables are now available twelve months out of the year doesn't mean we have to buy them before they are ripe and in season.

If you buy organic oranges, you will know for certain that they have not been degreened. USDA standards for the designation "organic" do not allow the forced ripening of oranges and most other fruit; what you see is what you get. As is true for all organically certified fruit, organic oranges also have few or no traces of pesticides or other potentially hazardous chemicals. Organic oranges may also be more flavorful and higher in nutrients than conventionally grown fruit, according to a 2006 European study.

HOW TO STORE ORANGES AND OTHER CITRUS FRUITS

Citrus fruits do not ripen after they've been harvested, so do not leave them on the kitchen counter in the hopes that their skins will turn a deeper color or that their flesh will become sweeter and less tart. Instead of ripening, the fruit will begin to shrivel, develop "off" flavors, and become coated with green mold. Eat them within a few days or store them in your refrigerator. They can be kept on a refrigerator shelf or in the crisper drawer. Do not store them in a plastic bag, however. The bag will trap too much moisture and promote the development of mold. Citrus fruits can be kept in the refrigerator for about two weeks. If you can't eat all the fruit in that amount of time, you can squeeze them and freeze the juice. You can also grate the peels and freeze them as well.

CARA CARA ORANGES

As I mentioned earlier, several varieties of oranges have more phytonutrients than Washington navel oranges. The Cara Cara is one of them. Cara Cara is a spontaneous mutant of the Washington navel. The fruit is about two-thirds the size of the original fruit. It, too, contains an undeveloped orange, but it is smaller in size. The fruit has few, if any, seeds, and it is easy to peel and segment.

The most important difference between the Washington navel and the Cara Cara is found inside. The flesh of the Cara Cara is a deep rose color, which is why it is also known as the red navel orange. Lycopene is the source of the red color. (There is no lycopene in Washington navel oranges.) Because of their high lycopene content, Cara Caras have two to three times more antioxidant activity than conventional navels. They are also sweeter and lower in acid. Until recently, this new variety was sold only in specialty stores; now you can find it in large supermarkets. The peak harvest season is from December to April. Supermarkets that carry Cara Caras are likely to identify them by name.

BLOOD ORANGES

Blood oranges (*Citrus sinensis* L. Osbeck) do the Cara Cara one better. Blood oranges—which are less than half the size of navel oranges—have thin skins and few, if any, seeds. The skin of these dainty citrus fruits can take on a pleasing purple blush as the fruit matures, and the flesh ranges in color from a pinkish orange to the deep red color of blood, thus their name. The color of the fruit comes from its high anthocyanin content, not lycopene (which is what colors Cara Caras). Blood oranges have been called the connoisseur's citrus because of their lively, nuanced flavor. Enthusiastic fans talk about "overtones of raspberry," "hints of grape," "a marriage between an orange and a plum," and "a Burgundy wine infused with orange zest." I call them delicious.

Climate plays a major role in determining the nutrient content of many fruits and vegetables, and this is especially true of blood oranges. In the United States, most blood oranges are grown in California, Texas, and Florida. California has cooler nights than the other two states, a condition that triggers more anthocyanin production. A 1990 study determined that blood oranges grown in California have a darker flesh color and as much as thirty-five times more anthocyanins than those grown in Florida and Texas.

Blood oranges are not well known in this country, but they are common throughout the Mediterranean. In fact, they are the most popular variety in Italy. We drink orange orange juice for breakfast; Italians drink red orange juice. American chefs are paving the way to greater acceptance of blood oranges by featuring them in salads and sauces, and using them as eye-catching garnishes. Their peak season is from January through mid-April, but most stores sell them for only a month or so. If you see them, buy them.

Do you live in orange-growing country? Consider planting a blood orange tree. The Moro variety has an unusually high level of anthocyanins. Buy a seedling tree this year and you will have your own supply of blood oranges in the years to come. You can also grow a tree in a pot in your office or home. With proper care, even these indoor trees will bear fruit.

VALENCIA ORANGES

The Valencia orange is a medium-size fruit that is grown primarily for its juice. It is the only orange that ripens in summer. The fruit was created in the backyard of a wealthy Californian named William Wolfskill, who started with cuttings from orange trees that he had imported from Valencia, Spain. Born in 1798, Wolfskill is famous for more than the Valencia orange. He is also known for selling lemons to California gold miners for a dollar apiece.

Valencias have seeds and a thin, tight skin that makes them difficult to peel. If you are willing to spit out the seeds and deal with the peel, you will get twice as many carotenoids as you would from a navel orange. The fruit is also sweeter, with a richer flavor. Valencias are available in most large supermarkets in limited quantity. Their peak season is from May to July, when other kinds of oranges are in short supply or not fully ripe.

Valencia oranges are unusual in that they can ripen, turn orange, then revert to green-colored skin later in the year. The green color makes them look immature even though they are fully ripe. When this occurs, many producers degreen the oranges with ethylene gas to restore the orange color. Unlike navel oranges, Valencias are already mature before they are exposed to the gas, so this is not such a deceptive practice.

TANGELOS

Tangelos (*Citrus* × *tangelo*) came into being in 1897, when a citrus grower applied the pollen of a tangerine blossom to the blossom of a grapefruit. The fruit does not look like either parent. Instead, it looks like a large orange with a nob on the top, giving it the shape of a bell—in fact, tangelos are often called honeybells. The flesh has the color and tang of a tangerine. Tangelos have more phytonutrients (especially flavanones) than most sweet oranges, making them a more nutritious choice. They are delightfully juicy.

MANDARINS

Mandarins (*Citrus reticulata*) comprise a large family of citrus fruits that includes satsuma oranges, Mediterranean mandarins, and tangerines. All fruits in this family have zip-off peels. Mediterranean mandarins have a lighter-colored peel and flesh than tangerines, which are reddish orange. The red tone in tangerines comes from lycopene. Tangerines are less acid than most oranges, but can be quite seedy. Mandarins, like oranges, become sweeter and less acid as they mature. Some growers pick them when they are immature and then degreen them. If you buy organic fruit or buy it from small-scale growers, you can be assured that it has not been degreened. Forced ripening is not allowed under USDA organic standards, and small-scale orchard owners can't afford to do it. If an organic mandarin has deep orange skin, it is ripe. Satsumas and clementines are seedless mandarins. Clementines are smaller than tangerines. Their flesh is a deep orange color and high in beta-carotene.

Preserving the Most Nutritious Part of an Orange

Surprisingly, the most nutritious part of an orange is not the pulp, the juice, or its bright neon skin. The greatest concentration of phytonutrients is in the pith, the spongy white tissue that lies just beneath the skin. The scientific name for the pith is albedo. The albedo is rich in pectin and has a high concentration of flavanones. It has a slightly bitter flavor and a dry texture, however, so most people remove it. When you buy processed orange products or canned orange segments, be aware that the citrus industry peels the fruit mechanically and then uses a chemical treatment to degrade the albedo and the inner membranes, which makes them easier to remove. The end result is a "naked" orange.

Consuming the albedo is good for your health. According to one study, a navel orange with some albedo left on the segments has four hundred milligrams of phytonutrients per serving. When all the white tissue is removed, it has only one hundred milligrams. The next time you peel an orange, leave as much of the albedo as you can without compromising your enjoyment of the fruit.

The membranes that encase the juice sacs are also good for you. Some recipes recommend that you "supreme" citrus fruit segments, a French technique that involves cutting off and discarding the membranes of each segment. If you slice the oranges, instead of separating them into individual segments, the membranes will be barely noticeable.

CHOOSING THE BEST OJ

By weight, we Americans consume six times more orange juice than we do whole oranges. Until about the early 1990s, most people made orange juice from frozen concentrate. Today we are confronted with a bewildering number of choices. One supermarket that I surveyed had a fifteen-foot-long orange juice section. The cartons, jugs, and bottles contained juice that was labeled "fresh-squeezed," "made from concentrate," "not made from concentrate," and "made from concentrate with calcium added"; there was also juice with "added pulp," "low-acid" orange juice, and juice with "added vitamin C and zinc"; one variety of juice was labeled "Premium Original" and another was labeled "Premium with Added Vitamin C"; and—curiously—one brand of commercial juice was described as "Home Squeezed."

The global soft-drink giants Coke and Pepsi have cornered 60 percent of the US orange juice market. Coca-Cola owns Minute

Maid and the newer, higher-priced Simply Orange brand. PepsiCo owns Tropicana and the premium brand Naked Juice. Both companies purchase oranges and orange juice from the United States and Brazil. A third and smaller company, Florida's Natural, is a cooperative of about one thousand Florida growers that makes all its juice from Florida oranges.

When you shop for orange juice, how do you know which one to buy? First, some basics. Orange juice retains more of the food value of the whole fruit than many other juices because it is less refined. Consumers accept the fact that you can't see through the juice and that most of it contains flecks of pulp.

Some brands and types of orange juice are more nutritious than others. Researchers at Texas A&M University analyzed twenty-six different brands of orange juice that they had purchased from local stores. To everyone's surprise, the juice that was made from concentrate had, on average, *45 percent more flavonoids* than juice that had never been concentrated. They made another unexpected find. Some of the least expensive juices in the study had more antioxidants than the most expensive brands. One premium brand of orange juice that sold for four dollars a quart had half the phytonutrients of the little known Donald Duck brand, which sold for less than two dollars a quart.

Many people buy "not from concentrate" juice because they prefer its flavor. That flavor is more likely to come from a chemical flavor packet, however, than the juice itself. Juice that is never frozen or concentrated is stored for weeks or months in million-gallon containers in order to spread the seasonal supply over the calendar year. Oxygen is removed from the juice to keep it from spoiling or turning rancid, but this process alters and diminishes its flavor. Before bottling the juice, the producers add back a mixture of chemicals in an effort to restore the natural flavor. If you prefer the flavor of one brand of "not from concentrate" juice over another, it may be because you prefer their patented mix of additives.

"Boutique" orange juice, which is often sold in pint-size plastic bottles, stands apart from the standard commercial varieties because it is made from organic, fresh-squeezed, flash-pasteurized juice. Sold by companies such as Odwalla (now owned by Coca-Cola) and Organic Valley, the juice is bottled and sold within days or weeks of squeezing. Because of this rapid turnaround, it does not have to be deoxygenated or stored in holding tanks. No flavor packets are needed, because the fresh flavor of the juice is retained. The flavor changes subtly throughout the year as different varieties of oranges come into season. Compare brands and choose the juice with the most intense orange color and the freshest flavor. The nutritional content of the juice will vary with the variety of oranges being used.

No matter what kind of juice you prefer, orange juice with pulp or extra pulp is better for you than filtered juice. New research has revealed that the pulp contains a number of phytonutrients, such as naringenin and hesperetin, that have antioxidant, antibacterial, antiviral, anti-inflammatory, and antiallergenic properties. It belongs in the juice.

THE BEST HOME-SQUEEZED ORANGE JUICE

The most flavorful and nutritious orange juice is the juice you squeeze at home—provided you select the right varieties. Most commercial orange juice is made from navel oranges, with varying amounts of Valencias added to deepen the color and sweeten the juice. If you make your juice from 100 percent Valencia oranges, it will be sweet and colorful and give you added phytonutrients as well. If you make it from Cara Caras, tangelos, or blood oranges, it will be even more colorful and nutritious. Consider mixing and matching citrus fruits to create your own house blend. There's another nutritional benefit to making your own juice: it does not require pasteurization. Pasteurization degrades some of the phytonutrients in orange juice, reducing their effectiveness by as much as 30 percent.

As a rough gauge, two or three large oranges make about six ounces of juice. To extract the most juice from the oranges, first roll them on the counter, pushing down hard enough to rupture the juice sacs. Cut the oranges in half, then remove the seeds. Squeeze the juice using a reamer, manual press, or electric juicer. Electric juicers extract the most juice and include more of the pith, increasing the nutritional content of the juice. Some electric juicers have a fast-spin cycle that squeezes the last drop of juice from the pulp. Do not strain the juice. Those bits of flotsam and jetsam have more phytonutrients than the juice itself. Add back any pulp that has been left behind in the juicer. Drink the juice right away. Food chemists have discovered that home-squeezed orange juice that sits in the refrigerator for just twenty-four hours loses most of its aroma and half of its antioxidant activity.

GRAPEFRUITS

Until the beginning of the twentieth century, all grapefruits had white flesh. Then, in 1905, a Florida grapefruit grower spotted some unusual-looking grapefruits on a limb of one of his trees. He cut one of the fruits open and saw that it had pink flesh. The bud that had developed on that limb had mutated, creating fruit of a different color. He took a bite and discovered that the fruit was also sweeter than the white grapefruits. He took a bud from the limb, cloned it, and went into business producing pink grapefruits. Consumers liked the pink grapefruits much better than the white ones. Within a decade, clones of the pink mutant were growing in citrus groves throughout Florida and Texas.

In Texas, about twenty-five years later, one of the trees that bore pink grapefruits underwent its own spontaneous mutation, and red-fleshed grapefruits were born. This new fruit, labeled Hudson Pink—a misnomer, because it is more red than pink—was sweeter than pink grapefruits and became very popular with consumers. Texas citrus breeders decided there was still room for improvement, so in 1959, the Texas A&M University Kingsville Citrus Center sent thousands of Hudson Pink seeds to the Brookhaven National Laboratory to be exposed to radiation: mutation on demand. One of those irradiated seeds grew into a tree that produced the Star Ruby variety. This fruit had fewer seeds and a deeper red color than the Hudson Pink. Buds from the Star Ruby were irradiated in 1963 to produce Rio Red, which is one of the darkest red grapefruits of all. These accidental and man-made mutants now dominate the US market.

Throughout the history of agriculture, many or most of our breeding efforts have reduced the nutritional content of our fruits and vegetables, but dark red grapefruits—which came from a mutant variety that was exposed to two bouts of radiation—are higher in anthocyanins and overall phytonutrients than the paler varieties. Their bounty of anthocyanins could have a significant impact on your health. In 1995, fifty-seven heart patients were enrolled in a month-long grapefruit study. All the patients were recovering from bypass surgery and were not responding to their prescribed triglyceride-lowering drugs. (High triglycerides are an independent risk factor for heart attack and stroke.) The patients were divided into three groups—a control group (no grapefruits), a group that consumed one white grapefruit a day, and a group that consumed one *red* grapefruit a day. After four weeks, both groups of grapefruit eaters had lower cholesterol levels than the control group, but only the people who had eaten the red grapefruits had lower triglyceride levels as well.

Grapefruits and Some Medications Don't Mix

Consuming grapefruit juice or fresh grapefruits can interfere with the action of some prescription drugs and a few nonprescription drugs. New findings suggest that consuming the fruit or juice several hours before or after you take your medications can increase the amount of the drug that enters your bloodstream. These higher amounts can in turn increase the severity of negative side effects linked with the drug or even put you at risk for liver damage and kidney failure.

Medications that are known to be influenced by grapefruits include some that lower cholesterol, reduce blood pressure, calm anxiety, and reduce the risk of the rejection of organ transplants. Talk with your health-care professional about these and other potentially dangerous interactions.

SELECTING THE BEST GRAPEFRUITS IN THE GROCERY STORE

As is true of oranges, many of the grapefruits that are harvested early in the season are degreened with ethylene gas. Although the fruit meets the legal definition of ripeness, growers degreen them anyway because consumers expect to see yellow, not green, skins. Grapefruits that are harvested after December are less likely to be degreened because they are closer to true ripeness. A ripe grapefruit is sweeter and more nutritious than semiripe fruit that has been degreened.

When choosing grapefruits, look for large, smooth-skinned fruits that are heavy for their size. (A large grapefruit that is relatively light has little juice and a thick rind.) The skin should be taut and spring back when you press it. Avoid grapefruits with dents, bruises, scars, or soft spots. When white grapefruits are ripe, their skin is yellow, not greenish-yellow. The ripest red grapefruits have a reddish blush.

If you don't like white grapefruits, you may be a supertaster (see pages 28–29). Most of the bitterness of the fruit comes from a compound called naringin. The more naringin in a variety of grapefruit, the more bitter it tastes, and the more supertasters dislike it. In order to make grapefruits appeal to more consumers, citrus breeders have done their best to remove the compound. Juice producers, meanwhile, have developed elaborate procedures to remove whatever remains. Late in the game, researchers have discovered that naringin has the potential to lower LDL cholesterol and slow tumor growth. Once again, our attempts to remove the bitterness from our food may have weakened our protection against some deadly diseases.

LEMONS AND LIMES

Lemons and limes are native to the mountainous regions of southern China and northeastern India. The parentage of the two fruits was in doubt until a 2010 DNA analysis unraveled the mystery: lemons are a natural cross between a citron and a sour orange; limes are a cross between a citron and a relatively unknown citrus fruit called a papeda.

Lemons and limes were cultivated at least four thousand years ago. In the fourth century BC, they were transported from Persia to Greece by—who else?—Alexander the Great. About eighteen hundred years later, Christopher Columbus brought their seeds to Haiti, where the fruits began to flourish. By the late 1500s, they were well established in Florida and the coastal regions of South Carolina.

Today, 90 percent of our US lemons are produced in California. The most common variety is the Eureka. The Meyer lemon (*Citrus × meyeri*) is not a lemon at all but a cross between a lemon and either a mandarin or another variety of orange. This thin-skinned, low-acid fruit was introduced into the United States in 1908, but did not become well known until recent years, when it was rediscovered by Alice Waters and other pioneering chefs.

Limes are no longer grown in this country in any quantity because they are vulnerable to the Asian citrus canker, a disease that devastates citrus trees. One hundred percent of our commercial lime crop now comes from Mexico. The dark green fruit you see in most stores is the Persian lime (*Citrus × latifolia*). Key limes (*Citrus aurantifolia*) are round and about the size of a golf ball.

(They are referred to as Key limes because the 1926 Miami hurricane destroyed most of Florida's lime groves except for those in the Florida Keys.) They are more aromatic, more bitter, and harder to find than Persian limes. Key lime pies are the best-known use of the fruit, although today, most people make the pie from bottled juice.

Ordinarily, we don't eat lemons and limes or drink their juice unless it's been highly diluted and flavored with sugar. The juice is about 5 to 6 percent citric acid—a 10 on the pucker scale. Instead, we use the juice and peels to flavor or preserve our food. Vitamin C was discovered as the result of a chemical analysis of lemons and limes performed by an early-twentieth-century Hungarian researcher named Albert Szent-Györgyi. Szent-Györgyi was awarded the 1937 Nobel Prize in Medicine for discovering this all-important vitamin.

Scurvy, a horrific and deadly disease, is caused by a vitamin C deficiency. Hippocrates described the symptoms of the disease as early as the fifth century BC. He wrote that it was characterized by bleeding gums and hemorrhage and could be deadly. When long sea voyages became common about two thousand years later, the disease was endemic among sailors, who had no access to fresh fruits or vegetables. The disease is said to have killed tens of thousands of men, including most of the original crew members who accompanied Ferdinand Magellan on his circumnavigation of the globe in the 1500s.

The fact that citrus fruits could prevent scurvy was known hundreds of years before the discovery of vitamin C. In 1564, a Dutch doctor by the name of Beaudouin Ronsse observed that "Dutch sailors who, returning from Spain, were attracted to the novel richness of the fruit [oranges] by their greed and gluttony, unexpectedly drove out the disease of scurvy." It wasn't until 230 years later, however, that lemon juice was officially approved as a treatment for the disease.

Like all citrus fruits, lemons and limes are more than good

sources of vitamin C. They are rich in compounds called flavanones, which can have important antioxidant and anticancer properties. In a test-tube study comparing the anticancer properties of individual fruits, lemons were second only to cranberries. Lemons also help preserve the phytonutrients in other foods. A little-known fact is that adding a squirt of lemon to your teacup or teapot *before* you brew green tea increases the amount of the phytonutrients in the brew and also enhances your ability to absorb them.

SELECTING AND STORING LEMONS AND LIMES

Only a few varieties of lemons and limes are available in this country, and there are few nutritional differences between them. You can concentrate your efforts on buying the juiciest, freshest fruits available. Fresh, high-quality lemons and limes are firm but not hard, and they have glossy skins with no soft spots. The juiciest fruits are heavy for their size. Both limes and lemons are harvested when immature to give them a longer shelf life. The riper the fruit is when harvested, the more juice it contains and the more nutritious it is. Look for lemons with a rich yellow color and no hint of green. Few people realize that ripe limes are yellow, not green. The darkest green limes in the store are the most immature and will have the least juice.

Citrus fruits of all types are quick to develop blue mold, which has been the bane of the citrus industry for a long time. In the 1940s, food scientists experimented with novel ways to preserve the fruit, including dipping it in the toxic pesticide 2,4-D. That practice, thank goodness, was outlawed a few decades later.

Lemons and limes, like other citrus fruits, can be kept at room temperature for about a week. Put them in your refrigerator if you plan to keep them longer than that. They won't stay fresh for more than two weeks, however. You can't freeze whole lemons, but you can freeze the juice. Freezing preserves the phytonutrient content of the juice and its flavor. Your home-frozen juice will taste much better than the bottled "fresh" juice sold in stores. I recommend freezing the zest as well.

BUY ORGANIC CITRUS FRUIT AND EAT THE PEELS

Ounce for ounce, the peel of citrus fruits has many times more phytonutrients than the flesh. Nutraceutical companies have been buying discarded peels from the citrus juice industry and turning them into high-antioxidant, high-priced supplements. You can save money by eating the peels of the fruit you bring home. However, I don't recommend that you do this unless you buy organic fruit. Most of the pesticide residues in citrus fruits are in the skin. Washing oranges still leaves between 16 and 57 percent of the pesticides on or in the fruit.

Grated citrus peels make a sprightly addition to pies, breads, cakes, marinades, sauces, and salad dressings. They add a refreshing flavor accent to cookies, cinnamon rolls, and brownies as well. Add them to your breakfast smoothie. When you add grated citrus peel to homemade or commercial salad dressings, you add flavor *and* nutrients. Make your own marmalade. Most commercial varieties are heavy on the sugar and light on the peels.

Do you have a citrus zester? A zester is an inexpensive hand tool that shreds the colored portion of the rind—the zest—into short, thin strings. Toss the colorful, aromatic zest on top of steamed vegetables and salads. Sprinkle orange zest on chocolate cake and lemon zest on apple pie. Add orange zest to carrot cake.

The following recipe for lemon pudding uses all parts of the lemon except the seeds. It is an easy, zesty dessert. The pudding does not have the silky texture of a lemon meringue pie because of the tiny bits of peel, but the intense lemon flavor is delightful. I recommend using organic lemons.

LEMON PUDDING WITH LEMON PEEL

PREP TIME: 15 MINUTES
COOKING TIME: ABOUT 30 MINUTES
TOTAL TIME: ABOUT 45 MINUTES YIELD: 5 SERVINGS

1 large or 2 small unpeeled lemons, seeded and cut into eighths
1 cup honey or 1¼ cups granulated sugar
4 large eggs
½ cup (1 stick) salted or unsalted butter, at room temperature
1 teaspoon pure vanilla extract
¼ cup finely chopped walnuts or pecans (optional)

Preheat the oven to 325°F. Grease five 6-ounce custard cups.

Combine all ingredients except the nuts in the bowl of a food processor. Process on high for 6 minutes. This will seem like a long time, so set a timer to make sure you blend it long enough. Scrape down the sides of the bowl halfway through. The mixture will be curdled at first, but will become smooth after about 5 minutes.

Pour the mixture into the custard cups and place on a baking sheet. Position the sheet on the middle shelf of the oven. Bake for 25 minutes, then check for doneness; if the pudding is not set, bake an additional 5 minutes, or until set. Remove from the oven and let cool. Sprinkle with the chopped nuts and serve warm, or transfer to the refrigerator and chill for 30 minutes or more before serving. (The pudding can also be made ahead and refrigerated overnight.)

VARIATIONS: Pour the pudding mixture into an 8-inch graham cracker or shortbread crust (or another kind of cooked pie shell) and bake for 30 minutes, or until set. To make lime pudding, use 2–3 limes instead of 1 lemon. Top the pudding with sweetened flaked coconut instead of nuts.

RECOMMENDED VARIETIES OF CITRUS FRUITS

Most of the varieties of citrus fruits recommended below are available in large supermarkets, specialty markets, and in farmers markets, so I have grouped all the locations together. I have also not given specific planting instructions for citrus fruits, because they are grown only in climate zones 9–10. If you live in those zones, you can get detailed tree-planting information from your local agricultural extension agent, fruit-tree nursery, library, garden club, or online.

SUPERMARKETS, SPECIALTY STORES, U-PICK FARMS, AND FARMERS MARKETS	
ORANGES	COMMENTS
Blood oranges	Blood oranges are small oranges with flesh the color of dark red wine. They have a sweet-tart flavor. The orange skin may have a purple blush. They are higher in antioxidants than all the other oranges. The Moro variety is the highest in anthocyanins. Peak season is from January to mid-April.
Cara Cara	Cara Caras are found in some large supermarkets and in many specialty markets. They are medium-size oranges with a rosy orange flesh. They have two to three times more phytonutrients than navel oranges and a sweeter, less acid flavor. Peak season is from December to April.
Valencia	A Valencia is a medium-size, seedy orange with thin, hard-to-peel skin. The fruit is sweeter and juicier than that of navel oranges and a good choice when making home-squeezed orange juice. Valencias are also higher in phytonutrients. They are available from February to October, but peak season is from May to July, when most other US varieties are out of season.

ORANGES	COMMENTS
Washington navel (also called navel oranges)	Ripe navel oranges are sweet and low in acid, and their skin and flesh are a deep orange color. Although other varieties are more nutritious, navels are high in vitamin C and phytonutrients and are one of the best choices in the supermarket. The new crop arrives in stores in October, but the oranges are more likely to be ripe after November.
TANGELOS	COMMENTS
Any variety	More nutritious than most oranges, tangelos have the tang and color of tangerines.
MANDARIN ORANGES	COMMENTS
Clementine	Clementines are an early-season mandarin orange. Free of seeds, they are similar to tangerines but somewhat smaller. Their deep orange flesh is rich in beta-carotene and other phytonutrients.
Satsuma	Satsuma is a variety of tangerine that is also known as satsuma mandarin and satsuma orange. It is seedless and very easy to peel.
Tangerine	Tangerines are small citrus fruits that are easy to peel. Their flavor is sweet, less sour, and more intense than most oranges. They are also higher in beta-carotene.
GRAPEFRUITS	COMMENTS
White varieties	White, or "blonde," varieties of grapefruit are more bitter than pink and red varieties, and they are lower in phytonutrients. Nonetheless, they have been shown to lower LDL cholesterol and to block the growth of several different types of human cancer cells.
Pink varieties	Pink grapefruit varieties are sweeter than white grapefruits and are slightly higher in antioxidant value.
Red varieties	Red grapefruits are the highest in lycopene and overall phytonutrient content of all grapefruit types. They are also the sweetest. The darker the red color, the more beneficial the fruit. The most nutritious varieties include Rio Star, Star Ruby, Rio Red, and Ruby Red, in that order. Grapefruits harvested after December are less likely to be force-ripened with ethylene gas.

CITRUS FRUITS: POINTS TO REMEMBER

1. ***The navel orange is both popular and nutritious.***
   Choose large navel oranges with deep orange skin and flesh. If all the oranges on display have a uniform, deep orange color, choose the largest fruits you see. Eat the membranes that surround the orange sections for added nutrition. If you slice the oranges rather than serve them as segmented wedges, the membranes are less noticeable.

2. ***Choose citrus fruits with the most colorful flesh.***
   The deeper the color of the flesh, the more phytonutrients the fruit contains. Varieties with extra-colorful flesh include Cara Caras, blood oranges, Valencias, mandarins, and tangelos.

3. ***Red and pink grapefruits are higher in phytonutrients than white grapefruits.***
   Red and pink grapefruits are sweeter tasting and better for your health than white grapefruits. Eating red grapefruits on a regular basis could lower your LDL cholesterol and triglycerides. Fruit with the deepest red color has the most phytonutrients.

4. ***Choose the most nutritious orange juice.***
   Deep orange-colored orange juice with pulp offers more nutrition than paler juices without pulp. Some inexpensive juices, including those made from concentrate, can have more phytonutrients than premium brands. Organic, flash-pasteurized orange juice is the most flavorful. Juice made from Valencia oranges, Cara Caras, or blood oranges is more nutritious than juice made from navel oranges. Use these varieties in your homemade juice as well. Drink your juice within a few hours of squeezing to get the most health benefits and flavor.

5. ***Choose the ripest lemons and limes.***
   Most lemons and limes are harvested and sold before they are ripe. Fully ripened fruit has the most juice. Select lemons that

are yellow without any traces of green. The most mature limes are beginning to turn yellow. The fruits should have glossy skins and be heavy for their size.

6. ***Store citrus fruits properly.***
   Citrus fruits can be kept on the kitchen counter for a week, but should be put in the refrigerator for longer storage. Do not store in plastic bags, as this promotes mold. If you have extra fruit, freeze the juice and the grated peels.

CHAPTER 16

TROPICAL FRUITS

MAKE THE MOST OF EATING GLOBALLY

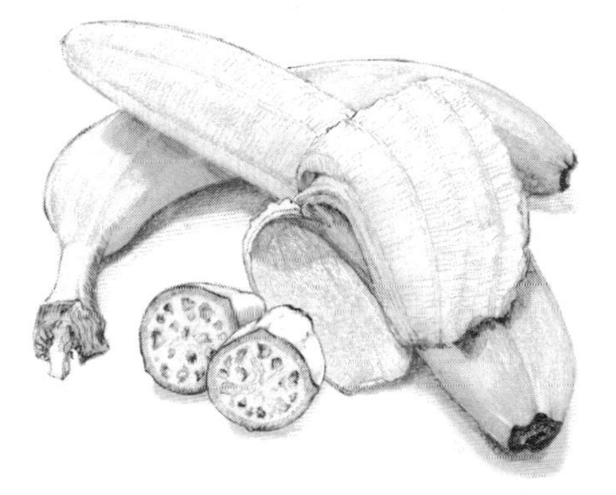

Modern and wild bananas

Thanks to global trade, we can now buy tropical fruit 365 days a year. The most popular tropical imports in this country are bananas, pineapples, and papayas. They come to us from thousands of miles away. The bulk of the bananas sold in Kansas City, for example, come from Ecuador, almost three thousand miles to the south. The pineapples in Manhattan fruit markets are shipped from Costa Rica and Hawaii. Most of our papayas come to us from Mexico and Hawaii. When we eat tropical fruit, we are eating globally, not locally, racking up thousands of miles on the "foodometer" and burning significant amounts of nonrenewable fuel. Our most popular tropical fruits are also significantly less nutritious than most of the fruits grown in the continental United States. When we choose the most nutritious types and varieties of the tropical imports, though, we are eliminating one of the strikes against them and increasing our odds of enjoying optimum health.

BANANAS

We eat more bananas than any other fruit—more than apples and oranges combined. We import twenty million tons each year to keep up with demand. The most popular variety by far is the Cavendish, the yellow, long-fingered banana that is the only banana available in most US supermarkets.

Bananas are native to Southeast Asia. In the wilderness, there are thousands of varieties, not just a few. There are round bananas, chunky bananas, two-foot-long bananas, and one-inch banana nubbins. Bunches of bananas can have from five to one thousand individual fruits. The skins can be red, black, green, pink, purple, or green with white stripes. Many of them are full of large, hard seeds. Some seeds are so large that people string them together and wear them as necklaces. The small amount of edible flesh on a wild banana might be red, ocher, white, or yellow, but it is usually starchy and dry. You wouldn't feed wild bananas to a baby or add them to your breakfast cereal.

Our Southeast Asian ancestors began taming the banana as early as 6000 BC, making it one of the first fruits to be domesticated. These early farmers planted the seeds of the banana or cloned them by propagating the stalks that sprang up from their underground roots. Generation after generation, careful selection made domesticated bananas more pleasing to the human palate.

At some point in time, someone stumbled upon a bush bearing mutant, nearly seedless bananas. The seeds had been reduced to a line of soft, black flecks running up the middle of the fruit. The seeds were not viable, so the fruit had to be propagated by cuttings, which was not difficult to do. The cuttings were poked into moist soil, and within two years they sprouted new roots, created a canopy of leaves, flowered, and began producing carbon-copy seedless bananas. Carrying a few cuttings from camp to camp required little effort, so before long, seedless bananas spread throughout the tropics and subtropics. The original seedless mutant became the template for all our modern bananas.

Today there are an estimated twelve thousand varieties of seedless bananas grown worldwide. There are two main categories: (1) starchy bananas (*Musa* × *paradisiaca*), which are called plantains or cooking bananas, and (2) sweet bananas (e.g., *Musa sapientum* and *Musa nana*), which are also known as dessert bananas. Genetically, there are few differences between them, but the differences in flavor and texture can be profound. Plantains are the primary source of carbohydrates for some twenty million people worldwide. Typically, the fruits are picked green, skinned with a knife, and then steamed, baked, or fried. In impoverished countries, some adults consume more than eight hundred pounds of plantains a year; they don't just like the fruit, they live on it. Few Americans eat plantains. Unless they are fully ripe, they are pithy, dry, and astringent. The first time I took a bite of one, I spit it out. Like most people, I favor our soft, sweet Cavendish.

People in Asian countries eat sweet bananas as well as plantains, and the sweet fruit comes in hundreds of varieties. Most of the varieties have at least ten times more beta-carotene than the Cavendish. The orange-fleshed uht en yap from Micronesia has 275 times more.

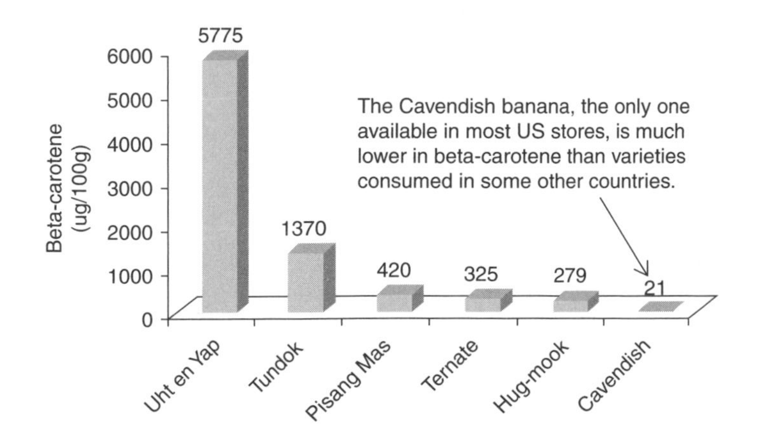

In addition to being low in beta-carotene, the Cavendish is lower in overall antioxidant value than almost all our fruits except for melons and two other tropical imports, papayas and pineapples. What's more, it is high in rapidly digested starch. The riper the banana, the greater its impact on your blood sugar. A ripe Cavendish has a glycemic load of 12; strawberries have a rating of 1.

The Cavendish banana began to dominate the US markets in the 1950s, following the devastating loss of the Gros Michel, or Big Mike, banana, which had been the most popular variety in the first half of the century. Big Mikes disappeared when a fungus infestation wiped out one hundred thousand acres of the fruit. The plantations were replanted with Cavendish bananas, a variety that was more resistant to the fungus. The Big Mike, according to those who can still remember eating it, had a richer flavor than the Cavendish.

The Cavendish does have nutritional merit, of course. A medium-size banana provides 3.5 grams of soluble fiber per serving. Although it is not among the top ten richest sources of potassium, it does have a goodly amount. Another vote in its favor is that the fruit is inexpensive and can be found in all grocery stores—even two-aisle convenience stores.

BEYOND THE CAVENDISH

What's life like beyond the Cavendish? It's worth finding out. Less common banana varieties have heady floral aromas, more intense flavor, and undertones of apple, pear, papaya, vanilla, cardamom, and lemon. They are also more nutritious. The color of the flesh is the key. The deeper and more vivid the color of the flesh, the better it is for you.

There's another reason to begin expanding our banana horizons. The iconic Cavendish is vulnerable to a nasty fungus called Tropical Race Four, which has destroyed banana plantations in Southeast Asia and Australia and could destroy crops in the Western Hemisphere as well. There is no known treatment for the disease, so there is a distinct possibility that our beloved banana will go the way of the Gros Michel. Banana researchers have identified a number of flavorful varieties that are resistant to Tropical Race Four, but they do not taste or look like the Cavendish. The scientists fear that they would be rejected by a population that is wedded to one particular clone.

Look beyond the Cavendish the next time you shop for bananas. In large supermarkets you will find the red banana, a red-skinned, pudgy fruit. The skin turns almost black when ready to eat, making it look like a miniature overripe Cavendish. When you peel back the skin, you will see the succulent, salmon-colored flesh, which is high in carotenoids and vitamin C. Take a bite and see if you can detect a touch of vanilla. If you have a toddler, consider adding red bananas to the menu. They're just the right size for young children, and they provide more nutrients than the Cavendish as well. Some supermarkets carry three-inch-long baby bananas, or niños—also called Lady Finger bananas. The flesh of this yellow-skinned variety is also richer in carotenoids than the Cavendish.

STORING BANANAS

Bananas are harvested and shipped when they are immature and dark green. In contrast to citrus fruits, they do ripen after harvest, typically with a little help from ethylene gas. The gas turns the skins yellow and also transforms the flesh from a hard, starchy food into a soft, sweet dessert. If you buy green bananas, you can store them at room temperature until they ripen, which takes about a week. To speed up the process, put the fruit in a closed paper sack with an apple, a natural producer of ethylene gas. Store ripe bananas in the refrigerator to keep them from spoiling. Although their skins will turn brown, their flesh will stay edible a few days longer than if you had kept them on the counter. Don't store unripe bananas in the refrigerator, however. The cool temperature will stop the ripening process. Even when the bananas are returned to room temperature, they are likely to stay green and starchy. This tropical fruit does not like the cold.

PINEAPPLES

Pineapples are our second-most-popular tropical fruit. Like bananas, they are relatively high in sugar and low in phytonutrients. They are a far cry from wild pineapples, which are bitter, seedy fruits guarded by spiky leaves to ward off predators. These undesirable traits motivated ancient farmers to create more pleasing varieties. They succeeded. By 1595, according to Sir Walter Raleigh, much friendlier fruit was growing in the area now known as Venezuela. This was the year that Raleigh journeyed up the Orinoco River and was greeted by men and women from the Maipure tribe, who were bearing baskets of ripe pineapples. It appears from Raleigh's description that the pineapples were very similar to the Cayenne, the variety that now dominates United States and world markets. If so, our present-day pineapples could be four-hundred-year heirlooms.

The first pineapple to challenge the Cayenne's worldwide dominion was developed in the 1990s by a consortium of Hawaiian pineapple growers. The growers were working with breeding stock that had been collected from the jungles of South America and Africa in the 1930s. After decades of crossing and recrossing the plants, one hybrid produced pineapples that were worthy of further attention. Labeled MD-2, the fruit was sweeter and less acidic than the Cayenne. It was also more pleasing to look at. Its skin was golden, not the mixed green-gold of the Cayenne, and its flesh was a deeper hue of gold.

The Del Monte company began growing and testing the MD-2 to gauge its commercial potential. Its first consumer taste test was encouraging. Consumers were blindfolded and given spears of the traditional Cayenne pineapple and the new extra-sweet variety in random order. Sixty-nine percent of the tasters preferred the new variety. This was a number the company could take to the bank. In 1996, the new variety was christened Del Monte Gold Extra Sweet and released on the market. Even though the new fruit sold for 50 percent more than the Cayenne, sales took off and increased year after year. By 2002, the company's pineapple sales had more than doubled. That was also the year that an international committee of food producers chose the extra-sweet pineapple as one of the most valuable new fruit products in the world.

Del Monte spent ten years in litigation trying to maintain its monopoly on the fruit. Although the company succeeded in knocking down a three-hundred-million-dollar class-action lawsuit, a federal judge ruled that other tropical fruit companies were free to market the MD-2 under different names. Two competing brands now on the market are Hawaii Gold and Maui Gold. All three brands come from the same genetic stock.

CHOOSING THE BEST PINEAPPLES IN THE SUPERMARKET

When you shop for pineapples in most large supermarkets, you will see the traditional Cayenne variety and at least one of the new super-sweet varieties. Paradoxically, the sweeter pineapples are the more healthful choice. Although they have 25 percent more sugar than the Cayenne, their glycemic index rating is the same. On the plus side, the MD-2 clones have 135 percent more beta-carotene and 350 percent more vitamin C than the Cayenne. One serving provides 95 percent of the recommended allowance of vitamin C, making them an excellent source of the antioxidant vitamin.

Once you have decided which variety to buy, concentrate on choosing the freshest pineapple in the market. Pineapples are harvested when ripe and do not continue to ripen once they've been harvested. If held too long, they begin to spoil. To choose a fresh pineapple, look for crown leaves that are a deep green color with no signs of fading or browning. If you can pluck a leaf from the crown, it may be over the hill. When you bring the pineapple home, eat it right away or store it in the refrigerator for no more than four days. Pineapples are not good keepers.

PAPAYAS

A bite of ripe papaya slips down your throat as smoothly as ice cream. Christopher Columbus, one of the first Europeans to taste a papaya, called it "the fruit of the angels." US consumers are becoming just as enamored with this angelic fruit. We now import more papayas than any other country in the world.

Papayas (*Carica papaya* L.) originated in the tropical forests of the Americas. The wild trees still flourish in gaps in the forest canopy caused by fire, fallen trees, or logging. It is believed that people living in southern Mexico and Central America were the first to domesticate the fruit.

Modern varieties range from pear-size to football-size. The flesh can be red, green, yellow, orange, salmon, or pink. The Solo is the most common variety in US supermarkets. Shaped somewhat like a pear, it weighs just over a pound. The pulp is a golden color. Some supermarkets now carry a much larger variety of papaya that has four aliases—Caribbean Red, Caribbean Sunrise, Mexican, and Maradol. Grown primarily in Mexico and Central America, the fruit is shaped like a truncated football and weighs between two and five pounds. This red-fleshed papaya has twice as many carotenoids as the golden Solos. It costs less per pound as well.

"I'd eat more papayas," said a friend of mine, "if I knew how to choose good ones." Color is the most important clue to ripeness. A ripe papaya is mostly yellow or orange-yellow. Press the rounded end of a papaya and it should have a slight give, but the stem end should be firm, not soft. A semiripe papaya will ripen very quickly. If the skin is equal parts green and yellow, it will become fully ripe in just two to four days at room temperature. If it is three-quarters yellow and one-quarter green, it will be ready to eat in one or two days. Brown "freckles" on the skin do not detract from the flavor or quality of the fruit. Once it's ripe, you can store the fruit in the refrigerator for up to three days.

A traditional way to serve papayas is to peel them, cut them into slices or cubes, and drizzle them with lime juice. For a Mexican flair, add a touch of chili powder and a sprinkle of finely chopped cilantro. For a wonderful summer dessert, cut the fruit in half, scoop out the seeds, and fill with ice cream or sherbet. Add sliced papaya to fruit salads and to your breakfast smoothie.

MANGOES

Most people in this country have never eaten a mango (*Mangier indicia*). But in other parts of the world, it is known as the king of fruits. In fact, worldwide, people eat ten times more mangoes than apples. The reason for this extraordinary volume is that the fruit is a staple in many of the most densely populated regions of the world—China, India, Southeast Asia, and Latin America. We should become better acquainted with this fruit. A ripe mango can be as sweet and creamy as a peach. Green mangoes, a traditional ingredient in southern Asian cuisines, add a sour tang to soups, salsas, salads, and sauces. The fruit offers nutritional rewards as well. Mangoes have five times more vitamin C than oranges, five times more fiber than pineapples, and more phytonutrients than papayas.

As is true for peaches and nectarines, the redness of a mango is not a good indicator of its ripeness. Some varieties blush red when they are still hard, while others are a solid green when ready to eat. Their aroma is a better guide. The fruit should have the distinctive aroma of a mango without any hint of ammonia, which is a sign of an overripe fruit. Their firmness is another clue. When you press the fruit gently between your palms, it should have a slight give.

Mangoes will ripen at room temperature after they've been harvested. If you bring home a semiripe fruit, you can speed the ripening process by putting it in a closed paper bag along with an apple or banana. Once the fruit is ripe, store it in the crisper drawer of the refrigerator to maintain its juiciness and prevent over-ripening. There are thousands of cultivated varieties of mangoes, but only a few are available in US supermarkets. For more variety, shop in Southeast Asian or Hispanic markets. No matter which mangoes you choose, they are guaranteed to be more nutritious than the varieties of bananas, pineapples, or papayas that are available in this country.

GUAVAS

The prevailing theory is that the wild ancestor of our present-day guava (*Psidium guajava* L.) is native to southern Mexico or northern Central America. The wild fruit is small, seedy, and sour. Modern varieties of the fruit are larger, less seedy, and range in flavor from sweet to sour. They're from two to four inches long and can be round, ovoid, or pear-shaped. Most varieties have a thin yellow skin.

In the United States, guavas are cultivated in Hawaii, Florida, Texas, and California. Despite the fact that the fruit has been modified to appeal to our modern sensibilities, it is more nutritious than most of our other tropical fruits, including mangoes. Red-fleshed guavas have an ORAC value 60 percent greater than white guavas, but white guavas are still highly nutritious fruits. In fact, they have twice the phytonutrient content of a ripe, red-fleshed papaya. A cup of sliced guava, red or white, has nine grams of fiber and a glycemic load of only 5. It has four times as much vitamin C as an orange. All this for fifty calories.

Fresh guavas are easiest to find in the states that produce them. To choose a ripe guava, look for one that yields to gentle pressure when pressed between your palms. It should be free of soft spots, dents, and scars. If the fruit is still green, store it on the kitchen counter until it ripens. Ripe guavas will keep in the crisper drawer of your refrigerator for three or four days.

Guava juice and nectar are available in large supermarkets, specialty stores, Hispanic markets, and on the Internet. The red juice has the most phytonutrients. You can drink it straight or add it to fruit punch. Red guavas make gorgeous cocktails. Mix red guava juice with vodka, a squirt of lime, and fresh mint. To your health!

Frozen guava puree (puré de guayaba) is available in many Hispanic markets. Add it to smoothies or use it in place of other fruit purees in recipes for ice cream, custard, and sorbet. On the Internet, you will find recipes for guava pies, cakes, puddings, sauces, ice cream, jam, butter, marmalade, relish, chutney, ketchup, and even guava crème brûlée.

FAIR TRADE TROPICAL FRUIT

Social injustice and the production of tropical fruit have gone hand in hand for hundreds of years. The connection continues today. Working conditions that most of us take for granted—a safe workplace, a forty-hour workweek, overtime pay, and adequate bathroom facilities—are uncommon. Many of the crops are sprayed with pesticides a dozen or more times a year, exposing workers to toxic chemicals on a routine basis.

There is an alternative. People in developed and developing countries are working together to create "fair trade" tropical fruit, fruit that is grown under conditions that are less harmful to the environment and less oppressive for the workers and small-scale producers. Some of the newest and best plantations are worker-owned companies. You can buy tropical fruits produced under fair trade guidelines in some farmers markets and specialty stores. If you can't find local sources, search the Internet. You pay more for fair trade fruit, but your dollars will help protect the ecosystem and improve the lives of field workers.

RECOMMENDED VARIETIES OF TROPICAL FRUITS

IN THE SUPERMARKET	
BANANAS	COMMENTS
Baby bananas (also called niños)	Compared to the Cavendish banana, niños have three times more vitamin C, plus more vitamin A, potassium, calcium, magnesium, manganese, and zinc. They are available in some large supermarkets.
Red bananas (also called red finger bananas)	Red finger bananas are sweet and creamy like the Cavendish, but they are higher in vitamin C and carotenoids. They are ready to eat when the skin is a dark magenta color with brown streaks. Add them to a breakfast smoothie or a fruit salad.
Burro	Let these fat and stubby bananas ripen until the flesh is yellow for the best flavor.
PINEAPPLES	COMMENTS
Golden, extra-sweet varieties	Gold-colored, very sweet pineapples are sold under a variety of brand names, including Del Monte Gold Extra Sweet, Hawaii Gold, and Maui Gold. They are sweeter and higher in beta-carotene than the traditional Cayenne variety.
PAPAYAS	COMMENTS
Caribbean Red (also called Caribbean Sunrise, Mexican, or Maradol)	This extra-large papaya can weigh between 2 and 5 pounds. Its red-colored flesh has twice the carotenoids and lycopene as the more common, golden-fleshed varieties. It is less expensive per pound as well. Most are grown in Mexico and Central America.
Solo	The Solo is the most popular papaya in US markets. It is an excellent source of vitamin C, but lower in carotenoids and lycopene than the Caribbean Red.
MANGOES	COMMENTS
Ataulfo, Haden, Francis, and Uba	All varieties of mangoes are more nutritious than bananas, pineapples, and papayas, but these four are the most nutritious varieties sold in the United States. In a 2010 study, Ataulfo and Haden had the most anticancer properties.

GUAVAS	COMMENTS
Red or pink	Guavas are the most nutritious tropical fruits in US supermarkets. Red- and pink-fleshed guavas are better for you than white-fleshed guavas. Guavas are high in fiber and have a low glycemic load. Look for red guava juice and frozen puree. If you can't find guavas in your supermarket, shop in ethnic markets.

HISPANIC, HAWAIIAN, AND ASIAN MARKETS	
BANANAS	COMMENTS
Brazilian Dwarf (also called apple banana and Dwarf Brazilian)	The Brazilian Dwarf is extra-high in vitamin C, lutein, beta-carotene, and alpha-carotene.
Hawaiian varieties	More than 50 different varieties of bananas are grown in Hawaii. If you live in Hawaii or vacation there, get to know some of these delightful fruits. The ones with the most highly pigmented flesh are the most nutritious.
PAPAYAS	COMMENTS
Rainbow	The most important papaya grown in Hawaii, the rainbow has orange-gold flesh. It has been genetically modified to resist the ring spot virus.
Sunrise	The Sunrise papaya has red-orange flesh, which translates into high levels of lycopene, beta-carotene, and a related carotenoid called beta-cryptoxanthin. It, too, has been genetically modified to resist the ring spot virus.

TROPICAL FRUITS: POINTS TO REMEMBER

1. ***Bananas are relatively high in sugar and low in phytonutrients.***
   The Cavendish banana is the most popular tropical fruit in the United States. It is lower in phytonutrients than all but a few of our fruits, such as melons, papayas, and pineapples, and it has a relatively high glycemic load. The Cavendish does provide some fiber, however, and it is a good source of potassium. Once the

fruit has fully ripened, store it in the refrigerator to prolong its palatability. Bananas with colorful flesh are more nutritious than the Cavendish.

2. ***Extra-sweet varieties of pineapples are more nutritious than the traditional variety.***
The Cayenne pineapple, our most widely sold pineapple, has a moderate glycemic load but also a relatively low phytonutrient content. The sweeter, more golden varieties of pineapple have more beta-carotene and vitamin C. Pineapples are harvested when ripe, so select the freshest fruits you can find. Fresh pineapples have dark green leaves on the crown with no signs of fading or browning.

3. ***Papayas are gaining popularity in the United States.***
Papayas have a glycemic load of 3 and are an excellent source of vitamin C. Red-fleshed papayas are more nutritious than golden-fleshed varieties and are beginning to show up in more supermarkets. You can finish ripening papayas on your kitchen counter. Eat them when they're ripe, or refrigerate them for a few days.

4. ***Mangoes deserve to be eaten in greater quantity.***
Mangoes have five times more vitamin C than oranges, five times more fiber than pineapples, and a moderate glycemic load. Mangoes with dark orange flesh give you extra phytonutrients.

5. ***The guava is one of our most nutritious tropical fruits.***
Guavas are more nutritious than bananas, pineapples, papayas, and mangoes. Red-fleshed guavas are the most nutritious of all, but even the white-fleshed varieties offer important health benefits. Eat fresh guavas and drink guava juice and nectar. Guava puree is available in some large supermarkets and most Hispanic markets and can be used in smoothies and to make ice cream, sherbet, pudding, chutney, relish, and jam.

CHAPTER 17

MELONS

LIGHT IN FLAVOR AND NUTRITION

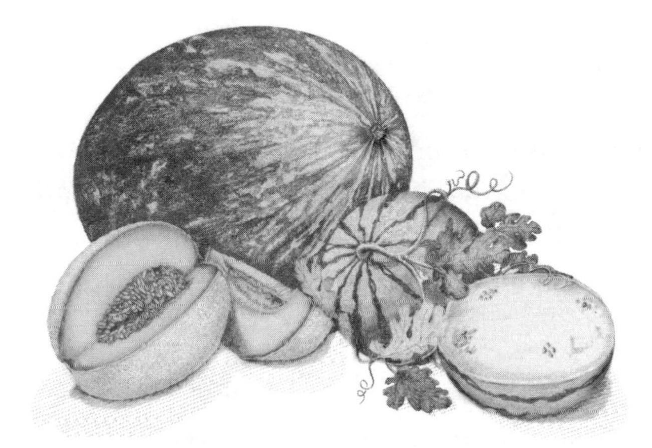

Modern and wild melons

For many people, melons are inextricably linked with summer. When I eat a great-tasting cantaloupe, I am transported back to the warm summer mornings of my childhood, when my parents and four siblings and I would eat breakfast on the patio. Cantaloupe was our favorite fruit. My dad would sprinkle his melon with salt, claiming it made it sweeter. (Science supports this.) My mom used a knife to cut her cantaloupe into cubes, then ate them with a fork. The five of us kids skipped the salt and dug into the fruit with our spoons. On warm summer evenings, we clamored for cantaloupe wedges topped with scoops of vanilla ice cream. I can still see the ice cream melting down the sides of the melon.

Most of the melons that are sold in the summer are grown in the United States, but in spring, fall, and winter they are imported from other countries. In 2010, we imported $478 million worth of melons, most of them from Mexico. The rest came from Guatemala, Costa Rica, and Honduras. We eat, on average, twenty-six pounds of melons a year, which puts them high on our list of favorite fruits. In fact, when all melons are combined, they come second to bananas in overall consumption.

Melons are about 95 percent water, so whatever nutrients they contain are highly diluted. This is one of the reasons they are lower in phytonutrients than almost all other fruits. Nonetheless, they are refreshing, juicy, low-calorie treats that provide a reasonable amount of vitamin C. If you know what to look for, you can get added phytonutrients as well.

WATERMELONS

The wild ancestor of the watermelon, the tsamma melon (*Citrullus lanatus*), is native to South Africa. The flesh of the fruit is whitish green, tart, and dry, and it has large brown seeds. The largest varieties are about eight inches in diameter. Lifelike illustrations of cultivated watermelons have been found in two-thousand-year-old Egyptian hieroglyphics, so we know that watermelons have been domesticated for at least four thousand years.

Today, wild watermelons serve as botanical canteens for the indigenous people of the Kalahari Desert. They poke a hole in the top of the fruit with a stick and twist the stick to mash the flesh. Then they upend the melon and drink the slurry. Years ago, some people on my island enjoyed a similar tradition, one they followed every Fourth of July. They, too, poked holes in watermelons, but they added a twist: they poured whiskey down the holes and used straws to slurp up the high-proof juice.

At some point in the domestication of watermelons, a red-fleshed mutant appeared. The red fruits were preferred over white-fleshed varieties and soon became more popular. Lycopene, we now know, provides the red color. Dark red watermelons are one of the best sources of this phytonutrient. In fact, some varieties have 40 percent more lycopene per ounce than ripe tomatoes.

Like most domesticated fruits, watermelons have gotten sweeter over the millennia. This trend has continued during the past one hundred years. Most heirloom varieties contain from 8 to 10 percent sugar; the sweetest hybrids approach 14 percent. We've also gotten rid of the seeds. This feat was accomplished by a Japanese scientist who—strange as it may seem—discovered that a chemical extracted from a crocus flower could alter the DNA of watermelons. The resulting change eliminated their seeds. The first seedless watermelons were bizarre-looking fruits. When these experimental fruits were crossed with conventional watermelons, however, their offspring were seedless and had a normal appearance and flavor. Today, "spitless" melons have captured 50 percent of the world market, even though they sell for a higher price.

SHOPPING FOR WATERMELONS IN THE SUPERMARKET

The most nutritious and delicious watermelons are fully ripe and have dark red flesh. A red-ripe melon can have three times more lycopene than a melon that is semiripe and pale in color. It will also have a richer, sweeter flavor. How do you know when a watermelon is ripe? Look for one that is beginning to lose its gloss. Then examine the "ground spot," the part of the melon that was in contact with the soil. It should be yellow, not green or white. When you tap the watermelon, listen for a hollow sound rather than a flat thump.

The foolproof way to pick a ripe watermelon, however, is to buy one that has been presectioned into halves, quarters, or wedges. This way you can see the color of the flesh at a glance. These cut sections are about as fresh as whole melons because the melons are cut up in the store. Watermelons that are cubed and packed into plastic cartons are not as fresh, however. They were chopped up in a distant processing plant and can be weeks old.

In recent years, "personal" watermelons have come on the market. These smaller fruits weigh about two pounds—the ideal size for one- or two-person households. Interestingly, they have more lycopene than most larger melons. Some of the large heirloom varieties, such as Black Diamond, have only a third of the lycopene content of small melons. One exception to the rule is the Dixie Lee, an heirloom variety with dark red flesh that is an excellent source of lycopene.

Watermelons are one of the rare foods that increase their antioxidant value after they've been harvested—provided you keep them out of the refrigerator. Keep a watermelon on your counter for several days and it will have 50 percent more lycopene than it did when you bought it. Chill before serving for a cool, refreshing treat.

Watermelons grow best in areas where the summer daytime temperatures are between 70 and 90 degrees and the nighttime temperatures stay above 60. If you want to grow them in cooler areas, start the seeds indoors or in a greenhouse, and then move them outdoors when the soil temperature is above 60 degrees.

CANTALOUPES

Cantaloupes (*Cucumis melo* L. var. *cantalupensis*) are second to watermelons in popularity. On average, each US adult consumes eleven pounds of cantaloupe per year. In recent years, plant breeders have created extra-sweet varieties because consumers prefer melons with a high sugar content. Genetic manipulation is one of the sugar-enhancing techniques now under investigation. Expect to see genetically modified supersweet varieties on the market in the years to come.

Meanwhile, if you're looking for sweet *and* more nutritious varieties, choose cantaloupes with deep orange flesh, which is an indication of their overall carotenoid content. The only way to determine the flesh color in a grocery store is to purchase melons that have been sectioned into quarters or halves.

When you're buying a whole cantaloupe, look for those that have no dents, fissures, or mold. To pick a ripe melon, look at the stem end. The fruit should have a slight depression, or an "innie." If it has a bit of a stub, or an "outie," it was probably picked while still green and won't have had time to develop its full flavor. Hold the stem end close to your nose and breathe deeply. A ripe melon will smell both sweet and a bit musky. Examine the opposite end, which is the "blossom" end. When you press it with your thumb, it should depress slightly.

Melons taste best when they are eaten as soon as possible after harvest. If a melon is not ripe when you buy it, store it at room temperature for one or two days. A ripe melon will keep up to five days in the crisper drawer of your refrigerator, but eat it as soon as possible.

If you're a gardener, scan the seed catalogs for cantaloupes with deep orange flesh. The images might not be representative of their true color, however, so look for words such as *deep orange* in the text. The Durango and Oro Rico varieties have been tested and found to be higher in beta-carotene than most other varieties. The beautiful French heirloom Charentais is a smooth, round melon with exquisite flavor and intensely orange-colored flesh. It does well in cool climates. If you want to leapfrog into even more exotic and historic varieties, I recommend you read *Melons for the Passionate Grower* by Amy Goldman. Whichever variety you choose, you will quadruple the health benefits you receive if you cut the melons in half and heap them with fresh or frozen berries before serving. Raspberries and cantaloupe are a good combination, as are blueberries and honeydews.

Melons grow in contact with the soil and can be contaminated by bacteria, including harmful salmonella and the potentially deadly E. coli 0157:H7. Cantaloupes, with their deeply netted skins, hold on to more bacteria than smooth-skinned melons. Before you slice a cantaloupe, scrub it thoroughly with a clean vegetable brush under running water. The use of soap or detergent is not recommended or approved for washing fruits and vegetables because fresh produce—especially porous foods such as cantaloupe—absorb detergent residues. Once you have sliced open a cantaloupe, cover it in plastic wrap and refrigerate. The cold temperature inhibits the growth of bacteria. Eat it within a day or two.

HONEYDEW MELONS

The green honeydew melon, our sweetest melon of all, is also the lowest in nutritive value. In recent years, melon breeders have crossed honeydews with cantaloupes to produce orange-fleshed honeydew melons. Surprisingly, these hybrids have even more beta-carotene than the cantaloupes. Two popular varieties are Orange Dew and Honey Gold. Because honeydews have smooth skins, they harbor fewer bacteria than cantaloupes and are easier to rinse clean.

A ripe honeydew melon feels heavy for its size, and its skin is cream-colored, not green. The stem end depresses slightly when you press it with your thumb. If it depresses too far, the melon is likely to be soft and mushy rather than ripe and crisp. Shake the melon. If the seeds rattle, it's overripe.

If you grow melons, there are two tricks that will make them more flavorful and nutritious. First, if a melon vine has multiple fruits, nip off a few of them and the remaining melons will be sweeter and more nutrient-dense. Second, if you stop watering the plants about a week before they ripen, their flavor will become more concentrated.

CASABAS

The casaba (*Cucumis melo* L. *inodorus*), a melon about the size of a honeydew, does not have the smooth skin of a honeydew or the netted skin of a cantaloupe. Instead, it has deeply wrinkled skin, which also requires extra scrubbing. Some varieties have bright yellow skin, whereas others are green or cream-colored. The flesh can range from light green to deep orange. As a rule, casabas are not as sweet as honeydews or as nutritious as cantaloupes. A standard serving has two grams of fiber and ten grams of sugar. Casabas have an extended shelf life, which makes them popular with producers and retailers.

FRUIT SALADS

A fitting way to end this section on fruits is with a nutritional makeover of the fruit salad. Throughout the history of this country, fruit salads have gone through many metamorphoses. Until the mid-1800s, most fruit salads were made exclusively from fresh or dried fruit, because freezing and home canning had not yet been invented. When John L. Mason invented the Mason glass canning jar in 1858, fruit salads began to be made from home-canned fruit as well.

In the late 1800s, fruit salad came under the sway of the home economics movement, a new school of homemaking that emphasized scientific home management, hygienic living, and rigid control. In keeping with this philosophy, progressive home cooks began to make highly structured fruit salads. Early-twentieth-century cookbook author Fannie Farmer enthralled the readers of *Woman's Home Companion* with her "Brazilian salad," which combined Brazil nuts, grapes, canned pineapple, celery, and mayonnaise, "stationing each serving in its own little pen of four saltines."

At the beginning of the twentieth century, the gelatin salad soared in popularity, thanks to the introduction of Knox gelatin. This prepackaged powdered gelatin could be dissolved in water and used in a recipe within five minutes, eliminating the need to spend an hour or more creating homemade gelatin by boiling calves' feet or knuckles. Entombing canned fruit in gelatin became the rage. Jell-O, introduced in the 1930s, combined gelatin, sugar, and artificial flavor and color, making gelatin salads even easier to make. All you had to do was add water and canned fruit. A 1940s kitchen was not complete without a set of decorative gelatin molds.

Canned fruit cocktail, a syrupy mixture of diced canned pears, peaches, pineapples, green grapes, and maraschino cherries, dominated home and restaurant tables in the 1950s. Introduced by Del

Monte as a stylish salad that was well suited for formal dinner parties, it became the most popular canned product the company ever made. Now it is known that the iconic fruit cocktail was created to find a use for culled fruit and misshapen pieces.

Gelatin salads continued to rule during the 1960s. In a recent search through my mother's faded and grease-stained recipe cards, I found a recipe entitled "Pineapple Cheese Salad" that was made from lemon Jell-O, cream cheese, crushed pineapple, whipping cream, miniature marshmallows, and Miracle Whip. A recipe entitled "Frozen Lime Butter-Mint Salad" called for lime Jell-O, crushed pineapple, a ten-ounce package of miniature marshmallows, one pint of whipping cream, and—strangely—a package of soft butter mints. The "7UP Salad" had just three ingredients: cherry Jell-O, canned applesauce, and one bottle of 7UP. "Lemon Daiquiri Salad," a more sophisticated offering, combined lemon Jell-O, frozen daiquiri mix, canned pears, cottage cheese, and sour cream. No rum.

Today, fruit salads made from fresh fruit and their natural juices are once again in the ascendancy. More often than not, however, the salads are made from some of the least nutritious varieties available, such as Thompson seedless grapes, Cavendish bananas, and Honeydew melons. To eat on the wild side, I recommend choosing the fruit from the following list of more nutritious varieties. Take the list with you to the market and see which varieties are fresh, ripe, and in season.

Recommended Ingredients for Fruit Salads

Apples with their skins

Berries of any kind, especially wild berries, blueberries, blackberries, strawberries, raspberries, cranberries, marionberries, loganberries, and boysenberries (fresh, dried, or frozen)

White-fleshed peaches or nectarines with their skins
Bing cherries, Royal Anne cherries, or sour cherries
Red-, blue-, or black-skinned plums
Dried currants
Red or black grapes
Navel oranges, Valencia oranges, Cara Cara oranges, blood oranges, or tangelos
Dark red grapefruits
Red papayas, mangoes (ripe or green), red guavas, or red bananas
Dark red watermelons, dark orange cantaloupes, or orange honeydew melons
Nuts or seeds, such as pecans, walnuts, pistachios, pumpkin seeds, or sunflower seeds (fresh or toasted)
Fresh mint or basil

Consider anointing your next fruit salad with the following dressing. A blend of sweet and tart, it will wake up any salad. The recipe was created by the talented Seattle chef and culinary instructor Pranee Khruasanit Halvorsen. Pranee travels to Thailand every year to visit her family. There, she harvests fruit from her family's tropical plantation and gathers exotic herbs and spices to bring back to the States.

I recommend that you use date sugar in this recipe, which you can find in the sugar section of large supermarkets or on the Internet. Date sugar is made from dehydrated dates. Dried dates are so sweet—from 50 to 70 percent sugar—there that there is no need for added sweetener. Its antioxidant value is very high, on a par with blackstrap molasses. Lemongrass, a quintessential ingredient in Thai food, is a tall, perennial grass that has a citrus aroma and flavor. It, too, is rich in antioxidants. You will find lemongrass in the produce section of many large supermarkets and in Asian markets.

SOM TUM POLLAMAI (MIXED SEASONAL FRUITS IN THAI HERBS AND LIME JUICE)

TOTAL TIME: 30 MINUTES YIELD: 5 CUPS (ABOUT 4 LARGE SERVINGS)

5 cups sliced or cubed assorted fresh fruit in season (see suggestions on pages 366–67)
3 tablespoons date sugar or firmly packed light or dark brown sugar
2–3 tablespoons freshly squeezed lime juice, to taste
¼ teaspoon salt
1 tablespoon finely chopped lemongrass
⅔ cup chopped fresh mint or 2 tablespoons dried mint
Grated zest of 2 limes

Place the fruit in a medium bowl. Combine sugar, lime juice, and salt in a small bowl and stir until the sugar dissolves. Pour over the fruit and toss until all the fruit is coated. Let stand for 30 minutes to blend the flavors. Just before serving, add the herbs and lime zest. The salad should be eaten the day you make it to preserve its fresh taste.

RECOMMENDED VARIETIES OF MELONS

IN THE SUPERMARKET	
WATERMELONS	COMMENTS
Small, seedless varieties	As a general rule, small, seedless varieties have more lycopene than large, seeded watermelons.
Precut watermelons	If watermelons are sold in halves or quarters, buy those that have the most intense red color – your guarantee of high lycopene content.
CANTALOUPES	COMMENTS
Precut cantaloupes	Because you cannot see the flesh color of whole cantaloupes, look for those that have been presectioned and displayed on ice. Choose cantaloupes that have the deepest orange flesh.
HONEYDEWS	COMMENTS
Orange-fleshed varieties	New varieties of orange honeydews are more nutritious than the traditional green varieties.
CASABAS	COMMENTS
All varieties	Casabas are not as nutritious as cantaloupes or as sweet as honeydews. They are very juicy.

FARMERS MARKETS, SPECIALTY STORES, U-PICK FARMS, AND SEED CATALOGS		
WATERMELONS	DESCRIPTION	INFORMATION FOR GARDENERS
Dixie Lee	Very large (up to 30 pounds), seeded, heirloom variety that has more lycopene than most old-fashioned melons.	Matures 90 days after transplanting outdoors. Best for zones 5–9.

WATERMELONS	DESCRIPTION	INFORMATION FOR GARDENERS
Extazy	Small, round, seedless watermelon with dark red flesh. Weighs 6–7 pounds. The skin has light stripes on a dark green background. Highest in lycopene in a recent review.	Matures 90 days after transplanting outdoors. Best for zones 5–9.
Lycosweet	Round, dark red, seedless watermelon with dark green skin. Weighs 6–7 pounds. Developed to be high in lycopene.	Matures 98 days after transplanting outdoors. Best for zones 5–9.
Millennium	Seedless hybrid melon. Weighs 9–11 pounds. Dark green skin without stripes. Dark red flesh. Higher in lycopene than Dixie Lee.	Matures 85 days after transplanting outdoors. Best for zones 5–9. Needs a seeded watermelon for a pollinator.
Mohican	Small, round, seedless watermelon about 7 inches in diameter. Indistinct stripes on a medium green background. High in lycopene. Noted for its excellent flavor and tender flesh.	Matures in 85 days after transplanting outdoors. Best for zones 5–9. Needs a seeded pollinator.
Summer Flavor #710	Large, great-tasting, dark red melon with seeds. Can reach 30 pounds. Light green skin with darker green stripes. Second highest in lycopene of the varieties in this chart.	Matures in 80–90 days after transplanting outdoors. Best for zones 5–9. Does not need a pollinator.
CANTALOUPES	DESCRIPTION	INFORMATION FOR GARDENERS
Bleinheim Orange	An heirloom cantaloupe with deep orange flesh.	Matures in 90–100 days. Best for zones 4–11. Does best in warm or hot growing conditions.
Charentais	A sweet, small French heirloom with very dark orange flesh. Great flavor. Not available in most markets because of its fragility.	Matures in 75–90 days. Can be direct-sown in warm climates when soil temperatures reach 70 degrees.
Durango	Firm, dark orange flesh. Extra-high in beta-carotene.	Matures in 90 days. Does better in cool conditions than some varieties.

CANTALOUPES	DESCRIPTION	INFORMATION FOR GARDENERS
Oro Rico	Sweet, firm, and crisp flesh. High in beta-carotene, but not as high as Durango. A California standby.	Matures in 90–95 days. Zones 5–11.
HONEYDEWS	DESCRIPTION	INFORMATION FOR GARDENERS
Honey Gold	Hybrid honeydew with dark orange flesh.	A vigorous vine with good yield. Does well in humid, tropical conditions and hot, dry conditions.
Orange Delight	Not as sweet or as high in beta-carotene as Orange Dew.	Matures in 100 days. Zones 5–11.
Orange Dew	Sweet, distinct flavor. Weighs about 6 pounds. Darker flesh than Orange Delight and slightly higher in beta-carotene.	Matures in 105 days. Zones 5–11.

MELONS: POINTS TO REMEMBER

1. ***Most melons are refreshing fruits with limited nutritional value.***
   All melons have a high water content, which dilutes the concentration of their nutrients. Melons with pale flesh have fewer nutrients than those with more intense colors.
2. ***Watermelons with deep red flesh are a good source of lycopene.***
   If you buy precut watermelons, you can see the inside color before you buy them. As a rule, small seedless watermelons are more nutritious than the large heirloom varieties. The skin of a ripe watermelon has lost its gloss, and the "ground spot" is

yellow. Listen for a deep sound when you thump it. Store watermelons at room temperature for a few days to increase their antioxidant value.

3. ***As a rule, honeydew and casaba melons are the sweetest and least nutritious of the melons.***
   An exception to this rule is the orange-fleshed honeydew, which has more beta-carotene than most varieties of cantaloupe.

4. ***Scrub melons thoroughly to remove surface bacteria.***
   Because melons rest on the ground, they come into direct contact with potentially harmful soil bacteria. Scrub them with a clean, soft brush under running water. Netted melons, such as cantaloupes, have more places in which to harbor bacteria and need an even more thorough scrubbing.

ACKNOWLEDGMENTS

I want to give my heartfelt thanks to Frances Robinson, my consultant, listening post, research assistant, business partner, and sister. I could not have written this book without her. I am indebted to Andie Styner of Roobiblue Studios for her exquisite illustrations and her ability to capture the essence of what I wanted to portray. My many years of research would have dragged on for yet more years without the research assistance of Moshe Rosenfeld, PhD. I give thanks to Arthur Agatston, MD, for his early interest in my work and his generous support. Dylan Bowen has been indispensable in helping to create and maintain my demonstration garden of exceptional fruits and vegetables.

Thank you to Richard Pine, my agent, who has, once again, been enthusiastic about my work and found a great publishing house to bring it out to the world. Tracy Behar, my editor at Little, Brown, has been a source of constant encouragement and has been instrumental in making *Eating on the Wild Side* more practical and accessible to readers. I also want to express my appreciation for the excellent publicity department at Little, Brown, especially Nicole Dewey, Carolyn O'Keefe, Heather Fain, Brittany Boughter, and Amanda Brown, for their determination to make the book a publishing success. Finally, I wish to thank Rick Mellen, friend and mate, who has been very patient with me as I have spent years immersed in the minutiae of human nutrition, plant chemistry, and anthropology.

SCIENTIFIC REFERENCES

The research citations are listed in the order of their relevance within each chapter. You can read a summary of any of these studies by going to http://www.ncbi.nlm.nih.gov/pubmed and entering the title of the article into the search field. You can also enter the title into any major search engine. The full text of some articles is free, but you will have to pay for the full text of the others. The cost ranges from twenty-five to forty-five dollars each, and most can be purchased online. You can also retrieve the articles from a medical or science library at a nearby college or university. The only cost will be the copying fee.

WILD NUTRIENTS: Lost and Found

Vafa, Mohammad Reza, et al. 2011. "Effects of Apple Consumption on Lipid Profile of Hyperlipidemic and Overweight Men." *International Journal of Preventive Medicine* 2 (2): 94–100.

Gibbons, Ann. 2006. "Ancient Figs Push Back Origin of Plant Cultivation." *Science* 312: 1292. The figs were a sterile variety that required human selection and propagation to grow.

Kreutzmann, Stine, Lars P. Christensen, and Merete Edelenbos. 2008. "Investigation of Bitterness in Carrots (*Daucus carota* L.) Based on Quantitative Chemical and Sensory Analyses." *LWT—Food Science and Technology* 41: 193–205.

1 | FROM WILD GREENS TO ICEBERG LETTUCE

Korcan, S. Elif, et al. 2012. "Evaluation of Antibacterial, Antioxidant, and DNA Protective Capacity of *Chenopodium album*'s Ethanolic Leaf Extract." *Chemosphere* 90: 374–79.

USDA National Nutrient Database for Standard Reference, Release 24. http://ndb.nal.usda.gov/ndb/foods/show/3233.

Tordoff, Michael G., and Mari A. Sandell. 2009. "Vegetable Bitterness Is Related to Calcium Content." *Appetite* 52: 498–504.

USDA Economic Research Service. Loss-Adjusted Food Availability: Spreadsheets. Fresh vegetable consumption. 2008.

Kang, Ho-Min, and Mikal E. Saltveit. 2002. "Antioxidant Capacity of Lettuce Leaf Tissue Increases After Wounding." *Journal of Agricultural and Food Chemistry* 50: 7536–41.

USDA Nutrient Data Laboratory. Oxygen Radical Absorbance Capacity (ORAC) of Selected Foods, Release 2 (2010). http://www.ars.usda.gov/Services/docs.htm?docid=15866.

Higdon, Jane V., et al. 2007. "Cruciferous Vegetables and Human Cancer Risk: Epidemiologic Evidence and Mechanistic Basis." *Pharmacological Research* 55: 224–36.

Ninfali, Paolino, et al. 2005. "Antioxidant Capacity of Vegetables, Spices, and Dressings Relevant to Nutrition." *British Journal of Nutrition* 93: 257–66.

Innocenti, Marzia, et al. 2005. "Evaluation of the Phenolic Content in the Aerial Parts of Different Varieties of *Cichorium intybus* L." *Journal of Agricultural and Food Chemistry* 53: 6497–6502.

McBride, Judy. 1999. "Can Foods Forestall Aging?" Agricultural Research Service News and Events. http://www.ars.usda.gov/is/AR/archive/feb99/aging0299.htm.

Gil, Maria I., Federico Ferreres, and Francisco A. Tomás-Barberán. 1999. "Effect of Postharvest Storage and Processing on the Antioxidant Constituents (Flavonoids and Vitamin C) of Fresh-Cut Spinach." *Journal of Agricultural and Food Chemistry* 47: 2213–17.

Pandjaitan, N., et al. 2005. "Antioxidant Capacity and Phenolic Content of Spinach as Affected by Genetics and Maturation." *Journal of Agricultural and Food Chemistry* 53: 8618–23.

Goltz, Shellen R., et al. 2012. "Meal Triacylglycerol Profile Modulates Postprandial Absorption of Carotenoids in Humans." *Molecular Nutrition & Food Research* 56 (6): 866–77.

Ghanbari, Rahele, et al. 2012. "Valuable Nutrients and Functional Bioactives in Different Parts of Olive (*Olea europaea* L.)—A Review." *International Journal of Molecular Science* 13: 3291–3340.

Tsimidou, Maria Z., et al. 2005. "Loss of Stability of 'Veiled' (Cloudy) Virgin Olive Oils in Storage." *Food Chemistry* 93: 377–83.

2 | ALLIUMS: All Things to All People

Moerman, D. E. 1996. "An Analysis of the Food Plants and Drug Plants of Native North America." *Journal of Ethnopharmacology* 52: 1–22.

Allard, H. A. 1955. "Chicago, a Name of Indian Origin, and the Native Wild Onion to Which the Indians May Have Had Reference as the 'Skunk Place.'" *Castanea* 20 (1): 28–31. *Castanea* was the name of the journal of the Southern Appalachian Botanical Society.

Gunther, Erna. *Ethnobotany of Western Washington.* Seattle and London: University of Washington Press, 1973. First published in 1945.

Mansell, Peter, and John P. D. Reckless. 1991. "Garlic: Effects on Serum Lipids, Blood Pressure, Coagulation, Platelet Aggregation, and Vasodilation." *British Medical Journal* 303: 379–80.

Rahman, K., and Lowe, G. M. 2006. "Garlic and Cardiovascular Disease: A Critical Review." *Journal of Nutrition* 136: 736S–740S.

Abdullah, Tariq, et al. 1988. "Garlic Revisited: Therapeutic for the Major Diseases of Our Times?" *Journal of the National Medical Association* 80: 439–45.

Ankri, Serge, and David Mirelman. 1999. "Antimicrobial Properties of Allicin from Garlic." *Microbes and Infection* 2: 125–29.

Choi, Hwa Jung, et al. 2009. "Inhibitory Effects of Quercetin 3-Rhamnoside on Influenza A Virus Replication." *European Journal of Pharmaceutical Sciences* 37: 329–33.

Boivin, Dominique, et al. 2009. "Antiproliferative and Antioxidant Activities of Common Vegetables: A Comparative Study." *Food Chemistry* 112: 374–80.

Song, Kun, and John A. Milner. 2001. "The Influence of Heating on the Anticancer Properties of Garlic." *Journal of Nutrition* 131: 1054S–57S.

Lee, J., and J. M. Harnly. 2005. "Free Amino Acid and Cysteine Sulfoxide Composition of 11 Garlic (*Allium sativum* L.) Cultivars by Gas Chromatography with Flame Ionization and Mass Selective Detection." *Journal of Agricultural and Food Chemistry* 53: 9100–9104.

Gorinstein, Shela, et al. 2007. "The Atherosclerotic Heart Disease and Protection Properties of Garlic: Contemporary Data." *Molecular Nutrition & Food Research* 51: 1365–81.

Yang Jun, et al. 2004. "Varietal Differences in Phenolic Content and Antioxidant and Antiproliferative Activities of Onions." *Journal of Agricultural and Food Chemistry* 52: 6787–93.

Lee, Seung Un, et al. 2008. "Flavonoid Content in Fresh, Home-Processed, and Light-Exposed Onions and in Dehydrated Commercial Onion Products." *Journal of Agricultural and Food Chemistry* 56: 8541–48.

Yang et al. 2004. "Varietal Differences."

Griffiths, Gareth, et al. 2002. "Onions—A Global Benefit to Health." *Phytotherapy Research* 16: 603–15.

Ioku, K., et al. 2001. "Various Cooking Methods and the Flavonoid Content in Onion." *Journal of Nutritional Science and Vitaminology* 47 (1): 78–83.

Lu, Xiaonan, et al. 2011. "Determination of Total Phenolic Content and Antioxidant Capacity of Onion (*Allium cepa*) and Shallot (*Allium oschaninii*) Using Infrared Spectroscopy." *Food Chemistry* 129: 637–44.

Yang et al. 2004. "Varietal Differences."

Bonaccorsi, Paola. 2008. "Flavonol Glucosides in *Allium* Species: A Comparative Study by Means of HPLC-DAD-ESI-MS-MS." *Food Chemistry* 107: 1668–73.

Stajner, D. 2004. "*Allium schoenoprasum* L., as a Natural Antioxidant. *Phytotherapy Research* 18: 522–24.

Guohua, H., et al. 2009. "Aphrodisiac Properties of *Allium tuberosum* Seeds Extract." *Journal of Ethnopharmacology* 122: 579–82.

Bonaccorsi, 2008. "Flavonol Glucosides."

Hsing, A. W., et al. 2002. "Allium Vegetables and Risk of Prostate Cancer: A Population-Based Study." *Journal of the National Cancer Institute* 94 (21): 1648–51.

3 | CORN ON THE COB: How Supersweet It Is!

Flint-Garcia, Sherry A., Anastasia L. Bodnar, and M. Paul Scott. 2009. "Wide Variability in Kernel Composition, Seed Characteristics, and Zein Profiles Among Diverse Maize Inbreds, Landraces, and Teosinte." *Theoretical Applied Genetics* 119: 1129–42.

Kingsbury, Noel. 2009. *Hybrid: The History and Science of Plant Breeding.* Chicago: University of Chicago Press.

Guohua, H., et al. 2009. "Aphrodisiac Properties of *Allium tuberosum* Seeds Extract." *Journal of Ethnopharmacology* 122: 579–82

Tsuda, Takanori, et al. 2003. "Dietary Cyanidin 3-O-Beta-D-Glucoside-Rich Purple Corn Color Prevents Obesity and Ameliorates Hyperglycemia in Mice." *Journal of Nutrition* 133: 2125–30.

Bradford, William. 1856. *Of Plimouth Plantation.* Boston: Massachusetts Historical Society. http://www.americanjourneys.org/aj-025/summary/.

Carter, G. F. 1948. "Sweet Corn Among the Indians." *Geographical Review* 38: 206–221. www.azwater.gov/Adjudications/documents/HopiContestedCaseDisclosures/Hopi%20Initial%20Disclosure/HP296%20-%20HP302.pdf.

Rea, Mary-Alice F. 1975. "Early Introduction of Economic Plants into New England." *Economic Botany* 29: 333–56.

Singleton, W. Ralph. 1944. "Noyes Darling, First Maize Breeder." *Journal of Heredity* 35 (9): 265–67.

Wilkinson, Albert E. 1915. *Sweet Corn.* New York and London: Orange Judd Company.

"Effects of an Atomic Bomb Explosion on Corn Seeds." Declassified Document 473888, published by the Armed Forces Special Weapons Project on July 6, 1951.

Maize COOP Information, by the Maize Genetics Cooperation and the University of Illinois, Urbana/Champaign. Published online: http://maizecoop.cropsci.uiuc.edu/mgc-info.php.

Laughnan, John R. 1953. "The Effect of the sh2 Factor on Carbohydrate Reserves in the Mature Endosperm of Maize." *Genetics* 38: 485.

Showalter, R. K. 1962. "Consumer Preference for High-Sugar, Sweet Corn Varieties." Florida State Horticultural Society.

Maize COOP Information.

Frank, Guido K. W., et al. 2008. "Sucrose Activates Human Taste Pathways Differently from Artificial Sweetener." *NeuroImage* 39: 1559–69.

Scott, C. E., and Alison Eldridge. 2005. "Comparison of Carotenoid Content in Fresh, Frozen, and Canned Corn." *Journal of Food Composition and Analysis* 18: 551–59.

Asami, Danny K., et al. 2003. "Comparison of the Total Phenolic and Ascorbic Acid Content of Freeze-Dried and Air-Dried Marionberry, Strawberry, and Corn Grown Using Conventional, Organic, and Sustainable Agricultural Practices." *Journal of Agricultural and Food Chemistry* 51: 1237–41.

Dewanto, Veronica, Xianzhong Wu, and Rui Hai Liu. 2002. "Processed Sweet Corn Has Higher Antioxidant Activity." *Journal of Agricultural and Food Chemistry* 50: 4949–64.

4 | POTATOES: From Wild to Fries

Smith, Andrew F. 2006. *Encyclopedia of Junk Food and Fast Food*. Westport, CT: Greenwood Press.

Iwai, Kunihisa, and Hajime Matsue. 2007. "Ingestion of *Apios Americana* Medikus Tuber Suppresses Blood Pressure and Improves Plasma Lipids in Spontaneously Hypertensive Rats." *Nutrition Research* 27: 218–24.

Im, Hyon Woon, et al. 2008. "Analysis of Phenolic Compounds by High-Performance Liquid Chromatography and Liquid Chromatography/Mass Spectrometry in Potato Plant Flowers, Leaves, Stems, and Tubers and in Home-Processed Tomatoes." *Journal of Agricultural and Food Chemistry* 56: 3341–49. The data for the accompanying graph came from this paper as well.

Soliman, K. M. 2001. "Changes in Concentration of Pesticide Residues in Potatoes During Washing and Home Preparation." *Food and Chemical Toxicology* 39: 887–89.

Friedman, Mendel. 1997. "Chemistry, Biochemistry, and Dietary Role of Potato Polyphenols. A Review." *Journal of Agricultural and Food Chemistry* 45: 1523–40

Foster-Powell, Kaye, Susanna H. A. Holt, and Janette C. Brand-Miller. 2002. "International Table of Glycemic Index and Glycemic Load Values: 2002." *American Journal of Clinical Nutrition* 76: 5–56.

Lewis, Christine E., et al. 1999. "Determination of Anthocyanins, Flavonoids, and Phenolic Acids in Potatoes. I: Coloured Cultivars of Solanum tuberosum L." *Journal of the Science of Food and Agriculture* 77: 45–57.

Thompson, Matthew D., et al. 2009. "Functional Food Characteristics of Potato Cultivars (*Solanum tuberosum* L.): Phytochemical Composition and Inhibition of 1-Methyl-1-Nitrosourea–Induced Breast Cancer in Rats." *Journal of Food Composition and Analysis* 22: 571–76.

"SCS Launches First Program to Certify Exceptional Nutrient Density in Fresh Produce." Annie Gardiner, Scientific Certification Systems, Director of Communications. May 2, 2006. http://www.marketwire.com/press-release/new-high-potency-antioxidant-purple-majesty-potatoes-make-national-debut-southern-california-685381.htm.

Vinson, Joe A., et al. 2012. "High-Antioxidant Potatoes: Acute in Vivo Antioxidant Source and Hypotensive Agent in Humans after Supplementation to Hypertensive Subjects." *Journal of Agricultural and Food Chemistry* 60: 6749–54.

Ek, Kai Lin, Jennie Brand-Miller, and Les Copeland. 2012. "Glycemic Effect of Potatoes." *Food Chemistry* 133: 1230–40.

5 | THE OTHER ROOT CROPS: Carrots, Beets, and Sweet Potatoes

Milton, Katharine. 1984. "Protein and Carbohydrate Resources of the Maku Indians of Northwestern Amazonia." *American Anthropologist* 86 (1): 7–27.

Silverwood-Cope, Peter. 1972. "A Contribution to the Ethnography of the Colombian Maku." PhD dissertation, Selwyn College, University of Cambridge.

Moerman, D. E. 1996. "An Analysis of the Food Plants and Drug Plants of Native North America." *Journal of Ethnopharmacology* 52: 1–22.

Banga, Otto. 1963. "Origin and Distribution of the Western Cultivated Carrot." *Genetica Agraria* 17: 357–70.

Metzger, Brandon T., and David M. Barnes. 2009. "Polyacetylene Diversity and Bioactivity in Orange Market and Locally Grown Colored Carrots (*Daucus carota* L.)." *Journal of Agricultural and Food Chemistry* 57: 11134–39. The data for the accompanying graph came from this paper as well.

Carlsen, Monica, et al. 2010. "The Total Antioxidant Content of More Than 3100 Foods, Beverages, Spices, Herbs, and Supplements Used Worldwide." *Nutrition Journal* 9: 3–23.

Hunter, Karl J., and John M. Fletcher. 2002. "The Antioxidant Activity and Composition of Fresh, Frozen, Jarred, and Canned Vegetables." *Innovative Food Science and Emerging Technologies* 3: 399–406.

Rock, C. L., et al. 1998. "Bioavailability of β-carotene Is Lower in Raw Than in Processed Carrots and Spinach in Women." *Journal of Nutrition* 128: 913–16.

Kobaek-Larsen, Morten, et al. 2005. "Inhibitory Effects of Feeding with Carrots or (-)-Falcarinol on Development of Azoxymethane-Induced Preneoplastic Lesions in the Rat Colon." *Journal of Agricultural and Food Chemistry* 53 (5): 1823–27.

Hornero-Méndez, Dámaso, and María Isabel Mínguez Mosquera. 2007. "Bioaccessibility of Carotenes from Carrots: Effect of Cooking and Addition of Oil." *Innovative Food Science and Emerging Technologies* 8: 407–12. The data for the accompanying graph came from this paper as well.

Li, Chaoyang, et al. 2011. "Serum Alpha-Carotene Concentrations and Risk of Death among US Adults: The Third National Health and Nutrition

Examination Survey Follow-Up Study." *Archives of Internal Medicine* 171: 507–15.

Poudyal, Hemant, Sunil Panchal, and Lindsay Brown. 2010. "Comparison of Purple Carrot Juice and β-Carotene in a High-Carbohydrate, High-Fat Diet-Fed Rat Model of the Metabolic Syndrome." *British Journal of Nutrition* 104: 1322–32.

Alasalvar, Cesarettin, et al. 2001. "Comparison of Volatiles, Phenolics, Sugars, Antioxidant Vitamins, and Sensory Quality of Different Colored Carrot Varieties." *Journal of Agricultural and Food Chemistry* 49: 1410–16.

Metzger and Barnes. 2009. "Polyacetylene Diversity."

US Census Bureau, Statistical Abstract of the United States: Table 104. Expectation of Life at Birth, 1970–2008, and Projections, 2010 to 2020.

US Department of Health and Human Services. National Diabetes Statistics, 2011.

Note on discussion of hunter-gatherer health: For more information about the health of hunter-gatherers, I recommend that you read *The Paleolithic Prescription* by S. Boyd Eaton, MD, Marjorie Shostak, and Melvin Konner, MD, PhD; *The Paleo Diet* by Loren Cordain, PhD; and "Paleolithic Nutrition—A Consideration of Its Nature and Current Implications," by S. Boyd Eaton and Melvin Konner, in *The New England Journal of Medicine* 312 (5): 283–89.

American Heart Association. Statistical Fact Sheet 2012 Update.

Carrera-Bastos, Pedro, et al. 2011. "The Western Diet and Lifestyle and Diseases of Civilization." *Research Reports in Clinical Cardiology* 2: 15–35.

Nielsen, F. H., et al. 1987. "Effect of Dietary Boron on Mineral, Estrogen, and Testosterone Metabolism in Postmenopausal Women." *Journal of the Federation of American Societies for Experimental Biology* 1 (5): 394–97.

Bor, M., F. Özdemir, and I. Türkan. 2002. "The Effect of Salt Stress on Lipid Peroxidation and Antioxidants in Leaves of Sugar Beet *Beta vulgaris* L. and Wild Beet *Beta maritima* L." *Plant Science* 164: 77–84.

Carlsen et al. 2010. "The Total Antioxidant Content."

Reddy, M. K., R. L. Alexander-Lindo, and M. G. Nair. 2005. "Relative Inhibition of Lipid Peroxidation, Cyclooxygenase Enzymes, and Human Tumor Cell Proliferation by Natural Food Colors." *Journal of Agricultural and Food Chemistry* 53 (23): 9268–73.

Lansley, Katherine E., et al. 2010. "Dietary Nitrate Supplementation Reduces the O2 Cost of Walking and Running: A Placebo-Controlled Study." *Journal of Applied Physiology* 110: 591–600.

Murphy, Margaret, et al. 2012. "Whole Beetroot Consumption Acutely Improves Running Performance." *Journal of the Academy of Nutrition and Dietetics* 112: 548–52.

Reynolds, Gretchen. 2012. "Looking for Fitness in a Glass of Juice." *New York Times,* August 8. Science section.

Jiratanan, Thudnatkorn, and Rui Hai Liu. 2004. "Antioxidant Activity of Processed Table Beets (*Beta vulgaris* var. *conditiva*) and Green Beans (*Phaseolus vulgaris* L.)." *Journal of Agricultural and Food Chemistry* 52: 2659–70.

Ravichandran, Kavitha, et al. 2012. "Impact of Processing of Red Beet on Betalain Content and Antioxidant Activity." *Food Research International.* http://dx.doi.org/10.1016/j.foodres.2011.07.002.

Nottingham, Stephen. 2004. *Beetroot.* Published online. http://www.stephennottingham.co.uk/beetroot.htm.

International Potato Center. 1988. "Exploration, Maintenance, and Utilization of Sweet Potato Genetic Resources: Report of the First Sweet Potato Planning Conference 1987."

Foster-Powell, Kaye, Susanna H. A. Holt, and Janette C. Brand-Miller. 2002. "International Table of Glycemic Index and Glycemic Load Values: 2002." *American Journal of Clinical Nutrition* 76: 5–56.

Carlsen et al. 2010. "The Total Antioxidant Content."

Teow, Choong C., et al. 2007. "Antioxidant Activities, Phenolic and β-Carotene Contents of Sweet Potato Genotypes with Varying Flesh Colors." *Food Chemistry* 103: 829–38.

Truong, V. D., et al. 2007. "Phenolic Acid Content and Composition in Leaves and Roots of Common Commercial Sweetpotato (*Ipomea batatas* L.) Cultivars in the United States." *Journal of Food Science* 72: C343–49.

6 | TOMATOES: Bringing Back Their Flavor and Nutrients

Smith, Andrew F. 1994. *The Tomato in America: Early History, Culture, and Cookery.* Columbia, SC: University of South Carolina Press.

Grolier, P., and E. Rock. 1998. "The Composition of Tomato in Antioxidants: Variations and Methodology." Proceedings of Tomato and Health Seminar. Pamplona, Spain.

Allen, Arthur. 2008. "A Passion for Tomatoes." *Smithsonian*: http://www.smithsonianmag.com/science-nature/passion-for-tomatoes.html?c=y&page=3#ixzz0mnaACMJ7.

Wolf, Gerhard, ed. 2012. *Colors Between Two Worlds: The Florentine Codex of Bernardino de Sahagún*. Florence: Villa I Tatti.

Cox, Samuel E. 2001. "Lycopene Analysis and Horticultural Attributes of Tomatoes." Master's thesis, Colorado State University.

Jefferson, Thomas. *Garden Book*. 1776–1824 Kalender. Available online at http://www.masshist.org/thomasjeffersonpapers/garden/index.html.

Sturtevant, E. Lewis. 1885. "Kitchen Garden Esculents of American Origin." *The American Naturalist* 19: 658–69.

Powell, Ann L. T., et al. 2012. "Uniform Ripening Encodes a Golden 2-Like Transcription Factor Regulating Tomato Fruit Chloroplast Development." *Science* 336: 1711–15.

Beckles, Diane M. 2012. "Factors Affecting the Postharvest Soluble Solids and Sugar Content of Tomato (*Solanum lycopersicum* L.) Fruit." *Postharvest Biology and Technology* 63: 129–40.

Unlu, Nuray Z., et al. 2005. "Carotenoid Absorption from Salad and Salsa by Humans Is Enhanced by the Addition of Avocado or Avocado Oil." *Journal of Nutrition* 135: 431–36.

Kuti, Joseph O., and Hima B. Konuru. 2005. "Effects of Genotype and Cultivation Environment on Lycopene Content in Red-Ripe Tomatoes." *Journal of the Science of Food and Agriculture* 85: 2021–26.

Shi, John, and Marc Le Maguer. 2000. "Lycopene in Tomatoes: Chemical and Physical Properties Affected by Food Processing." *Critical Reviews in Food Science and Nutrition* 40: 1–42.

Barrett, D. M., et al. 2007. "Qualitative and Nutritional Differences in Processing Tomatoes Grown Under Commercial Organic and Conventional Production Systems." *Journal of Food Science* 72: C441–51.

Toor, Ramandeep K., and Geoffrey P. Savage. 2005. "Antioxidant Activity of Different Fractions of Tomatoes." *Food Research International* 38 (5): 487–94.

Dewanto, Veronica, et al. 2002. "Thermal Processing Enhances the Nutritional Value of Tomatoes by Increasing Total Antioxidant Activity." *Journal of Agricultural and Food Chemistry* 50: 3010–14. The data for the accompanying graph came from this paper as well.

Gärtner, Christine, Wilhelm Stahl, and Helmut Sies. 1997. "Lycopene Is More Bioavailable from Tomato Paste Than from Fresh Tomatoes." *American Journal of Clinical Nutrition* 66: 116–22.

Stahl, Wilhelm, et al. 2000. "Dietary Tomato Paste Protects Against Ultraviolet Light-Induced Erythema in Humans." *Journal of Nutrition* 131: 1449–51.

7 | THE INCREDIBLE CRUCIFERS: Tame Their Bitterness and Reap the Rewards

Mitchell, N. D. 1976. "The Status of *Brassica oleracea* L. subsp. *oleracea* (Wild Cabbage) in the British Isles." *Watsonia* 11: 97–103.

USDA Economic Research Service. Food Availability (per Capita) Data System: Food Guide Pyramid Servings. 2011. Data as of 2009.

Johnston, Carol S., Christopher A. Taylor, and Jeffrey S. Hampl. 2000. "More Americans Are Eating '5 a Day' but Intakes of Dark Green and Cruciferous Vegetables Remain Low." *Journal of Nutrition* 130: 3063–67. The data for the accompanying graph came from this paper as well.

Vallejo, Fernando, Francisco Tomás-Baberán, and Cristina García-Viguera. 2003. "Health-Promoting Compounds in Broccoli as Influenced by Refrigerated Transport and Retail Sale Period." *Journal of Agricultural and Food Chemistry* 51: 3029–34.

Agricultural Marketing Resource Center. Broccoli Profile. Revised April 2012.

Cantwell, Marita, and Trevor Suslow. 1997. "Broccoli: Recommendations for Maintaining Postharvest Quality." *Perishables Handling* 92.

Lucier, Gary, Susan Pollack, and Agnes Perez. 1997. "Import Penetration in the US Fruit and Vegetable Industry." USDA Economic Research Service.

Nath, A., et al. 2011. "Changes in Post-Harvest Phytochemical Qualities of Broccoli Florets During Ambient and Refrigerated Storage." *Food Chemistry* 127: 1510–14.

Cieślik, Ewa, et al. 2007. "Effects of Some Technological Processes on Glucosinolate Contents in Cruciferous Vegetables." *Food Chemistry* 105: 976–81.

Vermeulen, Martijn, et al. 2008. "Bioavailability and Kinetics of Sulforaphane in Humans After Consumption of Cooked Versus Raw Broccoli." *Journal of Agricultural and Food Chemistry* 56: 10505–9.

Miglio, Cristiana, et al. 2008. "Effects of Different Cooking Methods on Nutritional and Physicochemical Characteristics of Selected Vegetables." *Journal of Agricultural and Food Chemistry* 56 (1): 139–47.

Zhang, Donglin, and Yasunori Hamauzu. 2004. "Phenolics, Ascorbic Acid, Carotenoids, and Antioxidant Activity of Broccoli and Their Changes during Conventional and Microwave Cooking." *Food Chemistry* 88: 503–09.

Yuan, Gao-feng, et al. 2009. "Effects of Different Cooking Methods on Health-Promoting Compounds of Broccoli." *Journal of Zhejiang University* 10 (8): 580–88.

Wang, Grace C., Mark Farnham, and Elizabeth H. Jeffery. 2012. "Impact of Thermal Processing on Sulforaphane Yield from Broccoli (*Brassica oleracea* L. ssp. *italica*)." *Journal of Agricultural and Food Chemistry* 60: 6743–48.

Boivin, Dominique, et al. 2009. "Antiproliferative and Antioxidant Activities of Common Vegetables: A Comparative Study." *Food Chemistry* 112: 374–80.

Cieślik et al. 2007. "Effects of Some Technological Processes."

Chun, Ock Kyoun, et al. 2004. "Antioxidant Properties of Raw and Processed Cabbages." *International Journal of Food Sciences and Nutrition* 55 (3): 191–99.

King, G. J. 2003. "Using Molecular Allelic Variation to Understand Domestication Processes and Conserve Diversity in *Brassica* Crops." *Acta Horticulturae* 598: 181–85.

Gratacós-Cubarsí, M., et al. 2010. "Simultaneous Evaluation of Intact Glucosinolates and Phenolic Compounds by UPLC-DAD-MS/MS in *Brassica oleracea* L. var. *botrytis*." *Food Chemistry* 121: 257–63.

Volden, Jon, Gunnar B. Bengtsson, and Trude Wicklund. 2009. "Glucosinolates, L-Ascorbic Acid, Total Phenols, Anthocyanins, Antioxidant Capacities, and Colour in Cauliflower (*Brassica oleracea* L. ssp. *botrytis*): Effects of Long-Term Freezer Storage." *Food Chemistry* 112: 967–76.

Volden, Jon, et al. 2009. "Processing (Blanching, Boiling, Steaming) Effects on the Content of Glucosinolates and Antioxidant-Related Parameters in Cauliflower (*Brassica oleracea* L. ssp. *botrytis*)." *LWT—Food Science and Technology* 42: 63–73.

Annual Report of the Agricultural Experiment Station, Michigan State University. 2003.

Olsen, Helle, et al. 2012. "Antiproliferative Effects of Fresh and Thermal Processed Green and Red Cultivars of Curly Kale (*Brassica oleracea* L. convar. *acephala* var. *sabellica*)." *Journal of Agricultural and Food Chemistry*. http://www.ncbi.nlm.nih.gov/pubmed/22769426.

USDA Economic Research Service. Data last updated February 27, 2009.

Dinehart, M. E., et al. 2006. "Bitter Taste Markers Explain Variability in Vegetable Sweetness, Bitterness, and Intake." *Physiology and Behavior* 87: 304–13.

Korus, Anna, and Zofia Lisiewska. 2011. "Effect of Preliminary Processing and Method of Preservation on the Content of Selected and Antioxidative Compounds in Kale (*Brassica oleracea* L. var. *acephala*) Leaves." *Food Chemistry* 129: 149–54.

8 | LEGUMES: Beans, Peas, and Lentils

Abbo, Shahal, et al. 2008. "Wild Lentil and Chickpea Harvest in Israel: Bearing on the Origins of Near Eastern Farming." *Journal of Archaeological Science* 35: 3172–77.

Dorsey, Owen J. 1884. "An Account of War Customs of the Osages." *The American Naturalist* 18:113–133.

Quinn, David B. 1967. "Martin Pring at Provincetown in 1603." *The New England Quarterly* 40: 79–91.

Sherwood, N. N. "Garden Peas." *Journal of the Royal Horticultural Society* XX, part 1 (1896): 117.

Bowles, Emily. 1888. *Madame de Maintenon.* London: Kegan Paul, Trench & Co.

Ou, Boxin, et al. 2002. "Analysis of Antioxidant Activities of Common Vegetables Employing Oxygen Radical Absorbance Capacity (ORAC) and Ferric Reducing Antioxidant Power (FRAP) Assays: A Comparative Study." *Journal of Agricultural and Food Chemistry* 50: 3122–28.

Murcia, Antonia, Antonia Jiménez, and Magdalena Martínez-Tomé. 2009. "Vegetable Antioxidant Losses During Industrial Processing and Refrigerated Storage." *Food Research International* 42: 1046–52.

Wu, Xianli, et al. 2004. "Lipophilic and Hydrophilic Antioxidant Capacities of Common Foods in the United States." *Journal of Agricultural and Food Chemistry* 52: 4026–37.

Campos-Vega, Rocio, Guadalupe Loarca-Piña, and B. Dave Oomah. 2010. "Minor Components of Pulses and Their Potential Impact on Human Health." *Food Research International* 43 (2): 461–82. The data for the accompanying graph came from this paper as well.

Flight, I., and P. Clifton. 2006. "Cereal Grains and Legumes in the Prevention of Coronary Heart Disease and Stroke: A Review of the Literature." *European Journal of Clinical Nutrition* 60: 1145–59.

Luthria, Devanand L., and Marcial A. Pastor-Corrales. 2006. "Phenolic Acids Content of Fifteen Dry Edible Bean (*Phaseolus vulgaris* L.) Varieties." *Journal of Food Composition and Analysis* 19: 205–11.

Adebamowo, C. A., et al. 2005. "Dietary Flavonols and Flavonol-Rich Foods Intake and the Risk of Breast Cancer." *International Journal of Cancer* 114: 628–33.

Phillips, R. D., and Bene W. Abbey. 1989. "Composition and Flatulence-Producing Potential of Commonly Eaten Nigerian and American Legumes." *Food Chemistry* 33: 171–280.

Xu, Baojun, and Sam K. C. Chang. 2008. "Effect of Soaking, Boiling, and Steaming on Total Phenolic Content and Antioxidant Activities of Cool Season Food Legumes." *Food Chemistry* 110: 1–13.

Floegel, Anna, et al. 2011. "Comparison of ABTS/DPPH Assays to Measure Antioxidant Capacity in Popular Antioxidant-Rich US Foods." *Journal of Food Composition and Analysis* 24: 1043–48.

Xu, Baojun, and Sam K. C. Chang. 2010. "Phenolic Substance Characterization and Chemical and Cell-Based Antioxidant Activities of 11 Lentils Grown in the Northern United States." *Journal of Agricultural and Food Chemistry* 58:1509–17.

National Soybean Research Laboratory at the University of Illinois.

Konovsky, John, Thomas A. Lumpkin, and Dean McClary. 1994. "Edamame: The Vegetable Soybean." In A. D. O'Rourke, ed., *Understanding the Japanese Food and Agrimarket: A Multifaceted Opportunity.* Philadelphia, PA: Haworth Press.

US Army Medical Research Institute of Infectious Diseases, Fort Detrick, Frederick, Maryland. AD-A221–05.

9 | ARTICHOKES, ASPARAGUS, AND AVOCADOS: Indulge!

Pinelli, Patrizia, et al. 2007. "Simultaneous Quantification of Caffeoyl Esters and Flavonoids in Wild and Cultivated Cardoon Leaves." *Food Chemistry* 105: 1695–1701.

USDA Nutrient Data Laboratory. Oxygen Radical Absorbance Capacity (ORAC) of Selected Foods, Release 1 (2007).

USDA National Nutrient Database for Standard Reference, Release 20: Fiber.

Eaton, Boyd S., Marjorie Shostak, and Melvin Konner. 1988. *The Paleolithic Prescription.* New York: HarperCollins.

USDA Economic Research Service. Data updated February 1, 2011. "Fresh Artichokes: Per Capita Availability Adjusted for Loss."

Lutz, M., C. Henríquez, and M. Escobar. 2011. "Chemical Composition and Antioxidant Properties of Mature and Baby Artichokes (*Cynara scolymus* L.), Raw and Cooked." *Journal of Food Composition and Analysis* 24: 49–54.

Ferracane, Rosalia, et al. 2008. "Effects of Different Cooking Methods on Antioxidant Profile, Antioxidant Capacity, and Physical Characteristics of

Artichoke." *Journal of Agricultural and Food Chemistry* 56 (18): 8601–8608. The data for the accompanying graph came from this paper as well.

Gil-Izquierdo, A., et al. 2001. "The Effect of Storage Temperatures on Vitamin C and Phenolics Content of Artichoke (*Cynara scolymus* L.) Heads." *Innovative Food Science & Emerging Technologies* 2: 199–202.

Halvorsen, Bente L., et al. "Content of Redox-Active Compounds (i.e., Antioxidants) in Foods Consumed in the United States." *American Journal of Clinical Nutrition* 84: 95–135.

Cato the Elder. *On Agriculture*. Loeb Classical Library, 1934.

Ferrara, L., et al. 2011. "Nutritional Values, Metabolic Profile, and Radical Scavenging Capacities of Wild Asparagus (*A. acutifolius* L.)." *Journal of Food Composition and Analysis* 24: 326–33.

Rosati, Adolfo. Personal correspondence. April 27, 2011.

Yamaguchi, Tomoko, et al. 2001. "Radical-Scavenging Activity of Vegetables and the Effect of Cooking on Their Activity." *Food Science and Technology Research* 7 (3): 250–57.

Lill, R. E., G. A. King, and E. M. O'Donoghue. 1990. "Physiological Changes in Asparagus Spears Immediately After Harvest." *Scientia Horticulturae* 44: 191–99.

Papadopoulou, Parthena P., Anastasios S. Siomos, and Constantinos C. Dogras. 2003. "Comparison of Textural and Compositional Attributes of Green and White Asparagus Produced Under Commercial Conditions." *Plant Foods for Human Nutrition* 58: 1–9.

http://www.ars.usda.gov/SP2UserFiles/Place/12354500/Data/ORAC/ORAC_R2.pdf.

http://www.ba.ars.usda.gov/hb66/032asparagus.pdf.

Eleftherios, Papoulias, et al. 2009. "Effects of Genetic, Pre-, and Post-Harvest Factors on Phenolic Content and Antioxidant Capacity of White Asparagus Spears." *International Journal of Molecular Sciences* 10: 5370–80.

Popenoe, Wilson. 1935. "Origin of the Cultivated Races of Avocados." *California Avocado Association Yearbook* 20: 184–94.

Galindo-Tovar, María Elena, Nisao Ogata-Aguilar, and Amaury M. Arzate-Fernández. 2008. "Some Aspects of Avocado (*Persea americana* Mill.) Diversity and Domestication in Mesoamerica." *Genetic Research and Crop Evolution* 55: 441–50.

Wu, Xianli, et al. 2004. "Lipophilic and Hydrophilic Antioxidant Capacities of Common Foods in the United States." *Journal of Agricultural and Food Chemistry* 52: 4026–37.

Lerman-Garber, Israel, et al. 1994. "Effect of a High-Monounsaturated Fat Diet Enriched with Avocado in NIDDM Patients." *Diabetes Care* 17: 311–15.

Unlu, Nuray Z., et al. 2005. "Carotenoid Absorption from Salad and Salsa by Humans Is Enhanced by the Addition of Avocado or Avocado Oil." *Journal of Nutrition* 135: 431–36.

10 | APPLES: From Potent Medicine to Mild-Mannered Clones

Stushnoff, C., et al. 2003. "Diversity of Phenolic Antioxidant and Radical Scavenging Capacity in the USDA Apple Germplasm Core Collection." *Acta Horticulturae* 623: 305–12. The data for the accompanying graph came from this paper as well.

Yoshizawa, Yuko, et al. 2004. "Antiproliferative and Antioxidant Properties of Crabapple Juices." *Food Sciences and Technological Research* 10 (3): 278–81.

Turner, Nancy J., 1995. *Food Plants of Coastal First Peoples.* Vancouver: University of British Columbia Press.

Stushnoff et al. 2003. "Diversity of Phenolic Antioxidant."

Ferree, D. C., and I. J. Warrington, eds. 2003. *Apples: Botany, Production, and Uses.* Oxfordshire, UK: CABI Publishers.

Rea, Mary-Alice F. 1975. "Early Introduction of Economic Plants into New England." *Economic Botany* 29: 333–56.

Schoolcraft, Henry Rowe. *Notes on the Iroquois.* 1847. Albany, NY: E. H. Pease & Company.

Parker, Arthur C. 1968. *Parker on the Iroquois.* Syracuse, NY: Syracuse University Press.

Hokanson, Stan C., et al. 1997. "Collecting and Managing Wild *Malus* Germplasm in Its Center of Diversity." *HortScience* 32 (2): 173–76.

Stushnoff et al. 2003. "Diversity of Phenolic Antioxidant."

"Apple Boosts Fight Against Cancer." *Otago Daily Times,* April 3, 2008. Online edition.

http://treecropsresearch.org/montys-surprise/.

Awad, Mohamed A., Patricia S. Wagenmakers, and Anton de Jager. 2001. "Effects of Light on Flavonoid and Chlorogenic Acid Levels in the Skin of Jonagold Apples." *Science of Horticulture* 88: 289–98.

Tarozzi, Andrea, et al. 2004. "Cold-Storage Affects Antioxidant Properties of Apples in Caco-2 Cells." *Journal of Nutrition* 134: 1105–09.

Liu, Rui Hai, Marian V. Eberhardt, and Chang Yong Lee, 2001. "Antioxidant and Antiproliferative Activities of Selected New York Apple Cultivars." *New York Fruit Quarterly* 9: 11.

Wolfe, Kelly, Xianzhong Wu, and Rui Hai Liu. 2003. "Antioxidant Activity of Apple Peels." *Journal of Agricultural and Food Chemistry* 51: 609–14.

Petkovsek, M., et al. 2009. "Accumulation of Phenolic Compounds in Apple in Response to Infection by the Scab Pathogen, *Venturia inaequalis*." *Physiological and Molecular Plant Pathology* 74: 60–67.

Van der Sluis, A. A., et al. 2002. "Activity and Concentration of Polyphenolic Antioxidants in Apple Juice. 1. Effect of Existing Production Methods." *Journal of Agricultural and Food Chemistry* 50: 7211–19.

Oszmianski, J., et al. 2007. "Comparative Study of Polyphenolic Content and Antiradical Activity of Cloudy and Clear Apple Juices." *Journal of the Science of Food and Agriculture* 87: 573–79.

Wojdylo, Aneta, Jan Oszmianski, and Piotr Laskowski. 2008. "Polyphenolic Compounds and Antioxidant Activity of New and Old Apple Varieties." *Journal of Agricultural and Food Chemistry* 56: 6520–30.

11 | BLUEBERRIES AND BLACKBERRIES: Extraordinarily Nutritious

Parker, Arthur C. 1968. *Parker on the Iroquois*. Syracuse, NY: Syracuse University Press.

Moerman, D. E. 1996. "An Analysis of the Food Plants and Drug Plants of Native North America." *Journal of Ethnopharmacology* 52: 1–22.

Zheng, Wei, and Shiow Y. Wang. 2003. "Oxygen Radical Absorbing Capacity of Phenolics in Blueberries, Cranberries, Chokeberries, and Lingonberries." *Journal of Agricultural and Food Chemistry* 51: 502–9. The data for the accompanying graph came from this paper as well.

Hosseinian, Farah S., et al. 2007. "Proanthocyanidin Profile and ORAC Values of Manitoba Berries, Chokecherries, and Seabuckthorn." *Journal of Agricultural and Food Chemistry* 55 (17): 6970–76.

Giampieri, Francesca, et al. 2012. "The Strawberry: Composition, Nutritional Quality, and Impact on Human Health." *Nutrition* 28: 9–19.

http://www.ers.usda.gov/data/foodconsumption/FoodAvailspreadsheets.htm.

White, Elizabeth. 1937. "Taming Blueberries." Radio Garden Club, Volume 6, Digest no. 50.

Castrejón, Alejandro D. R., et al. 2008. "Phenolic Profile and Antioxidant Activity of Highbush Blueberry (*Vaccinium corymbosum* L.) During Fruit Maturation and Ripening." *Food Chemistry* 109: 564–72. Note: The relationship between size and antioxidant levels in blueberries is true of *Vaccinium corymbosum,* but not all species.

Ehlenfeldt, Mark K., and Ronald L. Prior. 2001. "Oxygen Radical Absorbance Capacity (ORAC) and Phenolic and Anthocyanin Concentrations in Fruit and Leaf Tissues of Highbush Blueberry." *Journal of Agricultural and Food Chemistry* 49: 2222–27.

Gill, Sudeep. 2009. "Dementia: Cholinesterase Inhibitor Use Link with Syncope." *Archives of Internal Medicine* 169: 867–73.

Joseph, James A., et al. 1999. "Reversals of Age-Related Declines in Neuronal Signal Transduction, Cognitive, and Motor Behavioral Deficits with Blueberry, Spinach, or Strawberry Dietary Supplementation." *The Journal of Neuroscience,* 19: 8114–21.

Krikorian, Robert, et al. 2010. "Blueberry Supplementation Improves Memory in Older Adults." *Journal of Agricultural and Food Chemistry* 58: 3996–4000.

Joseph, James, Daniel Nadeau, and Anne Underwood. 2003. *The Color Code: A Revolutionary Eating Plan for Optimum Health.* New York: Hyperion.

Wallace, Taylor C. 2011. "Anthocyanins in Cardiovascular Disease." *Advances in Nutrition* 2: 1–7.

Erlund, Iris, et al. 2008. "Favorable Effects of Berry Consumption on Platelet Function, Blood Pressure, and HDL Cholesterol." *American Journal of Clinical Nutrition* 87: 323–31.

Lohachoompol, Virachnee, George Srzednicki, and John Craske. 2004. "The Change of Total Anthocyanins in Blueberries and Their Antioxidant Effect After Drying and Freezing." *Journal of Biomedicine and Biotechnology* 5: 248–52.

Oszmianski, Jan, Aneta Wojdylo, and Joanna Kolniak. 2009. "Effect of L-Ascorbic Acid, Sugar, Pectin, and Freeze-Thaw Treatment on Polyphenol Content of Frozen Strawberries." *Food Science and Technology* 42: 581–86.

Hatton, Daniel C. "The Effect of Commercial Canning on the Flavonoid Content of Blueberries." Report for the Canned Food Alliance by Oregon Health Sciences University. The data for the accompanying graph came from this paper as well.

López, Jessica, et al. 2010. "Effect of Air Temperature on Drying Kinetics, Vitamin C, Antioxidant Activity, Total Phenolic Content, Non-Enzymatic Browning, and Firmness of Blueberries Variety O'Neil." *Food and Bioprocess Technology* 3: 772–77.

Wang, Shiow Y., Hangjun Chen, and Mark K. Ehlenfeldt. 2011. "Variation in Antioxidant Enzyme Activities and Non-Enzyme Components Among Cultivars of Rabbiteye Blueberries (*Vaccinium ashei* Reade) and *V. ashei* Derivatives." *Food Chemistry* 129: 13–20.

Finn, Chad E., et al. 2010. " 'Wild Treasure' Thornless Trailing Blackberry." *HortScience* 45 (3): 434–36.

12 | STRAWBERRIES, CRANBERRIES, AND RASPBERRIES: Three of Our Most Nutritious Fruits

Wada, Leslie, and Boxin Ou. 2002. "Antioxidant Activity and Phenolic Content of Oregon Caneberries." *Journal of Agricultural and Food Chemistry* 50: 3495–3500.

Connor, Ann Marie, et al. 2005. "Genetic and Environmental Variation in Anthocyanins and Their Relationship to Antioxidant Activity in Blackberry and Hybridberry Cultivars." *Journal of the American Society of Horticultural Science* 130 (5): 680–87.

Gaustad, Edwin S. 2005. *Roger Williams.* Oxford: Oxford University Press.

Fletcher, Stevenson Whitcomb. 1917. *The Strawberry in North America: History, Origin, Botany, and Breeding.* New York: Macmillan.

Parker, Arthur C. 1968. *Parker on the Iroquois.* Syracuse, NY: Syracuse University Press.

Fletcher, *The Strawberry in North America.*

Wang, Shiow Y., and Kim S. Lewers. 2007. "Antioxidant Activities and Anticancer Cell Proliferation Properties of Wild Strawberries." *Journal of the American Society of Horticutural Sciences* 132 (5): 647–58.

Bertelsen, Diane. 1995. "The US Strawberry Industry." Commercial Agriculture Division, Economic Research Service, US Department of Agriculture Statistical Bulletin no. 914.

Olsson, M. E., et al. 2004. "Antioxidants, Low Molecular Weight Carbohydrates, and Total Antioxidant Capacity in Strawberries (*Fragaria* × *ananassa*): Effects of Cultivar, Ripening, and Storage." *Journal of Agricultural and Food Chemistry* 52: 2490–98.

Olsson, M. E., et al. 2007. "Extracts from Organically and Conventionally Cultivated Strawberries Inhibit Cancer Cell Proliferation in Vitro." *Acta Horticulturae* (ISHS) 744: 189–194.

Ayala-Zavala, J. Fernando, et al. 2004. "Effect of Storage Temperatures on Antioxidant Capacity and Aroma Compounds in Strawberry Fruit." *LWT—Food Science and Technology* 37: 687–95.

Holzwarth, Melanie, et al. 2012. "Evaluation of the Effects of Different Freezing and Thawing Methods on Color, Polyphenol, and Ascorbic Acid Retention in Strawberries (*Fragaria* × *ananassa* Duch.)." *Food Research International* 48: 241–48.

Pappas, E., and K. M. Schaich. 2009. "Phytochemicals of Cranberries and Cranberry Products: Characterization, Potential Health Effects, and Processing Stability." *Critical Reviews in Food Science and Nutrition* 49: 741–81.

Lian, Poh Yng, et al. 2012. "The Antimicrobial Effects of Cranberry Against *Staphylococcus aureus*." *Food Science and Technology International* 18: 179–86.

Greenberg, James A., Sara J. Newmann, and Amy B. Howell. 2005. "Consumption of Sweetened Dried Cranberries Versus Unsweetened Raisins for Inhibition of Uropathogenic *Escherichia coli* Adhesion in Human Urine: A Pilot Study." *Journal of Alternative and Complementary Medicine* 11 (5): 875–78.

Burger, Ora, et al. 2006. "A High Molecular Mass Constituent of Cranberry Juice Inhibits *Helicobacter pylori* Adhesion to Human Gastric Mucus." *FEMS Immunology & Medical Microbiology* 29 (4): 295–301.

Pappas and Schaich. 2009. "Phytochemicals of Cranberries."

Jennings, S. N., 2002. *Raspberries and Blackberries: Their Breeding, Diseases, and Growth*. London: Academic Press.

Deighton, Nigel, et al. 2000. "Antioxidant Properties of Domesticated and Wild *Rubus* Species." *Journal of the Science of Food and Agriculture* 80: 1307–13.

Lui, Ming, et al. 2002. "Antioxidant and Antiproliferative Activities of Raspberries." *Journal of Agricultural and Food Chemistry* 50: 2926–30.

Wada and Ou. 2002. "Antioxidant Activity and Phenolic Content."

Wang, Li-Shu, et al. 2007. "Effect of Freeze-Dried Black Raspberries on Human Colorectal Cancer Lesions." AACR Special Conference in Cancer Research. *Advances in Colon Cancer Research* B31.

Wang, Li-Shu, et al. 2011. "Modulation of Genetic and Epigenetic Biomarkers in Humans by Black Raspberries: A Phase 1 Pilot Study." *Clinical Cancer Research* 17: 598–610.

13 | STONE FRUITS: Time for a Flavor Revival

Hancock, James F., ed. 2008. *Temperate Fruit Crop Breeding: Germplasm to Genomics*. New York and Heidelberg: Springer.

Turner, Thomas Hudson. 1851. *Some Account of Domestic Architecture in England: From the Conquest to the End of the Thirteenth Century*. J. H. Parker, Publisher.

Hatch, Peter J. 1998. "We Abound in the Luxury of the Peach." *Twinleaf Journal* online.

Crisosto, Carlos H., Gayle M. Crisosto, and David T. Garner. 2009. "Quantifying the Economic Impact of Marketing 'Sensory Damaged' Tree Fruit." An annual research report submitted to the California Tree Fruit Agreement.

Crisosto, C. H. 2002. "How Do We Increase Peach Consumption?" Proceedings of the Fifth International Peach Symposium. *Acta Horticulturae* 592: 601–5.

Remorini, D., et al. 2008. "Effect of Rootstocks and Harvesting Time on the Nutritional Quality of Peel and Flesh of Peach Fruits." *Food Chemistry* 110: 361–67.

Gil, Maria I. 2002. "Antioxidant Capacities, Phenolics Compounds, Carotenoids, and Vitamin C Contents of Nectarine, Peach, and Plum Cultivars from California." *Journal of Agricultural and Food Chemistry* 50: 4976–82.

Metrics used in Environmental Working Group's Shopper's Guide to Pesticides. Compiled with USDA and FDA data.

Carbonaro, Marina, and Maria Mattera. 2001. "Polyphenoloxidase Activity and Polyphenol Levels in Organically and Conventionally Grown Peach (*Prunus persica* L., cv. Regina Bianca) and Pear (*Pyrus communis* L., cv. Williams)." *Food Chemistry* 72: 419–24.

Vizzotto, Marcia, Luis Cisneros-Zevallos, and David H. Byrne. 2007. "Large Variation Found in the Phytochemical and Antioxidant Activity of Peach and Plum Germplasm." *Journal of the American Society of Horticultural Science* 132: 334–40. The data for the accompanying graph came from this paper as well.

Parmar, C., and M. K. Kaushal. 1982. *Prunus armeniaca*. In *Wild Fruits*, 66–69. New Delhi, India: Kalyani Publishers.

Malik, S. K., et al. 2010. "Genetic Diversity and Traditional Uses of Wild Apricot (*Prunus armeniaca* L.) in High Altitude Northwestern Himalayas of India." *Plant Genetic Resources* 8 (3): 249–57.

Journal of the Royal Horticultural Society XX, part 1 (1896): 102.

Campbell, Oluranti E., Ian A. Merwin, and Olga I. Padilla-Zakour. 2011. "Nutritional Quality of New York Peaches and Apricots." *New York Fruit Quarterly* 19: 12–16.

Brunke, Henrich. 2006. "Commodity Profile: Apricots." University of California Agricultural Issues Center.

Hegedus, Attila, et al. 2010. "Antioxidant and Antiradical Capacities in Apricot (*Prunus armeniaca* L.) Fruits: Variations from Genotypes, Years, and Analytical Methods." *Journal of Food Science* 75 (9): 722–31.

Karabulut, Ihsan, et al. 2007. "Effect of Hot Air Drying and Sun Drying on Color Values and β-Carotene Content of Apricot (*Prunus armeniaca* L.)." *LWT—Food Science and Technology* 40: 753–58.

Moerman, D. E. 1996. "An Analysis of the Food Plants and Drug Plants of Native North America." *Journal of Ethnopharmacology* 52: 1–22.

Chaovanalikit, A., and R. E. Wrolstad. 2004. "Total Anthocyanins and Total Phenolics of Fresh and Processed Cherries and Their Antioxidant Properties." *Journal of Food Science* 69: 67–72.

Taylor, William Alton. 1892. "The Fruit Industry, and Substitution of Domestic for Foreign-Grown Fruits with Historical and Descriptive Notes on Ten Varieties of Apple Suitable for the Export Trade." Bulletin no. 7, US Department of Agriculture.

From *Iowa Journal of History* 27, no. 4 (October 1929); written by O. A. Garretson of Salem, Iowa, a family friend.

Wood, Marsha. 2004. "Fresh Cherries May Help Arthritis Sufferers." *Agricultural Research* 52: 18–19.

Simonian, Sonny S. 2000. "Anthocyanin and Antioxidant Analysis of Sweet and Tart Cherry Varieties of the Pacific Northwest." Bachelor of science in bioresearch thesis, Oregon State University.

Kuehl, K. S., et al. 2010. "Efficacy of Tart Cherry Juice in Reducing Muscle Pain During Running: A Randomized Controlled Trial." *Journal of the International Society of Sports Nutrition* 7: 17.

Gonçalves, Berta, et al. 2004. "Storage Affects the Phenolic Profiles and Antioxidant Activities of Cherries (*Prunus avium* L.) on Human Low-Density Lipoproteins." *Journal of the Science of Food and Agriculture* 84: 1013–20.

Hooshmand, S., et al. 2011. "Comparative Effects of Dried Plum and Dried Apple on Bone in Postmenopausal Women." *British Journal of Nutrition* 106 (6): 923–30.

14 | GRAPES AND RAISINS: From Muscadines to Thompson Seedless

Keoke, Emory Dean, and Kay Marie Porterfield. 2001. *Encyclopedia of American Indian Contributions to the World: 15,000 Years of Invention and Innovations,* s.v. "Grapes, Indigenous American." New York: Facts on File, Inc.

Hariot, Thomas. 1588. *A Briefe and True Report of the New Found Land of Virginia*. Ed. by Paul Royster. Electronic Texts in American Studies. http://digitalcommons.unl.edu/cgi/viewcontent.cgi?article=1020&context=etas.

Savoy, C. F., J. R. Morris, and V. E. Petrucci. 1983. "Processing Muscadine Grapes into Raisins." *Proceedings of the Florida State Horticultural Society* 96: 355–57.

Bohlander, Richard E., 1998. *World Explorers and Discoverers*. Cambridge, MA: Da Capo Press.

Pastrana-Bonilla, Eduardo, et al. 2003. "Phenolic Content and Antioxidant Capacity of Muscadine Grapes." *Journal of Agricultural and Food Chemistry* 51 (51): 5497–5503.

Stanley, Doris. 2007. "America's First Grape: The Muscadine." *News & Events Online,* published by the USDA Agricultural Research Service. http://www.ars.usda.gov/is/ar/archive/nov97/musc1197.htm.

Walker, Amanda R., et al. 2007. "White Grapes Arose Through the Mutation of Two Similar and Adjacent Regulatory Genes." *The Plant Journal* 49 (5): 772–85.

Breksa, Andrew P. III, et al. 2010. "Antioxidant Activity and Phenolic Content of 16 Raisin Grape (*Vitis vinifera* L.) Cultivars and Selections." *Food Chemistry* 121: 740–45.

Kanner, Joseph, et al. 1994. "Natural Antioxidants in Grapes and Wines." *Journal of Agricultural and Food Chemistry* 42: 64–69.

Seeram, Navinda P., et al. 2008. "Comparison of Antioxidant Potency of Commonly Consumed Polyphenol-Rich Beverages in the United States." *Journal of Agricultural and Food Chemistry* 56: 1415–22.

Krikorian, Robert, et al. 2012. "Concord Grape Juice Supplementation and Neurocognitive Function in Human Aging." *Journal of Agricultural and Food Chemistry* 60: 5736–42.

Chou, E. J., et al. 2001. "Effect of Ingestion of Purple Grape Juice on Endothelial Function in Patients with Coronary Heart Disease." *American Journal of Cardiology* 88 (5): 553–55.

Singletary, K. W., K. J. Jung, and M. Giusti. 2007. "Anthocyanin-Rich Grape Extract Blocks Breast Cell DNA Damage." *Journal of Medicine and Food* 10 (2): 244–51.

Kevers, Claire, et al. 2007. "Evolution of Antioxidant Capacity During Storage of Selected Fruits and Vegetables." *Journal of Agricultural and Food Chemistry* 55: 8596–8603.

Crisosto, Carlos H., and Joseph L. Smilanik. n.d. "Table Grapes: Postharvest Quality Maintenance Guidelines." http://kare.ucanr.edu/files/123831.pdf.

Parker, Tory L., et al. 2007. "Antioxidant Capacity and Phenolic Content of Grapes, Sun-Dried Raisins, and Golden Raisins and Their Effect on ex Vivo Serum Antioxidant Capacity." *Journal of Agricultural and Food Chemistry* 55: 8472–77. The data for the accompanying graph came from this paper as well.

Chiou, Antonia, et al. 2007. "Currants (*Vitis vinifera* L.) Content of Simple Phenolics and Antioxidant Activity." *Food Chemistry* 102: 516–22.

15 | CITRUS FRUITS: Beyond Vitamin C

Sun, Jie, et al. 2002. "Antioxidant and Antiproliferative Activities of Common Fruits." *Journal of Agricultural and Food Chemistry* 50: 7449–54.

Arias, Beatriz Álvarez, and Luis Ramón-Laca. 2005. "Pharmacological Properties of Citrus and Their Ancient and Medieval Uses in the Mediterranean Region." *Journal of Ethnopharmacology* 97: 89–95.

Janick, Jules. 2005. Purdue University Tropical Horticulture Lecture 32: Citrus. http://www.hort.purdue.edu/newcrop/tropical/lecture_32/lec_32.html.

Morton, Julia F. 1987. *Fruits of Warm Climates*. Miami, FL: Florida Flair Books.

Tarozzi, Andrea, et al. 2006. "Antioxidant Effectiveness of Organically and Non-Organically Grown Red Oranges in Cell Culture Systems." *European Journal of Nutrition* 45: 152–58.

Lee, Hyoung S. 2001. "Characterization of Carotenoids in Juice of Red Navel Orange (Cara Cara)." *Journal of Agricultural and Food Chemistry* 49: 2563–68.

Lee, Hyoung S., et al. 1990. "Chemical Characterization by Liquid Chromatography of Moro Blood Orange Juices." *Journal of Food Composition and Analysis* 3: 9–19.

Helebek, Hasim, Ahmet Canbas, and Serkan Selli. 2008. "Determination of Phenolic Composition and Antioxidant Capacity of Blood Orange Juices Obtained from cvs. Moro and Sanguinello (*Citrus sinensis* L. Osbeck) Grown in Turkey." *Food Chemistry* 107: 1710–16.

Gross, Jeana, Michaela Gabai, and A. Lifshitz. 1971. "A Comparative Study of the Carotenoid Pigments in Juice of Shamouti, Valencia, and Washington Oranges, Three Varieties of *Citrus sinensis*." *Phytochemistry* 11: 303–8.

Robinson, T. Ralph. 1952. "Grapefruit and Pummelo." *Economic Botany* 6 (3): 228–45.

Rapisarda, Paolo, et al. 2009. "Juice of New Citrus Hybrids (*Citrus clementina* Hort. ex Tan. × *C. sinensis* L. Osbeck) as a Source of Natural Antioxidants." *Food Chemistry* 117: 212–18.

Tomás-Barberán, F. A., and M. I. Gil, eds. 2008. *Improving the Health-Promoting Properties of Fruit and Vegetable Products*. Boca Raton, FL: CRC Press.

Vanamala, Jairam, et al. 2006. "Variation in the Content of Bioactive Flavonoids in Different Brands of Orange and Grapefruit Juices." *Journal of Food Composition and Analysis* 19: 157–66.

Gil-Izquierdo, Angel, et al. 2001. "In Vitro Availability of Flavonoids and Other Phenolics in Orange Juice." *Journal of Agricultural and Food Chemistry* 49: 1035–41.

Broad, William J. 2007. "Useful Mutants, Bred with Radiation." *New York Times,* August 28, Science section.

Gorinstein, Shela. 2006. "Red Grapefruit Positively Influences Serum Triglyceride Level in Patients Suffering from Coronary Atherosclerosis: Studies in Vitro and in Humans." *Journal of Agricultural and Food Chemistry* 54: 1887–92.

Drewnowski, Adam, Susan Ahlstrom Henderson, and Amy B. Shore. 1997. "Taste Responses to Naringin, a Flavonoid, and Acceptance of Grapefruit Juice Are Related to Genetic Sensitivity to 6-n-Propylthiouracil." *American Journal of Clinical Nutrition* 66: 391–97.

Li, Xiaomeng, et al. 2010. "The Origin of Cultivated Citrus as Inferred from Internal Transcribed Spacer and Chloroplast DNA Sequence and Amplified Fragment Length Polymorphism Fingerprints." *Journal of the American Horticultural Society* 135 (4): 341–50.

Waife, S. O. 1953. "Lind, Lemons, and Limeys." *American Journal of Clinical Nutrition* 1 (6): 471–73.

Sun et al. 2002. "Antioxidant and Antiproliferative Activities."

Zimmermann, Benno F., and Maike Gleichenhagen. 2011. "The Effect of Ascorbic Acid, Citric Acid, and Low pH on the Extraction of Green Tea: How to Get the Most of It." *Food Chemistry* 124: 1543–48.

Stewart, William S. 1949. "Storage of Citrus Fruits: Studies Indicate Use of 2,4-D and 2,4,5-T Sprays on Trees Prolong Storage Life of Citrus Fruits." *California Agriculture* 3: 7–14.

Li, Yuncheng, et al. 2012. "Effect of Commercial Processing on Pesticide Residues in Orange Products." *European Food Research and Technology* 234: 449–56.

16 | TROPICAL FRUITS: Make the Most of Eating Globally

Heslop-Harrison, J. S., and Trude Schwarzacher. 2007. "Domestication, Genomics, and the Future for Banana." *Annals of Botany* 100: 1073–84.

Englberger, Lois, et al. 2003. "Carotenoid-Rich Bananas: A Potential Food Source for Alleviating Vitamin A Deficiency." *Food and Nutrition Bulletin* 24 (4): 303–18. The data for the accompanying graph came from this paper as well.

USDA Nutrient Data Laboratory. Oxygen Radical Absorbance Capacity (ORAC) of Selected Foods, Release 2 (2010).

Gayosso-García Sancho, Laura E., Elhadi M. Yahia, and Gustavo Adolfo González-Aguilar. 2011. "Identification and Quantification of Phenols, Carotenoids, and Vitamin C from Papaya (*Carica papaya* L., cv. Maradol) Fruit Determined by HPLC-DAD-NS/MS-ESI." *Food Research International* 44: 1284–91.

Collins, J. L. 1951. "Notes on the Origin, History, and Genetic Nature of the Cayenne Pineapple." *Pacific Science* 5: 3–17.

Ramsaroop, Raymond E. S., and Aurora A. Saulo. 2007. "Comparative Consumer and Physicochemical Analysis of Del Monte Hawai'i Gold and Smooth Cayenne Pineapple Cultivars." *Journal of Food Quality* 30: 135–59.

17 | MELONS: Light in Flavor and Nutrition

Mahattanatawee, Kanjana, et al. 2006. "Total Antioxidant Activity and Fiber Content of Select Florida-Grown Tropical Fruits." *Journal of Agricultural and Food Chemistry* 54: 7355–63.

Wehner, Todd C. 2007. "Watermelon." In Jaime Prohens and Fernando Nuez, eds., *Vegetables I: Asteraceae, Brassicaceae, Chenopodiaceae, and Cucurbitaceae*, vol. 1 of *Handbook of Plant Breeding*. New York and Frankfurt: Springer. http://cuke.hort.ncsu.edu/cucurbit/wehner/articles/book16.pdf.

Kung, Shain-Dow, and Shang-Fa Yang. 1998. *Discoveries in Plant Biology*, vol. 1. Singapore: World Scientific Press.

Tlili, Imen, et al. 2011. "Bioactive Compounds and Antioxidant Activities During Fruit Ripening of Watermelon Cultivars." *Journal of Food Composition and Analysis* 24: 923–28.

Perkins-Veazie, Penelope, et al. 2006. "Carotenoid Content of 50 Watermelon Cultivars." *Journal of Agricultural and Food Chemistry* 54: 2593–97.

Goldman, Amy. 2002. *Melons for the Passionate Grower*. New York: Artisan.

Shapiro, Laura. 2008. *Perfection Salad: Women and Cooking at the Turn of the Century*. Berkeley: University of California Press.

INDEX

Note: Italic page numbers refer to charts.

agriculture
  avocados and, 9, 205–6
  corn and, 9, 76–83, 180
  flavor and, 11–13, 23
  legumes and, 178–80
  root crops and, 111–12
  Three Sisters tradition, 180, 182
  tomatoes and, 139–44
  transition to, 8, 111–12
  wild plants and, 8–11
Alexander the Great, 221–22, 277, 282, 336
alliums
  garlic, 50–57, 69–70
  hunter-gatherers and, 47–48
  leeks, 65, 66
  medicinal uses, 47–50
  onion chives and garlic chives, 67–68
  onions, 57–63, 71–72
  points to remember, 72–73
  scallions, 68–69
  shallots, 63–65
apios, 97–98
apples
  Apple Crisp with Apple Skins, 230–31
  apple juice, 231–32
  cider, 232
  clones, 220–22
  eating skins of, 228–29
  farmers markets, 235–37
  growing, 233–34
  health benefits of, 6–7, 215–16
  loss of diversity, 222–25
  points to remember, 237–38
  storage of, 12, 227–28
  varieties of, 14, 24, 217, 225–27, 232, 234–37
  wild ancestors of, 219–20
  wild apples, 216–19, *217*, 224
apricots
  cultivation of, 282–83
  dried, 284–85
  shopping for, 283–84
  varieties of, 283, 284, 297
  wild ancestors of, 282
aronia berries, 240, *241*
artichokes
  artichoke hearts, 200–201
  cooking, 198–200, *199*
  nutrients in, 14–15
  ORAC value, 196
  points to remember, 211
  varieties of, 197–98, 208–9
  wild ancestors of, 195–96
arugula, 32–34
asparagus
  cooking, 204–5
  farmers markets, 203
  growing, 204
  points to remember, 211
  shopping for, 202–3
  storage of, 203–4
  varieties of, 209–10
  wild ancestors of, 201–2
avocados
  agriculture and, 9, 205–6
  lettuce and, 26
  points to remember, 211

avocados *(cont.)*
storage of, 207–8
varieties of, 206–7
wild ancestors of, 205, 206

bananas
beta-carotene levels, 347–48, *347*
domestication of, 346–47
storage of, 349–50
varieties of, 346, 347–49, 356, 357
wild ancestor of, 3–4
beans, 179–80, 182–87, *184,* 192
beets
aphrodisiac properties of, 122–23
farmers markets, 126, 133–34
flavor of, 128–29
greens of, 122, 123, 125, 126
health benefits of, 123–25
preparation of, 126, 129
Steamed Beets with Sautéed Greens, Blue Cheese, and Balsamic Vinegar, 127–28
storage of, 126
varieties of, 125–26, 133–34
wild ancestor of, 10, 122
berries, 239–41, *241. See also specific berries*
bionutrients. *See* phytonutrients
blackberries
domestication of, 251
points to remember, 259
storing and freezing, 253
varieties of, 251, 252–53, 257–58
Blaxton, William, 222
blueberries
cooked, 248, *249*
domestication of, 242–43
dried, 249–50
farmers markets, 243, 250–51, 254–57
frozen, 247–48
growing, 250–51
health benefits of, 6, 244–46
ORAC value, *241, 249*
points to remember, 259
shopping for, 247
varieties of, 243, 250–51, 254–57
wild ancestor of, 3, 241–43, 286
Boldo, Bartolomeo, 197
Boysen, Rudolph, 253
boysenberries, 252–53, 257
broccoli, 15–16, 161–64, 171–72
Brookhaven National Laboratory, 334
Brussels sprouts, 159, 164–65
Bull, Ephraim, 308, 309
cabbage, 166–67, 172–73
cantaloupes, 362–64, 369, 370–71
cardoons, 195–96
carrots
colorful carrots, 114, 118–19
domesticated, 113–14
nutrients in, 4, *115,* 118
orange carrots, 114, 115–17
preparation of, 116–17, *117*
storage of, 119
varieties of, 131–32
wild ancestor of, 3, 10, 113–14
casabas, 364–65, 369
cauliflower, 167–68, 173–74
cherries
domestication of, 286–87
farmers markets, 288–89, 298–99
health benefits of, 288, 289
shopping for, 287–90
storage of, 289–90
varieties of, 287–89, 298–99
wild ancestors of, 285–86
chilling injury (CI), 279, 281, 283, 291
chokeberries, 240, *241*
chokecherries, 285–86
Christensen, Mark, 224–25
citron, 320, 336
citrus fruits
grapefruits, 321, 333–36, 342
health benefits of, 318, 319, 320
lemons, 38, 336–41
limes, 336–39
oranges, 318, 319, 322–33
pesticides, 338, 339
points to remember, 343–44
storage of, 325–26
varieties of, 341–42
wild ancestors of, 320–21
Cobo, Bernabé, 205–6
Colorful Cornbread, 90
Columbus, Christopher, 76, 129, 320, 336, 352
complex carbohydrate intolerance (CCI), 63
corn
agriculture and, 9, 76–83, 180
canned and frozen, 91
carotenoids in, *85*
Colorful Cornbread, 90
cooking, 87–88
cornmeal, 88–89, 90
farmers markets, 86–87, 93–94

genetics and, 79–83, 86
growing, 87
Laughnan's shriveled corn, 81–83, 87
organic, 86
points to remember, 95
sweet corn, 78–79
varieties of, 75–76, 85, 86–87, 92–94
wild ancestor of, 4, 74–75, 76
Cornè, Michele Felice, 137
cornmeal, 88–89, 90
Cortés, Hernán, 140
Coville, Frederick, 242–43
crabapples, 218–19
cranberries, 265–68, 273, 275
Cranberry Horseradish Relish, 268
crucifers
broccoli, 15–16, 161–64, 171–72
Brussels sprouts, 159, 164–65
cabbage, 166–67, 172–73
cauliflower, 167–68, 173–74
kale, 159, 168–69, 170, 174–75
ORAC value, 160, *160*
points to remember, 175–76
varieties of, 158–59, 171–75
wild ancestors of, 159–61
currants, 313–14, 317

dandelion leaves, 22–23
Darling, Noyes, 79
Democritus, 320
Dorsey, James Owen, 179–80
Durand, Peter, 187

edamame, 190–91
Environmental Protection Agency, 290
Environmental Working Group, 228, 310–11
ethylene gas
bananas, 349
carrots, 119
grapefruits, 335
oranges, 324, 325, 328
producers of, 105, 119, 207
tomatoes, 144, 324

FDA, 285, 290, 292, 324
flatulence, 185–86
flavor
of beets, 128–29
bitter foods, 27–29
hunter-gatherers and, 84–85
of legumes, 178
of peaches, 278–79
of strawberries, 262–63
of tomatoes, 139, 143–44, 145, 148, 150
umami response, 178, 181
of wild plants, 11–13
food supply industrialization, 11–13
Foolad, Majid, 145
fruit cocktail, 365–66
fruits. *See also specific fruits*
ripening guidelines, 321
storage of, 12
sulfur-treated fruits, 284–85, 310, 313
varieties of, 7, 14, 16–17, 40–41
wild ancestors of, 10
fruit salads
nutritional makeover of, 365–66
recommended ingredients for, 366–67
Som Tum Pollamai (Mixed Seasonal Fruits in Thai Herbs and Lime Juice), 368

garlic
convenience products, 56–57
farmers markets, 54–55, 69–70
nutrients of, 50–51
preparation of, 51–52
pressing, 52–53
softneck and hardneck, 55–56
storage of, 57
varieties of, 53–54, 69–70
garlic chives, 67–68
gelatin salads, 365, 366
Gilroy Garlic Festival, 54–55
glycemic index, 5, 40, 101–2, 103, 106, 351
Gold, Theodore Sedgwick, 142
Goldman, Amy, 363
grains, 9, 179
grapefruits
degreening of, 335
health benefits of, 334, 336
medications and, 334–35
shopping for, 335–36
varieties of, 333–34, 342
wild ancestors of, 321
grapes
comparison of nutrients, *307,* 309
currants, 313–14, 317
domestication of, 305, 306–7
Grape, Mint, and Feta Salad, 312
health benefits of, 304, 305–6, 308–9
ORAC value, 308, *313*
points to remember, 316–17
raisins, 306, 312–14, *313,* 316–17

grapes *(cont.)*
 shopping for, 309–11
 storage of, 311
 varieties of, 306–10, 314–15
 wild varieties of, 303–6, 308
guavas, 354–55, 357
Gunther, Erna, 48

Halvorsen, Pranee Khruasanit, 367
Hariot, Thomas, 304
Hass, Rudolph, 207
heirloom varieties
 of apples, 223, 224, 232
 of cantaloupes, 363
 of corn, 86, 87
 of grapes, 306
 of potatoes, 14
 of tomatoes, 138, 148–49
 of watermelons, 361, 362
 wild varieties compared to, 7
Hippocrates, 17, 47, 337
honeydew melons, 364, 369, 371
Honey Mustard Vinaigrette, 39
Hull, Henry, 266
hunter-gatherers
 alliums, 47–48
 apples, 218–19
 berries, 239–40
 bitter food and, 28
 corn, 74
 fiber consumption, 196
 grains, 9
 greens, 21–22, 23
 health and longevity of, 120–22
 legumes, 177–78
 potatoes, 97
 raisins, 312
 strawberries, 261
 sweet flavors and, 84–85
 transition to agriculture, 8, 111–12

iceberg lettuce, 23–24, 26
individually quick frozen (IQF), 247
insulin resistance, 101–2

Jamestown Colony, 260
Jefferson, Thomas, 141–42, 164–65, 182–83, 223, 277–78, 304–5
Joseph, James, 245

kale, 159, 168–69, 170, 174–75
Keller, Helen, 305
Knott, Walter, 253
Knott's Berry Farm, 253

lamb's quarters, 22
Laughnan, John, 81–83, 87
leeks, 65, 66
legumes
 agriculture and, 178–80
 beans, 179–80, 182–87, 192
 edamame, 190–91
 hunter-gatherers, 177–78
 lentils, 177–78, *184,* 185, 187–90
 ORAC value, *184,* 187
 peas, 182–87, 192
 points to remember, 193–94
 varieties, 192
Lemon Pudding with Lemon Peel, 340–41
lemons, 38, 336–41
lentils, 177–78, *184,* 185, 187–90
lettuce
 farmers markets, 31–32, 42–44
 freshness of, 26–27
 prepackaged, 29–30
 storage of, 30–31
 varieties of, 24–26, 32
limes, 336–39
Livingston, Alexander W., 142–43
Logan, James Harvey, 252
loganberries, 252, 257, 258
Luelling, Henderson, 287

mangoes, 353–54, 356
manioc, 112
marionberries, 253, 257, 258, 270
Mason, John L., 365
Mattioli, Pietro, 140–41
melons
 cantaloupes, 362–64, 369, 370–71
 casabas, 364–65, 369
 honeydew melons, 364, 369, 371
 importing of, 360
 points to remember, 371–72
 popularity of, 359
 varieties of, 369–71
 watermelons, 15, 360–62, 369–70
metabolic syndrome, 101, 118
microperforated bags, 30–31
Moerman, Daniel E., 47–48, 286

NASA, 318–19
nectarines
 domestication of, 277–78

farmers markets, 281, 295–96
flavor of, 278–79
shopping for, 279–80
varieties of, 280, 281, 295–96

olive oil, 37–38
olives, 9
onion chives, 67–68
onions
farmers markets, 61, 71–72
gastric distress, 62–63
preparing and cooking, 61–62
storage of, 61
varieties of, 57–61, *59,* 71–72
oranges
blood oranges, 326–27, 332
Cara Cara oranges, 326, 332
degreening of, 324, 325, 328, 329
health benefits of, 318, 319, 330, 332
home-squeezed orange juice, 332–33
identifying ripeness, 324–25
mandarins, 329, 342
organic, 325, 329, 332
pith of, 329–30, 333
shopping for orange juice, 330–32
storage of, 325–26
tangelos, 328, 332, 342
tangerines, 329
Valencia oranges, 328, 332
varieties of, 341–42
Washington navel, 322–23, 326
wild ancestors of, 320
Ottoman Empire, 306

Palladius, 268
papayas, 352–53, 356, 357
papoon, 78–79
parsnips, 10
peaches
color of flesh, 280, *281*
domestication of, 277–78
farmers markets, 281, 295–96
flavor of, 278–79
nutrients in, 14
shopping for, 279–80
varieties of, 278, 280, 281, 295–96
peas, 182–87, *184,* 192
Pesticide Action Network (PAN), 150
pesticides
apples and, 228–29
cherries and, 290
citrus fruits, 338, 339
corn and, 86
grapes and, 310–11
peaches and, 280
potatoes and, 102–3
strawberries and, 264
tomatoes and, 150
tropical fruits, 355
phytonutrients
in apples, 6–7, 14, 216–17, 219–20, 224–29, 231–33
in apricots, 283
in artichokes, 196
in asparagus, 201, 203–4
in avocados, 207
in beans, 180, 184
in beets, 123
in blueberries, 6, 243, 247, 248, 249
in broccoli, 161, 164
in carrots, 116
in cherries, 286, 288, 289
in citrus peels, 339
in corn, 75, 86, 89, 91
in cranberries, 266, 267
in currants, 314
in fruit varieties, 14
in grapefruits, 334
in grapes, 306, 313
in greens, 10, 22–24, 30–33, 35
in guavas, 355
in kale, 169
in leeks, 65
in lemons, 338
in lentils, 187
in lettuce, 24–26, 29, 30
in mangoes, 353
in manioc, 112
in melons, 360
in onions, 57, 58, 60, 62, 64
in oranges, 319, 323, 326, 328, 329–33
in peaches, 280
in pineapples, 350
in plums, 291
in potatoes, 6, 103
in raspberries, 269
in scallions, 68
storage and, 15–16, 30–31
in strawberries, 262, 263
in tomatoes, 6, 13–14, 138
in vegetable varieties, 14
in wild plants, 5–7, 10
Pieri, Peter, 57–58
Pilgrims, 77–78, 266

pineapples, 350–52, 356
plantains, 347
Pliny the Elder, 64, 286, 313
plums
  dried, 292–93
  health benefits of, 292, 293
  Savory Plum Sauce, 294
  shopping for, 291–92
  varieties of, 291–92, 299–300
  wild varieties, 291
pomelos, 321
potatoes
  farmers markets, 104–5, 108–9
  health benefits of, 14
  hidden pesticides, 102–3
  points to remember, 109–10
  Potato Salad with Sun-Dried Tomatoes and Kalamata Olives, 107
  preparation of, 96–97, 99, 105–6
  storage of, 12, 15, 99, 105
  varieties of, 99–100, *100*, 103–5, 108–9
  wild ancestors of, 6, 97–99, 104
prediabetes, 100–101
prunes, 292–93
purslane, 4

quinoa, 22

radiant energy vacuum drying (REV drying), 249
radicchio, 34
raisins, 306, 312–14, *313*, 316–17
Raleigh, Walter, 303–4, 350
Randolph, Martha, 277
raspberries
  black raspberries, 270–71
  points to remember, 275
  red raspberries, 268–69
  varieties of, 269, 270, 273–74
recipes
  Apple Crisp with Apple Skins, 230–31
  Armenian Lentil Soup, 189–90
  Baked Kale Chips, 170
  Colorful Cornbread, 90
  Cranberry Horseradish Relish, 268
  Grape, Mint, and Feta Salad, 312
  Honey Mustard Vinaigrette, 39
  Lemon Pudding with Lemon Peel, 340–41
  Potato Salad with Sun-Dried Tomatoes and Kalamata Olives, 107
  Sautéed Leeks with Mustard and Cumin, 66
  Savory Plum Sauce, 294
  Som Tum Pollamai (Mixed Seasonal Fruits in Thai Herbs and Lime Juice), 368
  Steamed Beets with Sautéed Greens, Blue Cheese, and Balsamic Vinegar, 127–28
  Tomato Salsa, 148
Rhodes, Ashby M., 83
Ronsee, Beaudouin, 337
Roosevelt, Theodore, 323
root crops. *See also* potatoes
  agriculture and, 111–12
  beets, 122–29, 133–34
  carrots, 3, 10, 113–19, 131–32
  points to remember, 135–36
  storage of, 112–13
  sweet potatoes, 129–31, 134–35
  varieties of, 131–35
Rosati, Adolfo, 201

Sahagún, Bernardino de, 140
salad dressings, 36–38, 39
salad greens
  arugula, 32–34
  lettuce, 24–32, 42–44
  points to remember, 45–46
  radicchio, 34
  at salad bar, 36
  spinach, 4, 34–35
  varieties of, 41–44
  wild ancestors of, 10, 22–24
Sautéed Leeks with Mustard and Cumin, 66
Savory Plum Sauce, 294
scallions, 68–69
Seed Savers Exchange, 87
sesame seeds, 9
Sforza, Ludovico, Duke of Milan, 290–91
shallots, 63–65
Silverwood-Cope, Peter, 112
Slow Food USA, 224, 262
Som Tum Pollamai (Mixed Seasonal Fruits in Thai Herbs and Lime Juice), 368
Southern Exposure Seed Exchange, 87
spinach, 4, 34–35, *35*
squash, 180
standard American diet (SAD), 118
Steamed Beets with Sautéed Greens, Blue Cheese, and Balsamic Vinegar, 127–28
stone fruits
  apricots, 282–85, 297
  cherries, 285–90, 298–99
  nectarines, 277–81, 295–96

peaches, 14, 277–81, 295–96
plums, 291–94, 299–300
points to remember, 301–2
shopping for, 276–77
Stoner, Gary, 270
strawberries
domestication of, 261–62
farmers markets, 265, 271–72
points to remember, 275
shopping for, 263–64
storage of, 264
varieties of, 262–63, 265, 271–72
wild strawberries, 260–61, 265
Sullivan, John, 78
supertasters, 28–29, 159, 169, 335
sweet potatoes, 129–31, 134–35
sweets, appeal of, 84–85
Szent-Györgyi, Albert, 337

Tang, 318–19
teosinte, 4, 74–75, 76
Theophrastus, 221–22
Thompson, William, 306
Tibbets, Eliza, 322–23
tomatoes
agriculture and, 139–44
farmers markets, 148–49, 154–56
flavor of, 139, 143–44, 145, 148, 150
health benefits of, 6
homegrown, 149–50
organic, 150
points to remember, 156–57
popularity of, 137–38
preparation of, 151–52, *152*
processed, 152–53
revival of, 144–45
storage of, 150–51
Tomato Salsa, 148
varieties of, 145–49, 154–56
wild ancestors of, 3, 13–14, 138–39, 145
tropical fruits
bananas, 3–4, 346–50, 356, 357
fair trade, 355
guavas, 354–55, 357
mangoes, 353–54, 356
papayas, 352–53, 356, 357
pineapples, 350–52, 356
points to remember, 357–58
popularity of, 345–46
varieties of, 356–57
Twain, Mark, 167
type 2 diabetes, 101

umami response, 178, 181
U.S. Department of Agriculture
apples, 216, 220, 224
asparagus grades, 202–3
blackberries, 251
blueberries, 242, 244, 251
consumption of fruits and vegetables, 12
corn, 86
fiber consumption, 196
grapes, 310
legumes, 184, 185
lettuce, 24
marionberries, 253
nutritional content, 10–11, 184
oranges, 325, 329
plant hardiness zones, 40–41
strawberries, 262, 265
tomatoes, 143

vegetables. *See also specific vegetables*
varieties of, 7, 14, 16–17, 40–41
Verrazano, Giovanni da, 304
Victoria (queen of England), 223
vinegars, 38
vitamins, in wild plants, 4

Washington, George, 78
watermelons
domestication of, 360–61
shopping for, 361–62
storage of, 15, 362
varieties of, 369–70
wild ancestor of, 360
Waters, Alice, 336
Welch, Thomas Bramwell, 308
White, Elizabeth, 242–43
wild plants
agriculture and, 8–11
flavor of, 11–13
as low-glycemic foods, 5
nutrients in, 4–5, 10–11, 13
phytonutrients in, 5–7, 10
redesign of, 3–4
Williams, Roger, 260–61
Winthrop, John, 77
Wolfskill, William, 328
Wood, William, 286

ABOUT THE AUTHOR

Jo Robinson is a health writer and food activist who is best known for her research into the benefits of raising pigs, poultry, cattle, and sheep on pasture rather than in large confinement operations. She has been a reliable source of information about grass-based production for dozens of major media, including *Time,* the *New York Times, USA Today, Men's Health, Mother Earth News,* National Public Radio, and the *Wall Street Journal.* Her website, http://www.eatwild.com, has attracted more than ten million visitors. With the publication of *Eating on the Wild Side,* Robinson expands her work to include fruits and vegetables as well as animal products. She lives and works on Vashon Island, a rural island close to Seattle, Washington, where she raises some of the delicious and nutritious varieties recommended in this book. Jo is the author or coauthor of fourteen books of nonfiction that have combined sales of more than two million copies.

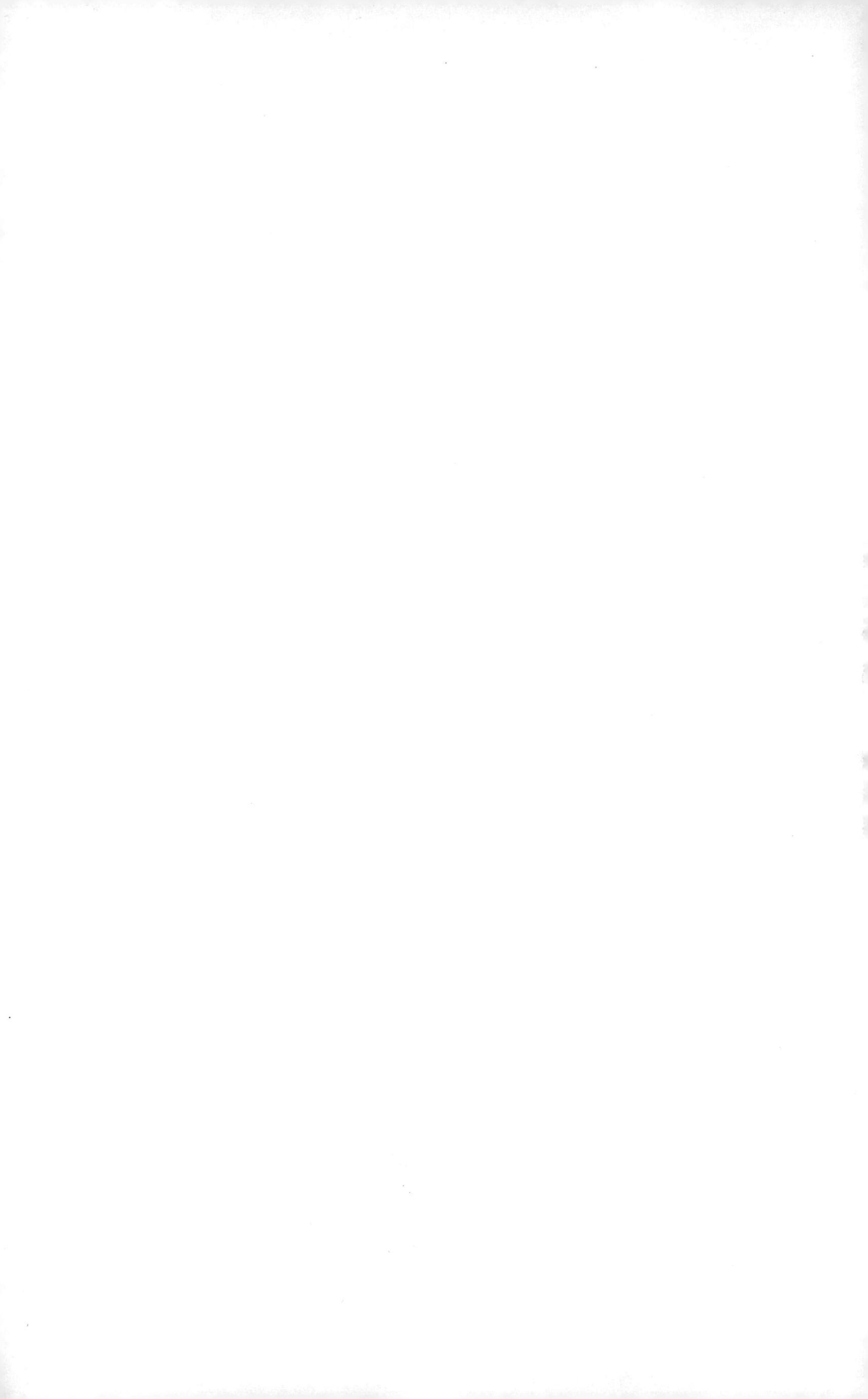